*This one is for Dave Mcdougle, Ralph Jessie,
Robb Coutinho, Monte Z. Ogle, Sarah Fitton,
and Heather Allen, readers and friends for a
long time now, and I hope
for a long time to come....*

www.brianlumley.com

Prologue

IN XANADU, JETHRO MANCHESTER HAD BUILT A pleasure dome, in fact the Pleasure Dome Casino. But that was some time ago, and since then Manchester's fortunes had changed. Now both the casino and the mountain resort of Xanadu belonged to another, to Aristotle Milan, and the new resident-owner's needs required that he make certain alterations.

The casino was a great dome of glass and chrome. It was a three-storey affair—or four-storey, if one included a smaller dome, which sat like a bubble or a raised blister on top of the main structure—that lorded its location at Xanadu's hub, on a false plateau in a high, dog-leg fold of the Australian Macpherson range of mountains.

Now it was night, but still the work on Mr. Milan's alterations continued. He wanted the work completed to his specifications before he reopened Xanadu to the public in just a few days' time. And in his private accommodation in the high bubble dome, Milan himself supervised the last of the work; or if not supervised, at least he was there to see it finished to his satisfaction. But Milan's presence—or more specifically the annoyance that accompanied it—wasn't to Derek Hinch's liking.

Hinch was a painter and decorator, but at times like this he tended to think of himself more as a steeplejack. Inside the bubble it wasn't so bad . . . there wasn't very far to fall if he made the classic mistake of stepping back a few paces to admire his work! But outside, some fifty or sixty feet off the ground: *that* had been nerve-wracking, and thank God he was done with it now.

But black? Painting perfectly good windows black, both

1

inside and out? It didn't make a lot of sense to Derek Hinch. And as for Mr Milan: he didn't make much sense either! The guy must be some kind of eccentric, a nut case, albeit a very rich, powerful one. The way he prowled through the glitzy false opulence of this place, apparently lost in some indefinable distance, in space and time; though mainly (Hinch suspected) lost in a world of his own, the extravagance of his thoughts.

And his music . . . his bloody terrible, interminable music!

There was a gleaming antique jukebox at one end of a small, gently curving, mahogany-topped bar on the perimeter of the bubble, and when Milan was taking it easy he would sit there in an armchair with a drink, just listening to the music . . . the same damn tunes or songs, or just, well, *music,* over and over again. And it was driving Hinch nuts, too!

Not that Hinch didn't care for the stuff; he liked—or he used to like, and he would have continued to like—all of this stuff just fine . . . if he hadn't been obliged to listen to each piece at least thirty or forty times in the space of just seven nights. So thank *God* he was almost finished here!

But nights! Why in hell couldn't this work be done in daylight hours? And why in hell couldn't Milan sleep nights—like any other mad millionaire? And why in double-damned *hell* did he have to play his bloody music like this!?

What was it that was playing now? Damn, the tunes had kind of run together in Hinch's head; he had heard them so often, he knew what was coming next. Mr. rich-foreign-handsome-bloody-bastard Milan kept playing them in sequence, in some kind of order of preference. But it was the order of disorder, totally *out* of order, to Hinch's way of thinking:

Oh, yes—now he remembered—*Zorba's Dance,* that was it! All bouzoukis, fast drumbeats, and Anthony bloody Quinn dancing on a beach! A Greek thing that was almost as much an antique as the machine that played it. One of those tunes that never dies, which as far as Hinch was concerned could die any time it fucking well liked! And of course as the tune ended, Hinch knew the next item in the circular, never-ending repertoire. And here it came yet again:

"Sunshine, you may find my window but you won't find me. . . ." Some kind of blues with a country-western flavour, and lyrics too deep for Hinch to understand. . . . Pleasing to listen to, even soothing, in a way . . . if you hadn't heard it half a dozen times already this very night! Some old black guy, singing his heart out about misery. But to Hinch's mind the only misery lay in having to listen to it over and over again.

"So, you don't care for my music, Mr. Hinch?" The voice was deep yet oiled; it seemed to rumble, or purr, yet was in no way catlike. On the other hand, Milan's movements *were* catlike as he came from the bar with a drink in his long-fingered hand, to gaze out on the night through an open window.

But if it wasn't painted black (Hinch thought,) *there'd be no need to open the fucking thing! Not that there's anything to see out there.* While out loud he said, "Er, did I say something about your music? I have a habit of talking to myself while I'm working. It doesn't mean anything." *Oh yes it fucking does! It means that I'm pissed to death with you, and your bloody music, and with bloody Xanadu, and all of this bloody black paint!*

He looked down on Milan from a height of some twelve feet, from a wheeled scaffolding tower where he had just put the finishing touches to the last pane of a high window. And that was it: the entire interior surface, every square foot of hundreds of square feet of glass, varnished for adhesion, painted black, and finally layered with polyurethane lacquer for durability. A double-dyed bastard of a job!

"Perhaps I don't pay you enough?" said Milan as Hinch put down his roller, wiped his hands, came clambering from on high.

"The money's fine," the bad-tempered Hinch said. He stood six feet tall, but still had to lift his head a fraction to look up at his employer. "And I'd like it now, for I'm all done."

"Then if the payment is fine," said Milan, "it can only be

that I was right and it's the music. Or perhaps it's me? Do you find my presence unsettling?"

While he was speaking, Hinch had checked him out—again. For Aristotle Milan was the kind of man you looked at twice. At a guess he'd be maybe forty, forty-five years old. Difficult to be more specific than that, because his looks were sort of timeless. He was probably sixty but topped-up with expensive monkey hormones or some such. Something was running through his veins, keeping him young, for sure. Spoiled, rich bastard!

But foreign? Even without the name to give him away, there could be no mistaking that: Italian with a touch of Greek—but in any case a mongrel, in Hinch's eyes. Milan's hair was black as night; worn long, it swept back from a high, broad forehead, and its shining ringlets curled on his shoulders. And handsome: he had the kind of Mediterranean looks that seemed to appeal to a lot of women. Hinch would guess that his bedroom crawled with all kinds of young, good-looking, dirty women.

His ears were fleshy—what could be seen of them—but he wore his sideburns thick and lacquered back to cover the upper extremities. Something odd about his nose, too: a flattish look to it, as if Nature had pushed it back a little to far, and his nostrils were too large and flaring. And then those arcing eyebrows over deep-sunken, jet-black eyes . . . those eyes that were Milan's most startling feature. Jet-black, and yet Hinch couldn't be certain. Catch them at the right angle, they'd sometimes gleam a golden, feral yellow. And despite the nose, those eyes loaned Milan the look of a bird of prey.

But handsome? Maybe Hinch was all wrong about that. It was simply the attraction of Milan's odd—his strange or foreign, his almost alien—features, that was all. And as for Mediterranean: well, that didn't seem quite right either, not with the cold pallor of his flesh, and the bloodred of his lips. He was something of a weird one, this Milan, for sure. Something of an enigma. An unknown or unspecified quantity.

"Payment when the job is done," Milan spoke again, the rumble lower than ever. "Which it isn't, not quite, not yet."

"What?" Hinch stared hard at him, tried to look hard, too—difficult with a man as sure of himself as Milan. Or as sure of his filthy money! But Hinch reckoned that for all his lousy millions, still Milan would be a cinch in a fight. Hinch was a powerful, brutal fighter, the victor of a dozen rough-house brawls. And Milan—he had the hands of a pianist, fingers like a girl! *Huh!* Hinch would bet his life that Milan had never felt a bunch of knuckles bouncing off that ugly nose of his. And the thought never occurred to him that he had already bet his life.

Cocking his head a little on one side, Milan looked at him curiously, sighed, and said, "First it's my music, and then it's because you've had to work late into the night, and now . . . now it's personal, to the point that you insult me and even measure your physical strength against mine, like an opponent . . . as if you could ever be an opponent. Or is it all just jealousy?"

And suddenly it sank into Hinch's less-than-enormous brain that while he'd *thought* all of these things, he hadn't actually voiced any of them—not even about the music! Was he that easy to read?

But he was tired of all this, and so, changing the subject, he said, "What's that about the job not being finished? I mean, you wouldn't be trying to avoid paying me—would you?" And the threat in his words, the way he growled them, was obvious.

"Not at all," Milan told him. "Payment is most certainly, very definitely due. And you shall have it. But out there— on the outside of the dome, just a little to the left of this open window here—there's a spot you missed. And I suffer from this affliction: I can't deal with too much sunlight. My eyes and my skin are vulnerable. And so you see, while sunshine may find my window, it must *never* find me. The work must be finished, to my satisfaction. That was our contract, Mr. Hinch."

God damn this weird bastard! Hinch thought as he paced to the window, leaned out (but carefully,) and looked to the left. But:

"God?" said Milan, from close behind. "Your god, Mr. Hinch? Well if there is such a being—and if his sphere of influence is as extensive as you suppose—I think you may safely assume that he 'damned' me a very long time ago."

"Eh?" said Hinch, looking back into the dome, surprised by and wondering at the sudden change in Milan's tone of voice.

Milan moved or flowed closer; his slim fingers were strong where they came down on Hinch's hand, trapping it on the window sill. And leaning closer still, with his face just inches away, he smiled and hissed, "You don't much care for heights, do you, Mr. Hinch? In fact you care for them even less than you care for me, or for my music."

"What the bloody . . . ?" Hinch looked into eyes that were no longer black or feral but uniformly red, flaring like lamps.

"Bloody?" the other repeated him, his voice a phlegmy gurgle now, full of lust, and his breath a hot, coppery stench in Hinch's face. "Ah, *yesssss!* But not your blood, not this time, Mr. Hinch. Your blood is unworthy. *You* are unworthy!"

"Jesus Christ!" Hinch gasped, choked, tried to draw away—and failed.

"Call on whom or whatever you like," Milan continued to pin him to the window ledge, and moved his free hand to the back of Hinch's thick neck. "No one and nothing can help you now."

"You're a fucking madman!" Hinch jerked and wriggled, but he couldn't pull free. The other's strength was unbelievable.

"And you . . . you are nothing!" Milan told him, continuing to smile, or at least doing *something* with his face.

Hinch saw it, but didn't believe it: the way Milan's lips curled back and away from his elongating jaws, the teeth curving up through his splitting gums, his ridged, convoluted nose flattening back, while his nostrils gaped and sniffed. And the red blood dripping from the corner of his mouth.

Then Milan freed Hinch's hand in order to clench his fist and hit him in his ribs—such a blow that Hinch, burly as he was, was lifted from his feet. At the same time, Milan hoisted him by the scruff of the neck and tilted him forward; concerted movements designed to topple him into space.

And as the shrieking Hinch flipped out into the night, so the Thing that looked like a man released him.

Hinch fell, but only for a moment. Then his shriek became a gasp as he came down on his belly and cracked ribs across the safety rail of a painter's platform slung between twin gantries. From above, seven or eight feet to the open window, Hinch heard Milan's cursing. And struggling to his feet inside the platform he looked up—to see that hideous, livid face looking down on him!

Then, moving like liquid lightning, Milan was up onto the window ledge, and light as a feather came leaping to the bouncing, rocking platform. His intentions were unmistakable, and as he landed Hinch went to kick him in the groin. Milan caught his foot, twisted it until the ankle broke, then reached out with a long arm to grab the other's throat. And without pause, lifting Hinch bodily into the air, he thrust him out beyond the rim of the safety rail—and let him fall.

As Hinch fell—grasping at thin air and failing to catch it—he was aware that Milan was speaking to him one last time. But whether it was a physical voice he heard, a chuckling whisper in his head, or simply something imagined, he couldn't have said. And he certainly didn't have time to worry about it.

Paid in full, the crazed voice whispered. *For your insults if not for your work. So be it!*

And below, crashing down headfirst, Hinch was dead before the pain had time to register. Like an egg dropped on the floor, the contents of his skull splattered at first. But the grey was soon drowned in a thick, night-dark pool that formed around his shattered head.

While up above, that terrible face continued to smile down on him . . . for a little while, until Aristotle Milan's features melted back into a more acceptable form, and he gave a careless shrug, and grunted again, "So be it!"

Then he returned to listening to his music, and no other's

thoughts to disturb him now, in the solitude of a strange place in a strange land. . . .

An "unfortunate accident" was how local newspapers would later report the matter. They also reported Milan's generous offer to pay all of the funeral expenses, and his very generous donation to Derek Hinch's widow. . . .

Part One
The How of It

1
See the Creechur

IT WAS HOT AS HELL, AND FLIES THE SIZE OF Jake Cutter's little fingernails had been committing suicide on the vehicle's windscreen for more than a hundred and fifty miles now, ever since they'd left Wiluna and "civilization" behind.

"Phew!" Jake said, sluicing sweat from his brow and out of the open window of their specially adapted Land Rover. The top was back and the windows wound down, yet the hot wind of passage that pushed their wide-brimmed Aussie hats back from their foreheads, tightened their chinstraps around their throats and ruffled their shirts still made if feel like they were driving headlong into a bonfire. And the "road" ahead—which in fact was scarcely better than a track—wavered like a smoke-ghost in the heat haze of what appeared to be an empty, ever-expanding distance.

Behind the vehicle, a mile-long plume of dust and blue-grey exhaust fumes drifted low over the scrub and the wilderness.

"That's your fifth 'phew,' " Liz Merrick told him. "Feeling talkative today?"

"So what am I supposed to say?" He didn't even glance at her, though most men wouldn't have been able to resist it. "Oh dear, isn't it hot? Christ, it must be ninety! 'Phew' is about all I'm up to, because if I do more than open my mouth a crack—*ugh!*" And he spat out yet another wet fly.

Liz squirmed and grimaced. "What the hell do they live on, I wonder? Way out here, I mean?" She swatted and missed as something small, black, and nasty went zipping by.

"Things die out here," Jake answered grimly. "Maybe

that's what they live on." And just when she thought that
was it, that he was all done for now: "Anyway, the sun's
going down over the hills there. Another half hour or so, it'll
be cooler. It won't get cold—not in this freaky weather—
but at least you'll be able to breathe without frying your
lungs." *Then* he was done.

She turned her head to look at him more fully: his angular
face in profile, his hard hands on the wheel, his lean outline.
But if Jake noticed her frowning, curiously intent glance, it
scarcely registered. That was how he was: hands off. And
she thought: *We make a damned odd couple!*

She was right, they did. Jake hard yet supple, like whip-
cord, and Liz soft and curvy. Him with his dark background
and current . . . condition, and Liz with her—

—Which was when they hit a pothole, which simultaneously brought Liz's mind back to earth while lifting her
backside eight inches off her seat. "Jake, take it easy!" she
gasped.

He nodded, in no way apologetically, almost absentmind-
edly. He had turned his head to look at her—no, Liz corrected herself—to look beyond her, westward where the
rounded domes of gaunt, yellow- and red-ochre hills marched
parallel with the road. They were pitted, those hills, pockmarked even from here. The same could be said of the desert
all around, including the so-called road. "These old mine
workings," Jake growled. "Gold mines. That was subsidence
back there, where the road is sinking into some old mine. I
didn't see it because of this bloody heat haze."

"Gold?" Squirming down into her seat, Liz tried to get
comfortable again. *Hah!* she thought. *As if I'd been comfortable in the first place!*

"They found a few nuggets here," he told her. "There was
a bit of a gold rush that didn't pan out. There may be gold
here—there probably is—but first you have to survive to
bring it up out of the ground. It just wasn't worth it. . . ."

"Because even without this awful El Niño weather, this
was one hell of an inhospitable place to survive in." She
nodded.

"Right." Finally Jake glanced at her—at *her* this time. And while he was still looking she grinned nervously and said:

"What a place to spend your honeymoon! I should never have let you talk me into it." A witticism, of course.

"Huh!" was his reply. Shielding his eyes, he switched his attention back to the rounded hills with the sun's rim sitting on them like a golden, pus-filled blister on the slumping hip of some gigantic, reclining, decomposing woman.

"Fuel gauge is low." Liz tapped on the gauge with a fingernail. "Are we sure there's a gas station out here?" In fact she knew there was; it was right there on the map. It was just the awful heat, the condition of the road, evening setting in, and a perfectly normal case of nerves. Liz's tended to fray a little from time to time. As for Jake's . . . well, she wasn't entirely sure about his, didn't even know if he had any.

"Gas station?" He glanced at her again. "Sure there is. To service the local 'community.' Heck, around these parts there's point nine persons per hundred square miles!" While Jake's sarcasm dripped, it wasn't directed entirely at Liz but rather at their situation. Moreover, she thought she detected an unfamiliar edge to his voice. So perhaps he did have nerves after all. But still his completely humourless attitude irritated her.

"That many people? Really?" For a moment she'd felt goaded into playing this insufferable man at his own game . . . but only for a moment. Then, shrugging, she let it go. "So what's it doing here? The gas station, I mean."

"It's a relic of the gold rush," he answered. "The Australian government keeps such places going with subsidies, or they simply couldn't exist. They're watering holes in the middle of nowhere, way stations for the occasional wanderer. Don't expect too much, though. Maybe a bottle of warm beer—make sure you knock the cap off yourself . . . yes, I know you know that—no food, and if you need the loo you'd better do it before we get there." Good advice, around these parts.

The road vanished about a mile ahead: an optical illusion,

just like the heat haze. As the hills got higher, so the road began to climb, making everything seem on a level, horizontal. Only the throb of the motor told the truth: that the Land Rover was in fact labouring, however slightly. And in another minute they crested the rise.

Then Jake brought the vehicle to a halt and they both went off into the scrub fifty yards in different directions. He got back first, was leaning on his open door, peering through binoculars and checking the way ahead when Liz returned.

"See anything?" she asked, secretly admiring Jake where he stood unselfconsciously posed, with one booted foot on the door sill, his jeans outlining a small backside and narrow hips. But the rest of him wasn't small. He was tall, maybe six-two, leggy and with long arms to match. His hair was a deep brown like his eyes, and his face was lean, hollow-cheeked. He looked as if a good meal wouldn't hurt . . . but on the other hand extra weight would certainly slow him down. His lips were thin, even cruel. And when he smiled you could never be sure there was any humour in it. Jake's hair was long as a lion's; he kept it swept back, braided into a pigtail. His jaw was angular, thinly scarred on the left side, and his nose had been broken high on the bridge so that it hung like a sheer cliff (like a Native American's nose, Liz thought) instead of projecting. But despite his leanness, Jake's shoulders were broad, and the sun-bronzed flesh of his upper arms was corded with muscle. His thighs, too, she imagined. . . .

"The gas station," he answered. "Sign at the roadside says 'Old Mine Gas.' There's a track off to the right from the road to the pumps . . . or rather, the pump. What a dump! Another sign this side of the shack says . . . what?" He frowned.

"Well, what?" Liz asked.

"Says 'See the Creature!' " Jake told her. "But it's spelled C-r-e-e-c-h-u-r. *Huh!* Creechur . . ." He shook his head.

"Not much schooling around here," she said. Then, putting a hand to the left side of her face to shut out the last spears of sunlight from the west, "That's some kind of eyesight you've got. Even with binoculars the letters on those signs have to be tiny."

"First requirement of a sniper," he grunted. "That his eyesight is one hundred percent."

"But you're not a sniper, or indeed any kind of killer, any longer," she told him—then caught her breath as she realized how wrong she might be. Except it was different now, surely.

Jake passed the binoculars, looked at her but made no comment. Peering through the glasses, she focussed them to her own vision, picked up the gas station's single forlorn pump and the shack standing—or leaning—behind it, apparently built right into the rocky base of a knoll, which itself bulged at the foot of a massive outcrop or butte. The road wound around the ridgy, shelved base of the outcrop and disappeared north.

And while she looked at the place, Jake looked at her. That was okay because she didn't know he was looking.

She was a girl—no, a woman—and a sight for sore eyes. But Jake Cutter couldn't look at her that way. There *had been* a woman, and after her there couldn't be anything else. Not ever. But if there could have been . . . maybe it would have been someone like Liz Merrick. She was maybe five-seven, willow-waisted, and fully curved where it would matter to someone who mattered. And to whom she mattered. Well, and she did, but not like that. Her hair, black as night, cut in a boyish bob, wasn't Natasha's hair, and her long legs weren't Natasha's legs. But Liz's smile . . . he had to admit there was something in her smile. Something like a ray of bright light, but one that Jake wished he'd never known—because he knew now how quickly a light can be switched off. Like Natasha's light . . .

"Not very appetizing," Liz commented, breathing with difficulty through her mouth.

"Eh?" He came back to earth.

"The dump, as you called it."

"The name says it all." Jake was equally adenoidal. "Probably the entrance to an old mine. Hence 'Old Mine Gas.' "

A great talent for the obvious, she wanted to tell him but didn't. Sarcasm again, covering for something else.

"So what do you think?" she finally said as they got into the Rover.

"Good time not to think," he answered, and Liz could only agree. At least he'd remembered what little he'd been told. So they tried not to think, and continued not thinking as he started up the vehicle and let her coast the downhill quarter-mile to the Old Mine Gas station . . .

Lights of a sort came on as they turned off the road to climb a hard-packed ramp to the elevated shelf that fronted the shack. The illuminated sign flickered and buzzed, finally lit up in a desultory, half-hearted neon glare; grimy windows in the shack itself burned a dusty, uncertain electrical yellow. In an ancient river valley like this, dry since prehistory, it got dark very quickly, even suddenly, when the sun went down.

It also got cooler; not cold by any means—not in this freakish El Niño weather—but cooler. After they pulled up at the lone pump, Jake helped Liz shrug herself into a thin safari jacket, took his own from the back of the Rover and put it on. In the west, one shallow trough in the crest of the domed hills still held a golden glow. But the light was rapidly fading and the amethyst draining from the sky, squeezed out by the descending sepia of space. To the east, the first stars were already winking into being over blackly silhouetted mountains.

Maybe twenty-five paces to the right of the main shack, a lesser structure burrowed into the side of the steep knoll. The SEE THE CREECHUR sign pointed in that direction. Liz wondered out loud, "What sort of creature, do you reckon?"

But now there was a figure standing in the shadow of the shack's suddenly open screen door. And it was that figure that answered her. "Well, it's a bloody *funny* one, I guarantee that much, miss!" And then a chuckle as the owner of the deep, gravelly voice stepped out into full view. "It's a bit late in the day, though, so if yer want ter see 'im, best take a torch with yer. Bloomin' bulb's blown again . . . or maybe 'e did it 'imself. Don't much care for the light, that creechur feller. Now then, what can I do fer you folks? Gas, is it?"

Jake nodded and tilted his hat back. "Gas. Fill her up."

"Ah!" The other's gasp seemed genuine enough. "Eh? What's this, then? Brits are yer? A pair of whingein' pommies way out 'ere? Now I asks yer, what next!?" He grinned, shook his head. "Just kiddin'. Don't yer be takin' no note o' me, folks."

To all appearances he was just a friendly old lad and entirely unaccustomed to company. His rheumy little pinprick eyes, long since abandoned to the wrinkles of a weathered face, gazed at his customers over a bristly beard like that of some garrulous stagecoach driver in an ancient Western. As he took the cap off the Land Rover's tank, his wobbly spindle legs seemed about ready to collapse under him. And as if to make doubly sure he'd said nothing out of turn: "Er, no offence meant," he continued to mumble his apologies.

"No offence taken," Liz gave a little laugh. And Jake had to admire her: her steady, give-away-nothing voice. She quickly went on, "Can we get a drink or something while you're filling her up? It's been a long and thirsty road, and a way to go yet. Maybe a beer? You do have beer, right?"

"Did yer ever meet up with an Australian" (but in fact he said *Orstrylian*) "who didn't have a beer close ter hand?" The old man grinned again, started the pump and handed the nozzle to Jake, then hobbled back and held open the inner door to the shack for Liz. "Just you 'elp yerself, miss. They're all lined up on the shelves back o' the bar there. Not a lot ter choose from, though—Foster's every one! It's my favourite. And since I'm the one who drinks most of it, it's my choice too."

"Well, good," said Liz. "It's my favourite, too."

Jake watched them go inside, frowned at the nozzle in his hand. Just like that, he'd accepted the bloody thing. Damn!

After that . . . but it seemed it was going to take forever to satisfy the Rover's greedy guzzling. So Jake quit when the tank was only three-quarters full, slammed the nozzle into the pump's housing, tried not to look too concerned as he followed Liz and the old boy into the shack. But he'd hated to lose contact with her, lose sight of her like that, even for a few seconds. And she'd looked back at him just before she passed from view, her green eyes a fraction too narrow, too anxious.

Inside, however, it wasn't as bad as he'd thought it would be. Or as it might have been.

It was the grime, the blown dust of the desert, clinging to the outside of the windows, that had shut the light in and made the place seem so dim from outside. But within—*this might be typical of any outback filling station a million miles from nowhere.* That was Jake's first impression. The bar was a plank on two barrels, with a bead curtain hanging from the plank to the floor in front and smaller barrels for seats. Liz was perched on one of them, and the old man had passed her a beer that she held unopened in her hand.

- She must have asked him if he was all alone out here, and he was in the process of answering: "Alone? Me? Naw, not much. And anyway I enjoys bein' on me ownsome. Oh, I got a couple o' boys to 'elp out. They 'aint 'ere right now, is all. It 'aint so bad, actu'ly. 'Ad a truck through just a day or so ago."

"A truck?" Liz said, all innocence and light. "Out here?"

And the old man nodded. "Gawd knows where they'd be goin'! But for that matter, where be *you* goin', eh? What're yer doin' out 'ere anyway?"

Having taken in much of the single room at a glance, Jake strode to the bar and asked for a beer. Without waiting for an answer from Liz, the old man reached for a bottle and turned to Jake. "Well now, *you* was a mite quick!" he said. "Yer just topped 'er up, am I right? I mean, yer'd never fill a big tank as quick as all that."

"Right," said Jake, accepting the beer. He gave the bottle a quick shake, forced the top off with a practiced thumb. Then, changing the subject as the warm beer foamed, "No cans?" he inquired. He passed the bottle to Liz, took hers, and repeated his trick with the same result. The beer wasn't

18

flat; these bottles were old stock, but they hadn't been opened previously.

And meanwhile: "Cans? I don't hold with 'em," the old-ster told him. "All this newfangled shite! But yer can trust a bottle." And turning to Liz again, "You were sayin'?"

"No," she answered, "*you* were saying. You asked what we're doing out here."

"Well, then?" he pressed.

She smiled. "Can you keep a secret?"

He shrugged his hunched shoulders, sat down on a barrel on his side of the plank and chuckled. "And who do yer reckon I'd be tellin'?"

Liz nodded. "We were visiting kin in Wiluna, decided to get married sort of quick. So here we are, run off where no one can find us."

"Eh? Honeymooners, yer say? Run off on yer ownsome and left no forwardin' address? All out o' touch, secret an' private in the Gibson Desert? *Huh!* Hell o' a place fer a honeymoon. . . ."

"I told him the very same thing." Liz nodded her agree-ment, shaking an I-told-you-so finger at Jake.

And Jake said, "Anyway, we're headed north. We thought we'd take a look at the lakes and—"

"Lakes?" the old fellow cut in, frowning. "Yer visitin' the lakes?" Then, with a knowing nod of his head, he muttered, "Big disappointment, that."

"Oh?" Jake lifted an eyebrow.

But the oldster only laughed out loud and slapped his thigh. "*Lake* Disappointment!" he guffawed. "Way up north o' here. Damn me, they falls fer it every time!" He sobered up, said, "Lakes, eh? Somethin' ter see, is it? *Huh!* Plenty o' mud and salt, but that's about all."

"*And* wildlife!" Liz protested.

"Oh, aye, that too," he said. "Anyway, what would I know or care? I 'ave me own wildlife, after all."

"The creature?" Jake swigged on his beer.

" 'Im's the one," the old boy nodded. "Yer wanna see 'im?"

Jake had done with studying the oldster. But he would certainly like to take a closer look at this shack—or what lay behind it or maybe beneath it. Liz could feel his curiosity no matter how hard he tried to keep it from the old boy. Moreover, she knew that between them they had to check this place out, and so decided to do her bit—create a diversion as best she could. And anyway (she told herself), the old man didn't seem much of a threat.

"I'd like to see him," she said. "I mean, what's the mystery? What kind of creature is it, anyway? Or is it just a con—some mangy, diseased dingo crawled in out of the desert—to pull in a few more travellers?" And to her partner, though she knew he wouldn't take her up on it: "What about you, Jake? You want to come and see this thing?"

Jake shook his head, took another pull at his bottle. "Not me, Liz. I've a thirst to slake. But if you want to have a look at some mangy dog, well go right ahead." Almost choking on the words, he got them out somehow. Damn it to hell— the idea was supposed to be that they *didn't* get split up! He hoped she knew what she was doing. There again, she'd been in this game longer than he had. And that pissed Jake more than a little, too: the fact that Liz was in effect the boss here.

"Torch," said the old boy, taking a heavy rubber-jacketed flashlight from the shelf and handing it to Liz. "Yer'll need it. I keeps 'im in out o' the sun, which would surely fry 'is eyes. But it's dark in the back o' the shack there. And this time o' evenin' even darker in 'is cage." When she looked uncertain, didn't move, he cocked his head on one side and said, "Er, yer just follers the signs, is all."

Liz looked at him, hefted the torch, said, "You want me to go alone?"

"Can't very well get lost!" he said. But then, grumblingly, he hobbled out from behind the makeshift bar. "It's these old pins o' mine," he said. "See, they don't much like ter go. But yer right—can't let a little lady go wanderin' about in the dark on 'er own. So just you foller me, miss. Just you foller old Bruce." And then they were gone.

Jake took a small pager out of his pocket and switched it

on. Now if Liz got in trouble she only had to press the button on her own beeper and he would know it . . . and vice versa. For in this game it was just as likely that he would be the one to make a wrong move.

Those were his thoughts as he stepped silently behind the bar and passed through a second bead curtain hanging from the timbered ceiling to the floor. And as easily and as quickly as that he was into a horizontal mineshaft, and almost as quickly into something far less mundane. . . .

Liz had followed the old man (*Bruce? Hell of a lot of Australians called Bruce,* she thought. *There have to be at least as many as there are Johns in London*) along the foot of the knoll to the lesser shack that leaned into an almost sheer cliff face.

It was quite dark now, and the torch he'd given her wasn't nearly working on full charge. The batteries must be just about dead. Of course, knowing the place as he did, that wouldn't much concern the old boy, but it concerned Liz. And despite following slowly and carefully in old Bruce's footsteps—mainly to give Jake the time he needed to look the place over—still she stumbled once or twice over large rocks or into this, that, or the other pothole. But in truth much of her stumbling was a ploy, too, so that it was perhaps a good thing after all that the torch was almost spent. She thought so at the outset, anyway.

Until eventually: "He we are," the old man said, turning a key in a squealing lock and opening an exterior screen door. Beyond that a second door stood ajar; and as old Bruce, if that really was his name, reached out an incredibly long arm to one side of Liz to push it fully open—at the same time managing to bundle her inside—so she recognized the smell of a lair.

It was a primal thing, something that lies deep in the ancestral memories of every human being: to be able to recognize the habitat of a dangerous animal or animals. The musty, feral smell of a cavern where something dwells—or perhaps an attic where bats have hibernated for untold years—or maybe the reptile house in a zoo.

But there are smells and smells, and this wasn't like anything Liz had ever come across before; or perhaps it was simply the tainted, composite smell of all of them. Until suddenly she realized that it wasn't *just* a smell—wasn't *simply* a smell—but her talent coming into play, and that the stench wasn't in her nostrils alone but also in her mind!

And then she had to wonder about its origin, the focus or point of emanation of this alien taint. Was it the shack—or the steel-barred, wall-to-wall cell it contained—or perhaps the night-black tunnel beyond the bars, with its as yet unseen, unknown "creechur" . . . or could it possibly be old "Bruce" himself?

There came a sound from the darker depths of the horizontal mine shaft. And just as there are smells and smells, so are there sounds and sounds. Liz gasped, aimed her torchbeam into the darkness back there, and saw movement. A flowing, gathering, *approaching* darkness in the lesser dark around; an inkblot of a figure, taking on shape as it came, bobbing, wafting on a draft of poisonous air from wherever and whatever lay beyond. And it had luminous yellow eyes—slanted as a beast's, and yet intelligent, not-quite-feral—that held her fixed like a rabbit in a headlight's beam!

But only for a moment. Then—

"You!" Liz transferred the torch to her left hand, dipped her right hand into a pocket and came out with a modified Baby Browning, used her thumb to release the safety and aimed it at the old man . . . or at the empty space where he had been. While from outside in the night, she heard the grating of his booted feet, his now obscene chuckle, and the squeal of a key turning in the exterior screen-door's lock as he shut her in.

Hell! But this could quite *literally* be hell! Along with her talent—held back far too long by her desire not to alert anyone or-thing to her real purpose here—Liz's worst fears were now fully mobilized, realized. She knew what the creature in the mineshaft was, knew what it could do. But even now she wasn't entirely helpless.

Tucking the torch under her arm, she found her beeper and pressed its alarm button . . . at the precise moment that it commenced transmitting Jake's own cry for help.

The shock of hearing that rapid *beep beep beep*ing from her pocket almost made Liz drop the torch; she somehow managed to hold on to it, held her hands together, pointed the gun and the torch both through the inch-thick bars of the cage. But as the weak beam swept the bars, it picked out something that she hadn't previously noticed; there had been little enough time to notice anything. The cage had a door fastened with a chain and stout padlock—but the padlock hung on the inside, the other side, where it dangled from the hoop of its *loose* shackle!

She knew what she must do: reach through the bars, drive home the shackle to close the padlock. A two-handed job. Again she put the torch under her arm, fumbled the gun back into her pocket. Then, in the crawling, tingling, living semi-darkness, Liz thrust her trembling hands between the bars . . . and all of the time she was aware of the thing advancing towards her, its slanted, sulphurous eyes alive on her . . . and the beeper issuing its urgent, staccato Mayday like a small, terrified animal . . . and on top of all this the sudden, nightmarish notion: *But what if this thing has the key to the padlock!?*

At that moment it was Liz Merrick who felt like some small, terrified, trapped animal—but a *human* animal. While the thing striding silently, ever closer to her along the shaft was anything but human, though it might have been not so long ago.

It was almost upon her; she smelled the hot stench of its breath! Liz had squeezed her eyes shut in a desperate effort to locate the padlock. Now she opened them . . .

. . . And it was there, it was there! Its face, caught in the upward-slanting beam of yellow light from the torch in her armpit, looked down on her. And:

"Ahhh!" It—or he, the "creechur"—sighed. "A girl. No,

a *woooman*. And a fresh one. How very *good* to meet you here! How very . . . provident. *Ahhh!"* And as simply as that his cold, cold hands took the padlock from hers, freed it from the chains, and let it fall with a clank to the dirt floor. . . .

2
Dark Denizens

MEANWHILE, JAKE CUTTER HAD PROCEEDED maybe a hundred yards down the gradually sloping shaft, deep into the earth. The shaft was quite obviously the entrance to an old mine; the walls and roof were timbered, and there were sleepers and rusty, narrow-gauge rails in the fairly uneven floor. In places there was some evidence of past cave-ins, where holes in the ceiling and boulders on the floor told their own story. Since the surviving supports seemed stout enough, Jake wasn't worried for his safety in that respect.

But in one other respect, he was. And he kept finding himself wishing that right now he wasn't some*where* but rather some*one* else—despite that he would usually prefer not to be. All very confusing and paradoxical, but it was something which had only ever happened twice, and then in the most extreme of circumstances. And for the time being Jake was *only* Jake Cutter.

Such were his thoughts when the narrow but adequate beam of his pencil-slim pocket torch picked out the first of several side tunnels, shafts that radiated off from the main, the original mineshaft.

Until now the floor had borne a thick coating of dust and sand, much of which had settled against the walls. Towards the centre, however, and between the rails, most of this had been scuffed away, presumably by the recent passage of several or many persons. But persons going where? Of course the old proprietor might be using this place as a warehouse or stock room; indeed, back where the shaft opened into the shack that fronted the mine, Jake had passed a jumble of old crates and cardboard boxes, and labels on the latter had declared their contents as wiper blades, fuses, various grades of motor oil, spark plugs, and spare parts and vehicle accessories in general. Of course, he would have expected as much that close to the entrance.

But all these signs of *recent* disturbance—or of occupation?—all this way back here? Why would anyone want to come back here, except perhaps on exploratory forays; maybe someone who was curious about old mine shafts? But recently? And how *many* someones? It was beginning to look like this might be the place. In which case he and Liz should never have split up and gone their own ways. Oh, he knew why she'd done it, all right, but now . . .

. . . *Now what was that?* Jake froze.

The side shafts weren't recent diggings; they were probably old exploratory digs from the days when prospectors sought an ultimately elusive "mother lode." Certainly quartz was present in the walls where the subsidiary tunnels had been hewn or blasted from the rock. It was here, too, that the scuff marks on the floor—in places actual footprints—were most in evidence, and it was from the first of these lesser branching diggings that the sound had issued. A sound like a sigh or a yawn, like someone waking up.

Jake knew that by now it would be night in the valley in the Gibson Desert, dark in the outside world. But not nearly as dark as it was in here. And Liz was back there somewhere, alone with the old man. Or maybe not alone. And hadn't his "Orstrylian" accent been a little too thick, and hadn't there been something—maybe just a trace—of the Gypsy about him?

Jesus! Jake was now aware of fumbling movements from the side tunnels—from more than one of them—and was immediately galvanized to action. But at a time and in a place such as this there was only one action he could take: flight.

Behind him, the main tunnel curved however slightly back towards the entrance. Setting off at a loping run, Jake played his torch beam on the ceiling in order to avoid the jagged ends of dangling timbers in a number of places where pressured beams had popped. And as he went he felt for his pager, making ready to send out his distress call. Not that he felt panicked or in immediate danger himself, but Liz might well be. If she wasn't already aware of the danger, the beeper would give her advance warning. He wouldn't use it just yet, though, because to do so would be to alert whoever she was with that he was on his way, perhaps precipitating some undesired activity.

In a matter of twenty seconds or so, when he was in sight of the bead-curtained rear entrance to the shack, Jake skidded to a halt. A figure, momentarily silhouetted by the light from the shack, had appeared on the other side of the curtain; Jake recognized it as that of the old proprietor. Switching off his torch, he flattened himself to the wall behind a support beam, took out his 9-mm Browning and soundlessly armed it. And none too soon.

Grumbling to himself in his fashion, the old man came on through the curtains and made straight for Jake; there was no other way he could go. But as he blotted out some of the light from the shack, so Jake noticed that his movements weren't any longer those of an old man. He came on at a sprightly, almost youthful lope, and his previously dim eyes were no longer hidden in wrinkled folds. Instead they were a glowing, feral yellow, and in their cores burned red as fire!

Jake needed no further warning or convincing. He now knew for a certainty what this place was if not exactly what he was up against. Going into a professional shooting stance, he took careful aim and squeezed the trigger.

But the other had seen or sensed Jake in the moment that he fired; seeming to flow to one side, he moved closer to the wall. Jake knew he'd missed and got off a second shot; the bullet whined where it ricochetted from the shaft's wall, hurling sparks and splinters of rock at the "old" man's face and neck.

He jerked at the impact of the stony fragments, then stood up straighter and stepped out into full view. And putting up a hand to his neck under the ear, he glanced at it almost curiously and said, "Blood?" That was all, *blood*. But his voice was no longer old, and his furnace eyes had turned uniformly crimson.

Knowing he couldn't afford to miss a third time, Jake moved forward. Behind him there was real activity now: voices calling out wailing questions, and the sounds of stumbling feet. And:

"Lead, is it?" said that low, growling, dangerous voice as the distance narrowed between them. "Oh, *ha! ha! ha!* Then come on, son, fire away. For as you'll discover, I've something of an appetite for lead."

"How about silver?" Jake said, squeezing the trigger again. His words were pure bravado for he was by no means sure of himself, but it was a nice line.

And perhaps in that last second the vampire sensed that his opponent had the advantage. He once more caused himself to relocate, used that weird flowing motion to move to one side. But not quickly and not far enough. The silver bullet hit him in the right shoulder, spun him around, and slammed his back against the wall. With a gurgling cry of, *"Ah! Ah!"* he clawed at his shoulder and fell to his right knee, and Jake leaped around him to carry on headlong through the bead curtains, taking them with him in a jangling tangle.

Maybe he should have stayed to finish the job. Certainly he would have if he had been that someone else—or half of someone else—but despite the danger Jake was still only Jake Cutter; he hadn't yet reached that point of uttermost desperation.

Free of the curtains he crashed through the makeshift bar and sent the plank flying from its barrel supports, and without pause he rushed out into the night, wheeling left to go sprinting towards the second shack. That was where the alleged "creechur" was, and Jake could scarcely doubt but that was where he would find Liz, too . . . where the lying, scheming, undead proprietor of this terrible place had left her. As he went, so he reached into his pocket to activate his pager. . . .

*   *   *

The thing's cold hands on Liz's hands . . . the beeper continuing to issue its endlessly repeating Mayday (or its cry of warning, she couldn't say which, but in any case the latter was far too late now) . . . and this thing from her worst nightmares, *smiling* at her through the stout iron bars. But bars that might as well be of paper, because the door in the cage stood ajar.

The creature freed her right hand, pushed at the door. Liz stood frozen; she let him get that far—but in the next moment was shaken from her paralysis on hearing Jake's shout of "Liz! Liz! Where in hell are you?" He was dead right: that was *exactly* where she was! But she guessed he already knew that.

All was total darkness now, all bar the glow of her monstrous adversary's eyes. Off-balance as the door swung squealingly open on her, carrying her with it, still Liz managed to snatch the Baby Browning from her pocket. Ramming it between the bars, she gritted her teeth and fired.

"Gah!?" said that shuddersome voice, sounding mildly surprised. And as the thing released its hold on her, she slammed the door shut again on its rusty hinges, and on him, turned, and groped fumblingly towards the inner door to the shack. She came across it, found the doorknob, and yanked it open. But the creature was behind her; she could feel its hot, fetid breath on her neck, its oppressive strength gathering in the darkness. Then:

"Liz?" came Jake's voice again. He'd heard her shot, had come to a halt beyond the locked screen door. She heard him cursing, rattling the lock, until: "Stand back!" he called out.

She should stand back? When right behind her something was rumbling, "Urgh—ah!—*argh!*" even now? And:

"Christ!" Liz said, quickly turning and firing again, and then a third time, until the grotesque black shadow of the creature was lifted from its feet and hurled bodily away, flailing its arms and spitting blood, back into the shack's more natural shadows—where it collided with yet *more* shadows that Liz hadn't been aware of until now.

Her shot had come simultaneously with Jake's as he blew the lock off the outer door. And a moment later she was out of the place, stumbling into his arms.

He steadied her, breathlessly told her, "This place. This is it! It's what we were looking for."

"Do you think I don't fucking know that?" she gasped.

And then they were running, both of them, heading for the Rover, for safety, and for sanity. But as yet safety, and especially sanity, seemed a long way off. Behind them, the smaller shack was spewing stumbling, dazed-seeming, zombielike figures into the night. A handful of them, four or five at least. While ahead of them . . .

"God almighty!" Jake breathed with difficulty.

The moon was up, a waxing moon that gave good light. Likewise the stars, very bright in a sky that was now black as jet and banded with varying degrees of purple on the hills. And so by moon and starlight the pair saw what waited for them close to their vehicle.

"We're in it up to here," Liz panted, choked. And: "God, I can't breathe!"

"Me neither," Jake told her. "But don't panic and keep the plugs in. This isn't over yet. Our beepers will have been heard by the others. They'll be on their way."

"We . . . we can't run forever," she answered, veering away with him towards the track back to the road. "How'll we get to the Rover with those damned things waiting for us?"

"Split up," Jake answered. "You head for the road. . . . Keep running like hell, north. . . . I'll try to lead the bulk of these bloody monsters on a wild goose chase."

Behind them the vampires were taking it easy. They weren't running; they ambled, arms hanging loose, some with their hands in their pockets, eyes aglow, kicking pebbles aside as they followed their intended prey. There was no great hurry—nowhere out here to hide that couldn't be sniffed out. The girl would be easier to handle when she was tired; they wouldn't have to damage her in order to have her one by one—or maybe two or three at a time—before they had her blood.

As for the man: his blood would be good, strong. But he'd caused Bruce Trennier no small amount of pain, and Bruce would be wanting him first. Oh, this one would be missing an arm or leg or both before Bruce gave him up to the rest of them. And the would-be "Lord" Trennier would wax fat on meat and marrow, while the hole in his shoulder slowly but surely healed. But:

Silver! came Trennier's voice in their minds, where they tracked the humans across the false plateau at the foot of the knoll. *These people are more than they appear to be. Their bullets are silver, which could mean danger for some of us in the short term, and for all of us in the long. Which in turn means I have to talk to them, question them. So be sure to take them alive, and do it quickly!* There was pain in his mental voice, quite a lot of it.

But . . . silver bullets? That took something of the arrogance out of the pursuit, while the rest of Trennier's sending served to speed it up.

Liz had almost reached the top of the ramp. Cut from the side of the plateau, the ramp would take her down to the road. But one of her pursuers had somehow managed to flank her and was drawing ahead. He would get there first, and the way was simply too narrow to avoid him. She cut right, heading for where she'd last seen Jake.

Meanwhile someone—or something—back at the shack had started up the Land Rover. Its lights came on, cutting a bright swath through the darkness as it bumped over the rough terrain. Whoever was at the wheel, Liz guessed he'd be looking for Jake. Since hiding or disguising her talent was no longer of benefit, finally she opened her mind to seek her partner's thoughts and perhaps discover his whereabouts.

Liz couldn't send, could only receive, but she knew that other minds—and especially enhanced vampire minds—might be able to detect her presence if not read her thoughts; this was a result of the germ of telepathy that was present in a majority of them. Thus vampires were frequently "spotters." Indeed, the best (or worst) of them could smell out an entirely human being much in the same way as a great hound. But what the hell . . . they already knew she was here.

Jake's mind was immediately accessible:

Fuck! he was thinking. *Oh, Jesus, they've got the vehicle! They're after me!* And yet even now there was very little of any real panic in him. He'd been in too many tight spots before.

But: *Do it!* Liz tried to send, to will him into action. *Do it now, for God's sake!* (Or if not for His sake, for Liz's most definitely!)

He couldn't hear her, of course not, but surely the *other* Jake, that other facet, would have to emerge now? Well, apparently not. And behind Liz her pursuer's footfalls sounded loud and clear, pebbles clattering as they squirted out from under his pounding feet.

She put on speed (one final burst, for her strength was on the wane now), took in great gulping drafts of air through her mouth, headed in the rough direction of Jake's thoughts, where they had led her to believe he was. . . .

Jake, too, was feeling stressed, but obviously insufficiently as yet. The nose plugs were killing him, but he'd been warned about the dangers of removing them. All well and good, but his throat was raw from drinking in dry, dust-laden air, and since he'd probably been splashed with blood it seemed likely he was already contaminated. God, how he could use a beer now, even a warm one—except he probably wouldn't have time to drink it.

The Rover was on his tail, right behind him, when Jake saw a flat-topped boulder. He spun to one side and the vehicle skidded and threw up a cloud of dust as its driver hauled the wheel over. Jake knew that if he had failed to get out of the way the Rover would have hit him. Not hard enough to kill him, maybe, but hard enough to put him out of business, certainly. This big boulder was his only chance.

Leaping onto the rim of the rock, he scrambled to its flat surface as the Land Rover came to a halt. There were two men in the vehicle; he could think of them as men, anyway. One seemed a little dazed: he must be a recent convert, recruit, or thrall. But the other, the driver . . . that one wore a grin like Satan himself. A lieutenant? Jake couldn't even hazard a guess. This was Jake's first time. *In at the fucking deep end!*

The driver was out of the vehicle in a flash, ducking and disappearing beneath the rim of the boulder before Jake could get a bead on him. The other was slower and Jake's first shot hit him in the head. Well, who or whatever he was, he wouldn't be getting back up on his feet again.

As for Jake: even with his record, still he felt sick knowing that he'd killed another man. Except this one hadn't been a man, not any longer. But the sight of the vampire's head exploding like that—the red wet spray, and whatever other colours there had been—just so much black slop in the moonlight . . .

. . . And then Jake asked himself, what moonlight? A cloud, just one damn cloud in an otherwise clear night sky, had drifted across the moon's three-quarters grimace. Just as quickly as that, the night was black as pitch, and the Rover's headlight beams were pointing the wrong way. Darkness favours the vampire, and Jake knew he had to make his move now.

There was room for just two short paces along the flat surface of the boulder. Jake took them, lifted his feet, and hurled himself up and outwards towards the Rover, his arms stretched forward for balance. But even as he cleared the boulder's rim a powerful arm and hand shot up, grabbed his left foot. Jake's impetus carried him forward, his balled-up body turning like a pendulum at the end of that oh-so-strong arm. And when he hit all of the wind was knocked out of him. He felt his nose plugs eject, trailing streamers of gritty snot, as his Browning flew from momentarily nerveless fingers.

Then that nightmare figure was standing over him, leering down at him, going to one knee and reaching for his throat with long, mantrap hands. "That's it," the thing that had been a man said. "The fun and games are over, friend. Well, *yours* are, for sure." With which he drew Jake effortlessly to his feet.

"But yours first!" said a small but resolute female voice. The moonlight came back, and Jake saw the vampire's yellow eyes go wide. As Liz stepped closer, the monster snarled and turned his awful head towards her. The muzzle of Liz's tiny weapon was almost in his astonished, gaping mouth when she pulled the trigger. In that same moment Jake turned his face away, but in any case the *debris* went the other way.

"The Rover!" Liz was pale as a ghost, stumbling where the moonlight picked out her softly feminine curves. She managed to run a few paces, but Jake caught up with her at the vehicle and almost threw her into the passenger seat. He had seen a handful of silent, flame-eyed figures approaching from the direction of the shack. They were the most immediate problem, obviously, but as yet Jake wasn't aware of the lone pursuer tracking Liz. She knew she hadn't lost him, however, and continued to urge Jake: "Let's go! Let's go!"

"Seat belts," he snapped. "It's going to be bumpy!"

Then the engine was roaring, the gears grinding, the Land Rover kicking up dirt as it wheeled for the service road. Which was when Liz's lone pursuer came aboard.

He came from the side, came vaulting into the rear seats in the moment before Jake picked up speed. And off-balance he staggered there, his eyes like hot coals in the night. Jake and Liz had seen him; Liz twisted her body, tried to fire her Baby Browning point-blank, and heard the *click* as the firing pin fell on a dud! The vampire grinned and reached for her, and Jake cursed, changed down, and floored the accelerator. In the back, the vampire was taken by surprise and thrown off-balance again, if only for a moment.

Then, falling to his knees on the back seat, he leaned forward, put his head between theirs, grinned first at Liz then at Jake—before taking the backs of their necks one in each hand. Which was exactly what Jake had hoped he would do. And:

"Hang on!" Jake yelled, and literally stood on the brakes.

Mercifully Liz had seen it coming; she leaned to the right even as Jake leaned left. And the loathsome thing gurgled, "Eh? What?" But the explanation was already forthcoming.

As he flew between them, he released their necks, tried to bring his hands forward to protect his face, didn't even nearly make it. With his arms forming a V behind him, he hurtled forward and smashed face-first through the windshield.

"Godawful—damn—*thing!*" Jake choked, slamming the Rover into first and crunching forward over something that was trying to stand up. They heard its body grinding and thumping, mangled between the Rover's underside and the stony rubble of the terrain.

"My God!" Liz gasped. "I think we might actually make it!"

"Never doubted it," her partner told her, lying for all he was worth.

Just as they turned onto the service track and headed for the ramp, a light commenced flashing on the dash. "Radio," Liz said, reaching under the dash to grab a hidden mike. Thumbing the transmit button, she said, "Hunter One for Zero. What kept you?"

"This is Zero One," a gravelly voice answered in a stutter of static to match the sudden throb of a chopper's rotors. "Is that you mobile down there?" And a searchlight beam swept down from above.

Jake leaned over and spat into the speaker, "Only *fucking* just! Zero—Trask, is that you?—we could use some help."

"Do you have a target?"

"If it's behind us and it's moving, it's a target," Jake said, straightening up in time to avoid a pothole. And as the adrenaline began to recede and his skin stopped prickling, he eased up a little so as not to send the Land Rover nose-diving off the rim of the ramp.

Then Liz said, "Stop!"

"Stop?"

"Stop the vehicle. I want to see."

"Feeling bloodthirsty?" Jake looked at her, frowning as he cautiously applied the brakes.

"Not me." She shook her head, shuddered her relief as she thumbed her nostrils one after the other to blow out her plugs. Then she half turned her head, inclined it to indicate the dark shelf of rock that they'd left behind. "And not them, not after this." And now her voice was a sigh.

They looked up and back. First at a sleek, black dragonfly shape under the gleaming blur of its fan, a shape that blotted the stars in its passing and turned the night to a whirling dervish dust-devil with its downdraft as it sped overhead, then at the torpedo-shapes that tumbled lazily, end over end, down from its belly like so many elongated eggs.

"Jesus!" Jake's sigh matched Liz's.

"Let there be light!" she said.

And there was light. The napalm hit a little way back from the top of the ramp. It lit up a widening path all the way back to the knoll, roared with the thunder of its all-consuming passion, washed the wall of the outcrop like a tsunami of fire. In the space of a few short seconds the scene might well have been that in the caldera of an active volcano; a small mountain burned in the night, with man-made lava flowing down its flanks.

For long moments there were running, leaping, screaming figures in the roiling smoke, blackly silhouetted against terrible balls of fire that seemed to roll across the shelf of the rocky outcrop with lives of their own. The spidery figures were there . . . and they were gone, cindered, rolled under. . . .

The unit was made up of two choppers, a giant support truck and various smaller vehicles, mainly Rovers. The truck and lesser vehicles wouldn't get here for some time yet. They had miles of rough road to cover.

The choppers landed on the shelf itself, one to the north and the other to the south. In half an hour their combat-suited, gas-masked, heavily-armed special forces crews were moving forward into the scorched zone. Meanwhile Jake and Liz had joined up with Ben Trask in charge of operations, also with Ian Goodly his second in command, and a "civilian," Peter Miller, of Australia's Rudall River National Park Administration—or "Mister" Miller, as he insisted on being called.

Obviously Miller hadn't been told too much, which was perfectly understandable; it was all on a need-to-know basis, and when E-Branch went out into the world it was standard procedure to avoid unnecessary rumour-mongering and the panic that might ensue. Miller was small, round and bouncy as a rubber ball; he was very excitable and utterly confused. And like many another small, insignificant man in a position of assumed "authority," he made a lot of noise. Right now he raved on at the tall, unflappable beanpole that was Ian Goodly, who kept steering him away from Ben Trask so that Trask could talk to Liz and Jake. But still Miller's yappy, little-dog voice could be heard over just about everything else that was going on. Right now he was flapping his arms, yelping about:

". . . This uttermost devastation? Damn it all, Mr. Goodly, I know that this is a wasteland, a useless desert region that you can't damage any worse than Nature herself. But . . . there were *men* in that blaze! I saw *men* burning in those hell-fires! What was that stuff, napalm? But in any case, what does it matter? What happened here tonight was sheer murder! There is no other word for it. I . . . I still can't believe what I witnessed here . . . cold-blooded *murder,* Goodly! And someone will be called to answer for it. In fact I demand an answer, right here and now!"

"Who is he?" Liz asked.

Trask frowned. "He's supposed to be our local liaison officer for the Western Deserts Region. A handful of top men in the Aussie Government know what we're doing, just how important our work is. Even so they couldn't simply let us loose, give us carte blanche to get on with things. We were obliged to accept an observer. But that doesn't make him one of us, and I've managed to keep him out of it . . . well, until tonight. Even now I don't intend to waste time with him on long explanations. What we're doing is impossible to explain anyway—not if we expect to be believed. But whether we want Miller or not we've got him, and maybe the best way to keep him quiet will be to let him see for himself something of what's going on."

"Well, he's seen it," Jake growled. "But he isn't quiet."

"He hasn't seen everything." Trask's face was grim. And to Liz, "What do you reckon?"

Knowing what he meant, she opened her mind, gazed intently through the smoke of the remaining fires at the burning shacks where they slumped in the lee of the knoll. And as lines of concentration formed on her brow, she said, "The worst of them—the 'old man,' Bruce Trennier—is still alive. Alive, afraid, and angry. He's still very dangerous, very clever, too. Despite that he tries to hide his thoughts, maybe because of it, I know he's there. His—what, mindsmog?— is as thick as the mist on a swamp, and it stinks a lot worse! He's the boss, but he isn't alone. Back where the fire couldn't reach, in the depths of the old mine, there's a handful of others. They're waiting for us."

Trask nodded. "Well, let's not keep them," he said, his lips twisting in a cold, cruel grimace and his eyes lighting with a vengeful fire of their own. And: "Mr. Miller," he called for the small and small-minded official. "If you will please accompany me? I hope to be able to answer some of your questions. . . ."

3
Firestorm

LOOKING AT BEN TRASK, JAKE CUTTER FOUND himself wondering what it was about the man. He knew some of it—that Trask was the head of a British Secret Service organization called E-Branch, based in London but with many other branches, affiliations, and powerful friends throughout the world—but not everything by any means.

One thing seemed certain, however: Ben Trask was a driven man. Moreover, Jake thought it likely that whatever was driving him was the same thing that caused him to look so much older than his years.

Not that Trask was young; in fact he could have been anything between fifty-five and sixty years old. But while his mousey hair was streaked with white, his skin pale, and his aspect in general aged and maybe even fragile, still the man inside, the mind, soul, and personality—the *id* itself—was diamond-hard. Jake sensed this, and felt a certain empathy for Trask, felt that he knew him, despite that the man had only recently become a factor in his life. But one hell of a factor!

For his height of about five-ten, Trask was maybe a couple of pounds overweight. His broad shoulders slumped just a little, his arms tended to dangle, and his expression was usually, well, lugubrious? Or maybe that, too, was as a result of ... of what? His loss? For that was the impression you got if you caught him unawares: the feeling that something had gone out of him, leaving him downcast, empty; his green eyes strangely vacant or far away, his face drawn, and his mouth turned down at the corners. As if he'd suffered a loss too great to bear. And Jake thought he knew something of how that felt.

On the other hand, if what little Jake had been told about Trask was true, then he might well be misjudging him; Trask's pain could have its origin in something else entirely. For in a world where the simple truth was becoming increasingly hard to find, it would be no easy thing to possess a mind that couldn't accept a lie. And that, allegedly, was what Trask was: a human lie-detector.

E-Branch: E for ESP. Telepaths, empaths, locators, precogs ... psychos? That's how Jake had thought of them just five days ago: as raving lunatics. No, as very quiet lunatics. For nary a one of them had actually raved. But that was five days ago, and in between he'd seen some stuff. And anyway, who was he to talk? What, Jake Cutter, who went on instantaneous, hundred-mile-long sleepwalking tours in broad daylight, and suspected that someone was hiding in his head?

All of these thoughts passing through Jake's mind as he and Liz followed Trask, Goodly, and Miller—who in turn followed a team of four armed-to-the-teeth special agents—between the stinking fires and towards the slumping, blazing ruin that had been the main shack. The lone pump had disappeared; now a column of shimmering blue fire roared its fury at the sky as fuel from the subterranean storage tank burned off. And as Trask's party advanced on the shack, so Miller went prattling on:

"Do you think there can ever really be an answer to this, Mr. Trask? Good Lord, man! But who gave you the authority to do such as this? I mean—*look!*" And his hand flew to his mouth. "A b-b-*body!*" he stammered. "For God's sake! A cindered body!"

In the lee of a clump of hip-high boulders where the blackened, smoking skeletons of cactuses and other once-hardy plants oozed bubbling sap, the clean-up squad had missed something. It was an arm and a hand, protruding from the molten mess of vegetation like a root among all the other exposed roots. Obviously someone had tried to escape the fire by diving for cover in the foliage . . . any port in a fire-storm.

Or rather *it had been* an arm and a hand. Now it was a smoking black twig-thing with four lesser twiglets and the remains of an opposing thumb. Yet even now it was twitching, vibrating, showing signs of impossible life, and the vile soup within the nest of rocks was heaving and bubbling.

"You there—you missed something," Trask called out. And one of the specialists came back with his flamethrower, playing its bright yellow lance on the shuddering mess until it seethed into a black liquid slop.

In the meantime, Miller had been sick. Trask looked at the little fat man unemotionally where he stood trembling, holding a handkerchief to his mouth, and said, "Best if you stay here." And to Liz and Jake, "You two keep Mr. Miller company. But make sure he gets a good look at it if . . . if anything happens." He turned away, moved off with Ian

Goodly. Both of them were equipped with vicious-looking machine-pistols.

"Oh my God!" Miller moaned, hanging half-suspended between Jake and Liz, swaying from side to side. "Oh my good God! Doesn't the man have a heart? I mean, doesn't he feel anything for these poor p-p-people?"

"Ben Trask is *all* heart," Liz told him. "And yes, he feels a great deal for people, for every man, woman, and child of us. For our entire—and entirely *human*—race. That's why we're here. Because these creatures aren't human, not any longer. . . ."

But Miller was bending over, being sick again, and Jake had got behind him, was holding on to make sure he didn't fall facedown in it.

The fires were burning lower now and the night was creeping in again. Long shadows danced like demons, turning the barren rock ledge into a scene from Dante's *Inferno*. Near the main shack the column of flame from the underground tank shrank down into itself, issued a final muffled blast, and then a fireball that rolled like a living thing up the face of the cliff.

Along the foot of the knoll, a second half-team of agents had killed the fire at the shack with the cage and gone inside to explore the secondary mineshaft. While fifty feet away from the main shack—which continued to burn, sending a column of smoke and the occasional lick of red and orange fire into the night sky—Trask brought his team to a halt.

"How about it?" he shouted at Goodly over the crackle of burning brush and scorched timbers. "What do you think? Do we burn him out?"

Not him, them! Liz wanted to yell, but Goodly was already doing it for her. "There's more than just him, Ben." (The precog's piping voice, carried on gusts of hot smoke).

"But we can handle them?" Trask seemed undeterred.

Goodly shrugged and said, "I'm not forecasting any casualties, if that's what you mean. But it won't be very pretty."

"It never is," Trask told him. He came to a decision, nodded, turned, and called for Liz. "Tell them we're going to bring the whole damn place down around their ears . . . and tell *him* he isn't getting out alive. I want you to taunt the bastard!"

"But . . . do you think that he'll hear me?" Liz seemed dubious, unsure of herself. "I mean, I'm only half a telepath. I can receive but not send, and—"

"We can't be sure about that," Trask cut her off. "That's one of the things we're here to find out. But we know your talent isn't fully developed yet, and just because you can't send to a *human* telepath doesn't mean Trennier won't hear you. He's in there, a vampire, and these things have skills of their own. Maybe this will give us some indication of what to expect from you when your talent is fully developed."

Liz gave an answering nod, moved forward. And Miller stood up a little straighter and asked Jake: "Who . . . who is he talking about? And how can that girl talk to someone in there?"

"Just take it for granted she can," Jake answered, despite that he wasn't too sure himself.

And now Liz was concentrating, concentrating, sending her thoughts into the main shaft, its entrance a smoking black hole glimpsed beyond the skeletal facade of the shack. There were no true telepaths on the team this time out, no one to "hear" her or even suspect that she was at work. But her thoughts—which weren't intended for the minds of common men—went out anyway:

We're coming for you, Bruce Trennier, she sent. *And if you think that what you've seen so far is hot stuff, wait till you see how hot it can really get! We have grenades that will bring the roof down on you and your thralls, burying you forever like fossils in the earth, and thermite bombs to melt the rocks into permanent cocoons for your molten bones. You're trapped, with no way out. So stay right where you are, hiding your face from the sun, and do your best to enjoy what little you have left of the rotten, parasitic half-life you call existence. . . .*

It was, of course, a taunt, a challenge, and coming from a

woman would be seen as even more of an insult. If Trennier answered, Liz didn't hear him. What she did hear, or more properly feel, was a sudden silence. A mental silence, a psychic serenity. Or was it more properly a *sullen* silence, the calm before the storm? Ian Goodly confirmed that last with his piped warning: "They're coming."

"How many?" As the combat-suited men fanned out a little, Trask swung his ugly-looking weapon up into the ready position and cocked it. Goodly followed suit, narrowing his eyes as his mind read the future's secrets.

He saw men staggering, crumpling to their knees, bursting into flames! Three of them. And he saw one other—more than a man, an animal, a Thing—leaping headlong to the attack! And:

"Three of them," he yelped. "On their way to hell. And one other who looks like he was born there! That'll be Bruce Trennier. And Ben, they're coming now!"

"Are they armed?" Trask snapped.

"No," Goodly piped. "But . . . do they *need* to be?"

The first three came like moon-shadows: dark and fleeting, seeming to flow with the wreathing smoke, out of the shack and into the open, so that Trask and Goodly could scarcely be sure what they were firing at—but they fired anyway. And in a matter of moments the scene became chaotic.

The nightmarish figures firmed into being as lethal silver bullets found their targets. They had been loping, flowing forwards with their arms and hands reaching, but now were brought up short in the stutter of gunfire, snapped upright and hurled backwards. The feral yellow eyes of the central figure turned red as blood—overflowed with blood—in the instant that the back of his head exploded in a crimson spray. He slumped, went to his knees and burst into flames as the agent with the flamethrower found the range and licked him with a tongue of cleansing fire. There on his knees, with his head half blown away, the vampire burned like a giant candle.

But astonishingly the other thralls recovered and came on. And driving them with the sheer force of his presence, flowing like a vast inkblot immediately behind them, came the last and the worst of them. Their master.

The two in front were Trennier's shields . . . he cared nothing for them or their undead existence . . . his leech was intent on only one thing: its own survival. And for the leech to survive its host must survive, too. But Ben Trask had other ideas.

"Ian, their legs!" he was shouting. "You men, aim at their legs—smash their bones—cut the bastards down!" He kept firing, his machine-pistol a stammering, jerking mad thing in his hands; Goodly's, too, as he followed his leader's example. Likewise from the flanks: a stream of gunfire that turned the night to an uproar as the weapons of the squad spat silver death.

Yet still the three came on. They seemed to float, drifting forwards in that dreadful, dreamlike, kaleidoscopic or strobing stop-motion manner of the vampire. It was hypnotic; it appeared to be slow-motion, but in fact was lightning fast. And now they were only thirty to forty feet away. At which Trask gave a nod to one of his men on the right flank. And:

"Down!" he shouted, as the man armed and lobbed a grenade.

Jake was young and fast, and his military training came in handy; Liz had already thrown herself flat when he took Miller off his feet, covering him with his own body. Then the brilliant flash, and a bang that echoed back from the valley walls.

The entire squad was on the deck; cordite stench came drifting, and with it the mewling of something utterly alien. Jake looked up, saw Trask getting to his feet and offering his hand to Goodly. But in front of the wrecked, smouldering shack: the scene was unbelievable.

One crumpled figure, a hump of broken flesh, shuddered and steamed in the flickering firelight. Another was sitting there, just a trunk with no arms. Smoke curled from his hair; his yellow eyes were dim, rolling vacantly in their orbits. But Trennier was still on his feet. And Jake thought:

This is the "old man," Bruce. A pitiful wreck of a man was what we saw, but this was the reality!

With his clothing in rags, blood-spattered, his awful face sliced open to the bone, still Trennier stumbled forward. Crying out his agony he came on, hands like claws reaching, blood spurting from his gums as his jaws cracked open, and open, and open! His eyes were scarlet . . . his great ears curved and scalloped like the wings of a bat . . . and those *teeth*, scything up through his riven gums!

The man with the flamethrower was on the ground. His weapon lay where he'd let it fall. Trask grabbed it up. And still Trennier came on, weaving towards Liz, reaching for her where she'd managed to get to her knees. "You," the thing rumbled, spitting blood. He seemed dazed; his flickering forked tongue licked tattered lips; finally his eyes focussed and he smiled a monstrous smile. "You, woman . . . thought-caster? You thought to fool me—you even taunted me. Very well, and so you'll *die* with me!"

Jake was up on his feet now, and Miller was on his fat backside, scrabbling away from the horror for all he was worth. But Trennier was concentrating on Liz. He was almost upon her, his oh-so-long hands dripping blood as they reached for her.

Jake caught her round the waist and ran with her, made only two or three paces before tripping and falling. But they didn't hit the ground. No, for it was as if they fell in slow-motion, and in Jake's mind a voice saying: *Now! The numbers—the formula! Read it! Use it!* But his own voice, or some other's?

Numbers rolled on the screen of Jake's mind . . . an endless mathematical progression displaying itself on his brain's computer. Numbers, yes, and he knew them—or *someone* did! Still holding on to Liz, still falling, Jake (or the unseen, unknown someone) stopped the numbers at a certain combination, an impossible formula that at once formed into a door.

They tumbled through it, into a place of negative gravity, a place of nothing at all, and in another moment—or perhaps no *time* at all—through a second door, and only *then* hit the ground. And rolling in the dust full fifty feet away from where they had been, so Jake heard Peter Miller babbling his terror, Trask's cry of triumph or vengeance or both, and the unmistakable roar of the flamethrower.

Even at that distance, still Jake and Liz felt something of the heat and drew back from it, and a moment later spied Miller where he came crying like a child, dragging his fat body along the scorched earth. Then they looked back.

Trennier danced there: the hideous, agonized dance of the true death. Vampire that he was, he beat his arms and screamed his wrath. Or was the awful sound something else? Like the hissing and popping of air- or gas-filled body-cavities when live lobsters are dropped in the pot? Maybe it was the nerve-rending fire-screech of the flamethrower, or perhaps a mixture of both? Jake wasn't sure, couldn't rightly say. He didn't see how Trennier *could* scream—not in the airless inferno that surrounded his melting body.

His stumbling dance went on for many a long second, there in the heart of that blue-white blast of superheated chemicals, until finally he succumbed. But the Thing inside him fought on—or at any rate caused Trennier to fight on—for a while longer yet. And that was the proof, the undeniable proof, of just how long he had been a vampire.

For as his body began to melt and his legs gave way, letting him collapse onto his backside, so at last his meta-morphic flesh answered the call of his vampire nature. It was one last, desperate attempt by Trennier's leech to escape the fire—by using his altered flesh and liquids to damp down the flames.

His scraps of clothing had drifted free of his blackened body to waft aloft on the vile updraft. Now his fingers elon-gated into writhing worms, and his stomach bulged and burst into a nest of lashing purple tentacles. And all of these ap-pendages were like penises that pissed into the fire, but use-lessly. For this was a fire they couldn't put out. Only Ben Trask could do that, and he wouldn't until there was nothing left to burn. Or nothing left that could be considered injurious, anyway. Or at least until his weapon ran out of fuel.

But now the members of the other half-team were back from the ruins of the lesser shack. One of them had a flame-thrower; turning his liquid fire on the vampire and his fallen thralls, he finished what Trask had started. . . .

Eventually it was over, and Trask wanted to know:

"Were there no weapons? Why didn't they have weapons?" Now that it was done he seemed half-mazed, drained, as if there had been fires in him also, and they, too, were now extinguished.

"Weapons?" The second team's leader answered him. "There's a small armory in the mine shaft behind the lesser shack! Maybe they didn't think they'd need guns against just two humans. Anyway, we've set charges well back inside the mineshaft. Thermite, too. When that blows, the whole place will go with it. If there's anything still in there, it won't be getting out."

"Good!" Trask gave himself a shake and took a deep breath. And to the leader of the first team: "Let's get to work on this end, too. I want the main shaft rigged good and deep. Okay, gentlemen, let's move it. The night's not over yet." But it soon would be. By then, too, Trask would be his old self again, hard and businesslike. At least on the surface. . . .

Within the hour the charges were triggered. The ground trembled underfoot, and the deep rumble of man-made thunder sounded from the mouths of the mine shafts. And even though the team's members were standing safely back from the face of the knoll, still they felt the flurry of hot air that rushed out of those night-dark pits, and smelled stenches other than those of chemicals.

Then there were clouds of dust, erupting as from blowholes, as the shafts gave way to countless tons of solid rock and lesser debris that came avalanching from on high. But even then it wasn't quite over, for now the effect of the thermite was seen: white gasses escaping in high-pressure jets, and smoking liquid that filled even the smallest crevices, running over the rocks to seal them.

Finally someone said, "In there, right now, it will be much like a blast furnace—the entire mine, cooking itself. I would sooner take my chances in a cellar in World War II Dresden than in there!"

To which no one gave argument, or even made reply. . . .

The backup vehicles started to arrive and secondary clean-up could now commence. An old man, apparently plagued by rheumatism, hobbled here and there, examining the ashes of fires that were already cooling. Like Trask and Goodly, he wasn't especially protected; he wasn't wearing a gas mask, seemed to breathe freely (which indicated the absence of nose plugs), and didn't appear too concerned with contamination. His only weapons were a wicked-looking machete, hanging in its sheath under his left arm, and an antiquated hand-fashioned crossbow.

While this final phase of the operation got underway, Jake and Liz waited for Trask's instructions. By no means fully recovered from the night's events—lost in private and personal thoughts—they leaned against the side of the Land Rover where Jake had driven it back up onto the shelf to clear the way for the articulated ops vehicle. And they were mainly silent.

But finally Jake shook off his mood of introspection—a worrying, morbid train of thought where he questioned his sanity and pondered the seeming unreality of certain things that had happened and were continuing to happen to him—and fixed his attention on the hobbling old man, who apparently had more than a little authority here. Limping between the flamethrower teams, he appeared to be pointing out areas they had missed in their "scorched earth" mission.

"Burn here," Jake heard him growling over the hiss and roar of searing lances of fire. "And over there, too. Oh, it's charred, I'll grant you that, but charred isn't enough. It must be burned right through. Then, when it's smoke and ashes drifting on the wind . . . *then* it's done with. Not before."

His accent was strange, hard to place: European Mediterranean area, though, definitely. Italy, Sicily, Romania? There was something of a romance language in it, anyway. But in fact, Jake couldn't have been more wrong. Or rather, his conclusion was too "mundane" in the literary sense of the word.

"Who is he?" he asked Liz. "The old boy there? Look at him. He reminds me of nothing so much as a bloodhound . . . the way he stops every now and then to sniff the night air! The only thing *I* can smell is smoke and fire . . . and death. And what about his clothing? Just what does he think he is: some kind of frontiersman out of the wild west?"

And for a fact the old man might well have been a frontiersman—and was, of sorts—but a wilder west than any Jake might have imagined.

"You know," Jake went on, "I got the impression that there was something of the Romany, something Gypsyish about the vampire Bruce Trennier. Well, now I have the same kind of feeling about this fellow. Hell, he even jingles when he moves!"

But the oldster had spotted them even as Jake spoke, and he came hobbling in their direction. Ben Trask came, too; probably to make introductions, Jake thought. And meanwhile Liz was answering at least one of his queries:

"You said he reminded you of a bloodhound," she said. "And you're just about right. A human bloodhound is exactly what he is. What you've seen tonight, he's seen so many times he can't count them. So I've gathered, anyway. His name is Lardis, sometimes called the Old Lidesci."

"Liz." The old fellow nodded his greeting and smiled a gap-toothed smile, but in the next moment he was frowning, stepping closer, turning his head on one side to look up into Liz's face. *"Huh!"* he grunted, spitting in the dirt. "No plugs! What, and are you imp—imper—er, imperv . . ."

"Impervious?" she helped him out.

"Yes!" he snapped, pointing an accusing finger at her. "And you, too!" He turned to Jake. "Cutter, is it? Jake Cutter?"

"We *were* wearing plugs," Jake answered. "Then we got involved in a lot of activity. My plugs were knocked out of me, but Liz had hers to the end. And anyway, who the hell—?"

"Decon—!" the other abruptly cut him short. "Er, decontam—contam . . ."

"Decontamination," Liz said.

"Right!" the old man snapped, jerking his thumb in the direction of the command truck. "Both of you. Now!"

"Who on earth—?" Jake started again. But by then Ben Trask was there to stop him.

"Jake Cutter," Trask said, "this is Lardis Lidesci. I heard you asking who on earth? Well, nobody on *Earth*, actually. Originally he's from . . . oh, a different place entirely." Trask had almost let something drop, stopped himself at the last moment. "Lardis was in the Greek Islands with another team," he changed the subject. "When they didn't find what they were looking for, I asked that he be sent here. He came in this afternoon by chopper from Perth." And turning to the Old Lidesci, he said "Well? How about it?" Obviously there was something between the two of them that Jake and Liz weren't privy to.

"Him?" Lardis looked at Jake, frowned, gave a shrug. "Can't say. Could be, I suppose. Fit and young . . . and stubborn! Won't listen to good advice, and doesn't respect his elders too much, either! Makes him a funny choice if you ask me. But if it's so it's so, and who are we to fathom the ways of the Necroscope?"

"Nothing certain, then?" Trask seemed disappointed.

Lardis shrugged again, and said, "Well, the proof could be right here in the slime and the stink where these bastards burned . . . that's if you *really* want to test your theory?"

Trask knew what Lardis meant even if Jake didn't. He shook his head, said, "No, he's not ready for that yet. And probably not for quite some time to come."

Jake had been studying Lardis. The Old Lidesci was short, barrel-bodied, almost apelike in the great length of his arms. His lank black hair, beginning to grey now, framed a leathery, weather-beaten face with a flattened nose that sat uncomfortably over a mouth that was missing too many teeth. As for the ones that remained: they were uneven and stained as old ivory. But under shaggy eyebrows, Lardis's dark brown eyes glittered his mind's agility, denying the encroaching infirmities of his body. Jake guessed he'd been a leader, and rightly so.

If Jake examined Lardis Lidesci, it was certainly no less of an inspection that the old man was giving him. And suddenly, feeling uncomfortable, Jake went on the defensive. Frowning, he said, "I wish you'd talk *to* me, you two, instead of *about* me! I mean, you were talking about me, weren't you?"

"About you and about someone else," Trask told him. "We're talking about the fellow that you think—and that we think—might be in your head. Talking about a man called Harry Keogh."

"I never heard of him," said Jake, but wondered if in fact he had. The name did seem somehow familiar . . . and *felt* familiar, too, in a weird sort of way. Which only served to confuse him and make him angry. "Anyway, what has he to do with me?"

Trask rubbed his chin, said, "There's something he used to do that . . . well, that you seem to do, too. When Liz was under threat, you . . . you *moved* her away from Trennier. And I know I don't need to remind you that that's how you first came to our attention. It's how you brought yourself to our attention: by moving in on us."

Jake shook his head. "That wasn't deliberate," he said. "I mean, I didn't have anything to do with it. It wasn't me."

"Exactly," Trask told him.

Jake frowned again. "I don't see the connection."

"Neither do we," Trask said. "Not just yet. But if there is one, we're going to find out about it." His eyes were speculative, bright with some strange emotion—hope, perhaps?—where they studied Jake's face. But then he shrugged it off and said, "Meanwhile, Lardis is right. Decontamination time for you two. And I do mean right now."

And Liz and Jake both knew enough—they had seen enough now—not to argue; and so headed for the command vehicle. . . .

When they had left:

"I missed it," the Old Lidesci spoke to Trask. "But he did actually do it, then, this Jake? He used the Möbius Continuum?"

Trask nodded. "And that makes three times now that we know of."

"Then we must accept that he is what he is," Lardis shrugged. "It seems obvious to me."

"And I wish it seemed as obvious to me," said Trask. "It's just that I don't like the coincidence—that at a time such as this he turns up."

"But what better time?" Lardis asked him.

"Or what worse?" Trask countered. "The point is, we know what he *might* be, but we don't know what he *is*. The only thing I know for sure, it isn't an act. He really doesn't know what's going on."

"And you haven't told him?"

"What do you want me to tell him, Lardis? That part of him has been occupied by someone who talks to dead people? Someone who can even call the dead up out of the earth, to walk again? Someone who, at the end of 'life as we know it,' was himself a vampire—and not only him but two of his sons, too? Should I tell him that in Starside, in your world, one of Harry Keogh's sons was a Lord of the Wamphyri, while another was The Dweller, a werewolf? And if Jake didn't think I was a madman, if he actually believed me, what then?"

Again Lardis's shrug. But then, perhaps grudgingly: "I see what you mean," he growled. "If it was me, I'd run like all the devils of hell were after me!"

"And so might he," Trask nodded. "And in the Möbius Continuum, he can run a very long way. We can't afford that, can't afford to lose him. Which is why we'll just let this thing develop for a while, and see what happens. . . ."

*   *   *

Some little distance away, as Jake and Liz passed a patch of blackened, tarry ground and a slumped mound that still gave off the stench of roasting flesh:

"What?" Jake paused, his face very pale. "What? Do you hear that, those screams? Jesus, what the hell *is* that?" He turned in a circle, looked all about, but no one was there.

For a moment Liz said nothing. She had heard nothing and couldn't imagine what he was talking about—or maybe she could but didn't want to. But it was plain to see that Jake was badly shaken. "Screams?" she said. "The hiss and sputter of sap, perhaps, boiling out of a scorched branch?"

"Well, maybe," Jake shuddered. "Maybe."

But he really didn't think so. What he *knew* he'd heard had sounded much more like the screaming soul of a sinner, roasting in his own private hell. Or perhaps someone shrieking his final denial from a world beyond the flames, a world beyond life.

And the bubbling patch of scorched earth continued to give off steam and smoke. . . .

4
Gadgets and Ghosts

THE DECONTAMINATION BOOTHS REMINDED JAKE of those antique telephone kiosks so treasured by collectors. They weren't red and didn't have those small glass panes for windows, but they were much the same size and even smelled bad. Not of urine, no, but of garlic; Jake couldn't make up his mind which was more nauseous.

Situated in the back of the rearmost articulated trailer section, and fitted with doors as small as the toilet doors on an airplane, there were three booths on each side. Inside each booth was a disposal unit for soiled clothing; discarded items were sucked away, irradiated and microwaved, spat from an exterior chute and burned. The procedure covered *all* clothing.

Which meant you were left buck-naked in the waterproof and airtight booth, where the rest of the process was entirely automatic. And that was when you discovered why these claustrophobic little shower-units—for that's what they were—smelled so foul. At first it was just hot water, stinging like BB shot where it blasted down on you from overhead jets, but in a few seconds it was something else: a mixture of something chemical and antiseptic, and something vegetable and oily. The chemical saturated and then evaporated, but the oil stayed. And—damn it to hell!—you were supposed to rub it into your pores. But if there was one thing Jake especially hated, it was garlic!

There was an intercom system; you could talk to people in the ops section, or to other agents undergoing decontamination in the booths. The uppermost sections of the booths were glass-panelled on the sides from the neck up, and from there down stainless steel. This last was simply a matter of common decency; there were female as well as male agents.

Jake had chosen a central booth and Liz had taken the one to his left. Switching on her booth intercom, she said, "I see you picked the middle one. You could have taken the one on the end, so there'd at least be a booth between us!" Looking sexy as hell (for all that Jake could only see her face, her long slender neck and shoulders), she pulled an impish face at him through the glass.

But he only grinned—a rare occurrence in itself where Jake Cutter was concerned—and answered, "Oh, really? And why didn't you choose one on the other side of the vehicle, so you wouldn't have to be near me at all?" Then on the spur of the moment he leaned forward, flattened his hawk nose to the glass panel, and made as if to look down inside her booth. There was no way; the glass was misted at the edges and it was all gleam, steam, and cream down there. "Oblige me and stand on your toes, will you?" he grunted— and was so astonished at himself that he bit his tongue—and

53

was equally amazed at Liz when, for a single instant of time, she actually seemed to consider doing it.

It was the look on her face: a not-quite innocence, a curiosity, a magnetism that worked both ways. She looked beautiful like that: hair plastered down, makeup all washed away, and her skin shiny with oil yet still beautiful. Jake was drawn by it—and repulsed. There was something he'd vowed to himself, and he would stick by it to the end, until it was done. And anyway, Liz didn't stand on her toes but simply blushed. Or maybe that was as a result of the steam. In which case it would be hiding his colour, too . . . thank the Lord!

"Anyway, what are you doing here?" she said. And maybe it was his imagination, but her voice sounded just a little husky. Must be the intercom. "I mean, you've made it amply clear that you don't want to be with us. So why are you?"

Jake glanced at the intercom panel. Liz's button was the only that was lit up. No one else was listening, so their conversation would be completely private. That was assuming he wanted to talk, of course. And suddenly he did. "I didn't have any choice," he said. "I could be here or I could be locked up. Well, I've been in jail, and here is better. But after tonight, I can tell you it's not *much* better." There he stopped short, reconsidered. Why bother? Why try to get close to anyone? He'd been close to someone before, and she'd paid for it. Once was enough.

"They . . . they jailed you for murder?" Liz said, and her face was very serious now. "That's what I've heard, anyway."

"I killed some people," Jake nodded. "And if I get half a chance there are still two more who I want to kill." He admitted it oh so matter-of-factly, and for a moment his brown eyes were very nearly black; they were bleak, too, almost vacant in their intensity. Liz felt that Jake's eyes looked at something a thousand miles away, perhaps a scene from memory, his as yet undisclosed past. Or maybe it was just an effect of the misted glass.

But then he smiled, however wanly, and was animate

again. "So, there you go. That's me, Mr. Bad Man. So what's your story, Liz? What's a nice girl like you doing in a freaky outfit like this?"

She felt cheated, because she knew he hadn't told it all. Not nearly. "Tell me just one more thing," she said, shivering because the spray was cooler now, and also because of the look she'd seen in his eyes. "About you, or about those men you say you killed. Did they deserve it?"

He looked at her, then answered her with a question of his own. "What about those creatures tonight: did *they* deserve it?"

"But they were vampires, monsters!"

He simply nodded, left it for her to figure out. . . .

By which time the spray had become shampoo, and they knew it was nearly over, this part of it, anyway. As he soaped himself down Jake reminded her, "I'm waiting." Despite his doubts, his resolve, still his interest couldn't be denied.

"Hmm?" she said. Then, "Oh! Why am I here? That's easy. I was doing some work for a psychic research group. Looking back, I suspect it was an E-Branch recruiting ploy. They haven't said as much, not yet, but I gather they're pretty hush-hush until a person is well established with them. Anyway, the job was easy, the money was good and I needed the work. My office was in central London; I interviewed people, allegedly for *Mind Magazine*, and if they responded positively to a certain set of questions, then I was supposed to work with them and carry out a series of tests." She shrugged, and through the misted glass Jake saw her shoulders give a little twitch, the suggestive movement of her underarm flesh as the weight of her ample breasts settled.

"Anyway," she went on, "I used an old German Prismaton 70 in the tests, and—"

"A what?" Jake cut her off.

"It's a machine that chooses psi symbols at random."

"Psi symbols?"

Liz sighed. "Five designs: a star, a circle, a square, a plus sign, and wavy lines."

"I'm with you now," Jake said. "The machine picks the

symbol, and the test subject has to guess which one it is."

"Except it's not supposed to be a guess," Liz told him. "I mean, they're supposed to concentrate and try to *know* what symbol it is! That's what ESP is all about."

"Go on."

"Well, at first I would get a few lucky guessers . . . they might come up with two or three correct symbols in a row and I would get all excited. But in the long run it never worked out to anything, and I'd be disappointed because, you know, I wanted to *earn* my money. But for me to be successful, obviously my test subjects had to be successful, too. And so I found myself willing them to get it right. Someone would say, "Square!" And I would be telling myself, "No, no, *no!* That's wrong! It's the wavy lines!" Until I reached the stage when I was saying, "No, that's wrong," or, if someone got lucky, "yes, that's right," *before* they named their choice, before they even spoke!"

"Let me guess," said Jake. "You didn't know what was going on. You thought that either you were mistaken, or the machine—the, er, Prismaton 70?—was playing tricks with you, or—"

"But it couldn't be the machine," Liz cut him short, "because it's *only* a machine."

"—Or that you yourself," Jake went on, "must somehow be 'in tune' with your subjects. Mental telepathy, right?"

She nodded. "It was me. It wasn't that my subjects, an incredibly high percentage of them, were good at sending—which is E-Branch parlance for telepathic transmissions—but that *I* was good at receiving. I *was* a receiver, a mind-reader. I could 'tune in' to other people's thoughts, yes. Not all the time and not without a lot of effort and concentration, but sometimes."

"Which was something you'd never noticed before?" Despite the events of the night—the fact that he'd observed for himself her obvious effect on Trennier—still Jake was a little skeptical. "I mean, that you knew what people were thinking?"

She grinned. "Well, I frequently knew what *men* were

thinking!" Slowly her grin disappeared. "No, seriously, I hadn't the foggiest idea. But as soon as I *did* know, then it was like Topsy."

"It just growed and growed. . . ." Jake thought it over.

"And then there's you," Liz said pointedly. But he wasn't having any and simply looked away.

The soap had stopped and it was plain water now, and cold. Just as they might have started complaining, the system closed itself down and a light began flashing on the intercom. It was Trask, wanting to know, "Are you people done? Good! So get out of there and make room for someone else." The rest of the team, all of them, would go through a less intensive cycle. But Jake and Liz weren't finished yet.

Dry towelling robes dispensed themselves from compartments in the rear of the booths, with plastic bag "booties" for their feet. Then the doors concertinaed of their own accord, and outside in the corridor other agents were coming aboard and making ready. But Jake and Liz stayed apart from them and went on into the body of the ops vehicle and the next stage, where Trask himself administered hypodermic injections while the old man, Lardis Lidesci, stood watching. Until finally they were obliged to drink something vile.

"God!" Jake gasped, clutching his throat. And again: "*God,* but if I'm not going to be sick as a dog . . . !"

"If you *are,*" said the Old Lidesci, "I'll take it as a very bad sign." And Trask grinned, however coldly, as Lardis fondled the grip of his machete.

"He won't be sick," Trask said then. "And even if he is it won't mean anything. I remember I was sick myself, desperately, the first time I tasted that stuff."

"Garlic?" Still Jake felt like gagging.

"Derived from," Trask shrugged. "Anyway, it's good for you . . . or so I'm told." Turning, he led the way down the corridor, past doors to a half-dozen cramped bunks, and through a telescopic conduit and hatch into the vehicle's forward trailer section. Then at last they were there: in the ops room itself, the mobile nerve-centre. . . .

* * *

Ian Goodly was in the hollow oval that formed the central desk. He swung round the oval on a tracked chair, studying the various illuminated wall-charts and monitor screens. The place was hi-tech heaven, well in advance even of anything else that AD 2011 had to offer. In complete contrast to the articulated shell of truck and trailers—indeed, utterly contradicting that outer façade, with its mundane and easily identifiable "Castlemaine" and "XXXX" legends—this interior was something out of speculative fiction. And never a can of beer in sight.

Goodly was wearing what looked like a virtual reality headset that was constantly tuning itself to whatever event or location he was observing. But as he swung into a new position and Trask and company came between the precog and the ever-changing screens, so Goodly brought his chair to a halt and took off the headset.

The Old Lidesci shook his grizzled head in astonishment and grunted, "After all this time working with you people, I'm still not used to it! Not used to . . . to this."

Trask nodded his understanding. "I know what you mean," he said, "but you won't get too much sympathy from me. Hell, it's been more than thirty years for me—and I *still* feel the same about it! What was it Alec Kyle used to say? How did he put it? Or was it Darcy Clarke?" He shrugged. "But what difference does it make, eh? It could have been any one of us. 'Robots and romantics. Super science and the supernatural. Telemetry and telepathy. Computerized probability patterns and precognition. *Huh!* Gadgets and ghosts!' Well, that's it. That's E-Branch."

But Jake wanted to know: "Just what *is* E-Branch? What's it all about? Don't you think it's time we saw the whole picture?" He glanced at Liz. "Well, me at least . . . especially after what you threw me into tonight?"

"Threw *us* into," said Liz. "I'm not as much in the dark as you, Jake, but it's still pretty murky around here." She looked at Trask, perhaps accusingly. "And after all, while tonight was one of the first things we've done, it might also have been the last."

But Ian Goodly shook his head. "No," he said. "You have a way to go yet, you two."

"Precog," Jake said, sourly. "That's how I've heard people refer to you. But how can you possibly know for sure?"

And Trask said, "Because he hasn't let us down yet."

"And what if tonight had been the first time?" Jake wasn't convinced.

But Trask only raised a white eyebrow. "So what's your big problem, Jake? Are you trying to kid us you haven't been doing your best to get yourself killed these last three years?"

"Maybe," Jake snapped. "But on *my* terms!"

"Well, now it's on my terms," Trask growled. "Or E-Branch's terms." Then he relaxed a little, looked less severe, and said, "Okay, I'll tell you. It was a test. Oh, it served its purpose, too, but it was nevertheless a test. And you both passed it. We saw enough tonight—enough happened—to convince us we were right."

"About me?" Jake said.

"About both of you," Trask replied. "Liz did her thing, and we all saw Trennier's reply. She sent and he received—and he reacted!"

"Did he ever!" said Liz with a shudder. "But you're the one who told me to taunt him."

Trask nodded and said, "And you made a damn good job of it, too, and satisfied our best expectations. So, if you still want in, welcome to the club. You're one of us. And having seen what you've seen—even with what little we've allowed you to learn—we've no doubt but that you'll join us. So that's that. And in any case you have time to think about it."

"And do I have time to think about it, too?" Jake said testily. "If so you can have my answer right now. It's no, I'm out."

Trask frowned, narrowed his eyes, and said, "Well, that's a damn shame because *you* don't have a choice. And that's because you, too, did your thing tonight. Something I haven't seen the likes of in, oh, five years. And when I did last see it . . . it was in another world, a vampire world, Lardis's world."

Jake looked at the three men in turn—Trask, Goodly, Lardis Lidesci, the way they looked back at him: sincere, serious, speculative?—and shook his head in mock despair. "I've been telling myself that it's all a dream, one from which I'll soon be waking up," he said. Then his voice hardened. "But it isn't and I won't—not from any dream of *mine*, anyway. This is your dream, your fucking nightmare, and I've had it up to here!"

"Oh no, this is everyone's nightmare," Trask told him, and then pressed on: "But which part do you think is a dream, Jake? The strange work we do, or the fantastic thing that you do?"

"I don't *do* anything!" Jake turned on him, and for a moment looked like he might hit him. "It just . . . it just happens." He clenched his fists, unclenched them, stood lost for words.

Trask shook his head. "But things don't just happen, Jake," he said. "They happen for reasons. And we've got to figure out why they're happening to you." He turned to Ian Goodly. "Do we have his file?"

The precog nodded, swung his chair to a filing cabinet set in a section of the oval desk, took out a slim folder and handed it over.

There were chairs that folded into the walls. Trask let one down, sat in it, and invited the others to do the same. Then he opened the file. And:

"Jake Cutter . . ." he began.

But Jake's voice was harsh as he interrupted: "Do you intend to read it all? Even the nasty bits? With a woman present?" The others had taken chairs, but he was still standing.

"Brief details," Trask said, staring up at him. "Why do you ask? Is there something you're ashamed of?"

"What has that got to do with it?" Jake blurted. "That's my life you're holding in your hands. It's private—or it used to be."

"The newspapers didn't think so." Trask didn't even blink.

"Hell, no, they didn't!" Jake said. "They held me one hundred percent responsible for my 'crimes'! And do you intend to detail those, too? Is this how you're going to keep me in line, working for you, for E-Branch: by holding a bloody axe over my head every time I voice an opinion or refuse to cooperate?"

Trask shook his head. "That has nothing to do with it. The object of the exercise is to get to the root of your talent. As for your so-called 'crimes,' it's the opinion of this Branch that you don't have too much to be ashamed of."

For a moment Jake was taken aback, but then he said, "What if I don't much care about the opinion of this Branch?"

"But you do," said Trask. "You believe in justice, and you couldn't get any. So you provided your own rough justice, which was just a little *too* rough for our modern society. In E-Branch, Jake, we understand rough justice. It's sometimes the only kind that will fit. And we were taught by an expert, someone who believed in an eye for an eye almost as much as you do. Well, now we wonder if that's all you have in common with him, or if this talent of yours is something else. And what's more, there might even be other talents. We want to explore that possibility, too—indeed, every possibility—and you can help us or hinder us. In which case . . . eventually we'd be obliged to give up on you. And there's still an empty cell waiting for you, remember?"

Jake's hard-frozen shell was coming apart now. Not his resolve but the icy sheath that covered it, without which he wouldn't have been able to face his own atrocities. For that was how he secretly viewed some of his past deeds, as atrocities. Everyone else had seemed to think so anyway. Yet in his heart, still Jake believed that what Ben Trask had said was right: sometimes an eye for an eye was the only way. And suddenly Jake found himself believing everything else that Trask was telling him, that E-Branch really did care and was on his side. It was just that it had been such a long time since anyone was on his side.

And now Trask was saying, "So can we get on?"

Jake drew a chair out from the wall, sat down heavily, and

said, "Why do I get this feeling this isn't a con? You're what they call a human lie-detector, right? Well, Mr. Trask, if you ask me, I'd say *your* talent works both ways. I get the impression that you really do want to help me, even if it's only so I can help you."

Trask actually smiled then, and said, "Jake, you're exactly right. I hate all lies and liars, and I instinctively know when something isn't true, isn't right. Don't ask me how, I just do. But it's equally hard for me to *tell* a lie as to listen to one. I just thought you might like to know that."

Jake nodded, and feeling a little more in control now said, "Okay, so if you think there's . . . something wrong with me and you can maybe fix it, I suppose I'd be a fool to object."

Trask sat back and issued an audible sigh. "Very well. But you have to understand. It's not that we think there's anything wrong with you, but that something may be right. From our point of view, anyway."

And then he returned to the file. . . .

"Your father was a USAF pilot," Trask began. "As a rookie, Joe Cutter served at an American air-base in southern England. That was where he met your mother, an English girl from a well-to-do family. Janet Carson's folks objected; they got married anyway; for a while Janet was a camp-follower, living wherever Joe was based. Then you came along, doing your bit to stabilize a frequently stormy relationship . . . well, for a little while, anyway. But the marriage didn't last. Your father was too often away, and your mother . . . took lovers." Trask lifted his gaze from the file, looked at Jake. "If this is too personal I can skip forward . . . ?"

"You're doing okay." Jake shrugged. "Since my parents left me nothing in the way of great memories, what does it matter?"

And so Trask continued. "Your mother had friends in what's called 'high society.' Eventually she married a French businessman, with whom she lived in Saint-Tropez, until . . . well, until she died five years ago."

Again Jake's shrug, though not as careless as he might

have tried to make it seem. "It's nice in Nice," he said.

"So as a baby you went to your British grandparents," Trask went on, "who were maybe a little on the wrong side of fifty to take on your upbringing. As for your father: Joe Cutter died on aerial manoeuvres in Germany in 1995, piloting a way-beyond-its-sell-by-date airplane known 'affectionately' to its pilots as a 'Flying Coffin.' Joe was coming to the end of his service when it happened, and you were just fifteen years old.

"You were an unruly kid, Jake. Too much money, courtesy of your then aging and indeed doting grandparents, too many opportunities to smoke 'funny' cigarettes, and probably to try other 'controlled' pharmaceuticals? Too much time on your hands, and nothing much to look forward to, not to your way of thinking at least. So you dropped out of school, spent some time with your mother in France; but she had quite a few bad habits of her own and wasn't a very good influence. And anyway, you didn't get on with her. You said you might join the army and your grandfather was delighted. He said, 'Excellent! The Brigade of Guards! The old school tie and all that, wot? Wot?' So you joined the parachute regiment because you wanted to jump out of airplanes. And in just two years you transferred to the SAS. Well, so much for parental guidance.

"When they kicked you out of the SAS your final report said you were incapable of taking orders. Also, and this is a damned strange thing for the SAS, the report said you were too much of a loner. This from an outfit that prides itself on self-dependence, or total *in*dependence! So there you were, five years ago: back to the good life, a life of luxury in the South of France, where you lived off your ma's money."

Jake shrugged, but he looked more than a little uncomfortable. "Her second husband left her a packet," he said. "And her third was even richer. So why should I break my back working?"

"I'm not criticizing you, Jake," Trask told him. "I'm just pointing out what you were then, in order to find a comparison with what you later became in the eyes of society.

Which is to say a criminal. More than that, a brutal murderer."

"Now just you wait a minute!" Jake started to say, "Didn't you tell me that you—" until Trask cut him off with:

"In the eyes of *society*, anyway. But society has been known to make the odd mistake here and there. And E-Branch . . . well, we're sometimes called in to clean up the mess; though as often as not we just jump in feetfirst regardless. Very well, now we can get away from your story for a minute or so. . . ." And after a brief pause he went on:

"For the last fifteen to twenty years—or even longer than that, indeed ever since the fall of Communism—Europe has been in one hell of a mess. Recessions, revolutions, coups one after the other; nuclear black spots where Russian power-stations and weapons dumps are left rotting down to so much atomic rubble; little wars, and not so little wars left, right, and centre as nations take their revenge, engage in racial vendettas that should have been settled, probably would have been settled, a hundred years ago if Soviet expansionism and Communism hadn't called a temporary halt to them. Power struggles in political systems that are *still* sorting themselves out, in Rome and Moscow and elsewhere; ethnic cleansing in and around the Slavic and Baltic countries, and regular revolutions in Turkey, Bulgaria, and Romania. Italian, French, and German governments coming and going as regular as the ticking of a clock, and lasting about the same length of time, never long enough to do anyone any good. And as for the Near and Middle East, Africa, Asia . . ." Trask sighed and shook his head. "Have I painted a sufficiently gloomy picture?" And without waiting for an answer:

"Well, thank God we're an island—England, I mean—and also that we've maintained and strengthened our ties with America and Australia. Because the rest of the world seems like no-man's-land. In a word, it's chaos.

"It seems an ideal scenario for the end of life as we know it, right? Even as I speak the depletion of the ozone layer continues, we're into yet another El Niño—the fourth in fifteen years—and there's a rip-roaring plague spreading west out of an ideologically and financially exhausted China. But there are worse plagues than a new strain of the bubonic, believe me."

Again a brief pause, until: "And so back to you," Trask continued, staring at Jake.

"Your mother died of an overdose, left you some money—"

"The money was about the only decent thing she ever did for me," Jake nodded, his husky tone betraying his true emotions.

"—But you and money together spelled more trouble," Trask chose to ignore the interruption. "So maybe you didn't have too much going for you, you and your ma—still, her death affected you badly. You went on a long drinking spree in all the Mediterranean resorts from Genoa to Marseille, wrecked your car on the Italian Riviera; the paparazzi took your photograph during several fist-fights in Cannes. Also it's not at all unlikely that you returned to your drug-taking habits."

"I never had much of a habit," Jake told him. "Oh, I tried just about every brand, that's true, but they only made me ill. Those 'funny' cigarettes were about as bad as it ever got, and where I've spent the last three months even they were far too expensive. I'm used to my asshole the shape and size I've always known it." He looked at Liz and said, "Sorry, but if you insist on being here . . ."

She shook her head, answered, "I'm not a child, Jake. After tonight I thought you'd know that much at least."

Trask went on just as if no one else had spoken. "Then you met a girl. There'd been women in your life—quite a few—but this one was something else. She was special."

"This is the bit you can skip," Jake told him gruffly.

"Unfortunately not," Trask answered. "If Liz is to be your partner, and the rest of E-Branch is to work with you, they'll need to know that you aren't quite the savage that the world—and probably you, too, Jake—thinks you are. They'll need to know you had your reasons."

And Jake sat silently now, his head lowered. . . .

5
Jake's Story

"HER NAME WAS NATASHA," TRASK WENT ON. "AND she was working for the Moscow Mafia. She was a courier for the Mob in the guise of a fashions artist, but in fact the only designs that interested her were the designer micro-drugs in her sports car's roll bars. Natasha was also the Mob's collection agent and ferried lots of high denomination francs and lire back to a vastly depleted Russian economy . . . or rather, to the thugs who were in large part responsible for that depletion."

Trask shook his head in disgust. "God! Hoods of the world, unite! We thought it was over and done with when the Mafia took a couple of bad falls back in 1984 to '87. In America, the families really suffered. When Gotti went down everyone thought it was the end of that kind of corruption, at least in the USA. In Sicily, '87, nearly four hundred of these lizards were convicted of murder, extortion, graft, racketeering, prostitution, you name it. Surely that was the end of it? Oh, really?

"But the Russian Mafia were just starting out, and with the collapse of the European immigration laws ten years ago and the removal of border controls on the continent . . . Well, as I said, thank the Lord that the U.K.'s an island. We kept our border controls, our immigration laws, and for once we got it dead right. Even so, the illicit drug trade is hard to beat and we're suffering our fair share, though not nearly as badly as the rest of the world. And of course hardcore survivors of police activity and 'old' Mafia-style gang wars in Italy, Sicily, and the States have formed liaisons with the ever-more-powerful Russian gangs, which means that in common with the world's terrorist organizations, they're now pretty much integrated.

"Marseille has always had a big drug problem. The Riviera, with its jet-setters and high-roller socialites, has been drug-dealer heaven for a long, long time. Natasha Slepak's mobility—the routes she used—were several, but mainly she would fly from Moscow to Budapest and then drive down into Italy or over into France. Or she might use another route into France, driving into Genoa, then taking a yacht to the French Riviera. The Mob have contacts, keep boats, in most Italian seaports.

"Jake met Natasha in Marseille. According to a statement he made later—much later—to the Italian police, she wanted out of the drugs business. She was being pestered for sex by one of the Italian Mob's top men, one Luigi Castellano, a young Sicilian who ran the French side of the action from a sprawling villa on the outskirts of Marseille. Castellano was Natasha's top contact in France, and he was also the man she most feared and hated. . . ."

As Trask paused, Jake—who had been looking more and more agitated—burst out, "If it has to be told, let me do the telling from here on in." Trask pursed his lips, then nodded.

"We met in a bar," Jake began. "What you've just heard is true: Natasha wanted out. But there was nowhere she could run, not on the Continent, anyway. No border controls; the Mob would find her wherever she went. Maybe that's why she went for me—because I had British nationality—but that's only a maybe. I prefer to think . . . well, otherwise. Anyway, we got on famously. For a couple of days I wined and dined her; she was a very good reason for staying sober, staying clean. We roomed at different hotels . . . so I thought. But in fact she was staying at Castellano's villa, and all the time fending the bastard off! She wouldn't come anywhere near my place. In short, she wasn't any kind of pushover. And I knew she was worried about something.

"Eventually she told me just about everything. And all the time—all through our 'romance,' if you want to call it that— I was aware that she was being watched; even when I'd first met her, there was this tall guy watching from the shadows. I didn't tell her about it, but I knew I wasn't mistaken. Finally she told me why we couldn't be together. It was for my sake: she didn't want me to get into trouble.

"The time came when she said she'd have to be moving on. I knew I loved her, even though it had been less than a week. Maybe I needed someone to love. My mother was recently dead, and I guessed that at the rate I was burning myself up it wouldn't be too long before I'd be joining her. And now there was Natasha to fill a void I had never thought would exist, and I just couldn't see anything to stop us being together. But she could: the Mob. So I asked her why shouldn't we go and tell her story to the local police, the Surete? She said they were in Castellano's pocket. So I said she should think about something: next time she'd be in Marseille, let me know beforehand and I would be there to take her out of it; to England where she'd be safe. Or comparatively safe, anyway. And she said okay.

"So on our last night together I was in a pretty frustrated mood. And wouldn't you know it? Her tail was there as always. I would know him anywhere: this tall man with his thin white face and dark eyes. But we had made our plans and the next time Natasha was in town would be the last time. She would come with me into England on a tourist visa, we'd get married, and she would stay on as my wife. It seemed more than likely she'd be lost to the Mob for good. So maybe she thought we should seal our pact. Or perhaps it was more than that; maybe she simply wanted to be with me on what would be our last night for some time to come.

"Anyway, she said yes, she would come back to my hotel with me. But there was no way I intended to have the tall fellow for company."

"We took a taxi to a bar a stone's throw from my hotel, and when Natasha went to the ladies' I waited just inside the door. Sure enough a car pulled up and the tail got out. And that finally did it for me; I'd had it up to here. So stepping outside I didn't bother to introduce myself but simply lashed out and knocked him down. Some of the stuff the SAS had taught me was finally coming in handy. And before he was even nearly ready to get up again, I took Natasha off to my hotel.

"Looking back on it now—oh, I was some kind of clown! To actually believe I could get away with it. Worse, I hadn't considered the repercussions where Natasha was concerned. Though I certainly did the next morning. . . .

"After breakfast, when I took her down to catch a taxi, the heavies were there. And this time I didn't see them, didn't see it coming—didn't even feel it until I woke up at Castellano's villa. Not that I knew where I was at the time; my location was something I found out later. Anyway:

". . . I was tied to a chair in one of the bedrooms. And Natasha was tied to a bed. We were both in our underwear. I seem to remember windows with thick drapes, so that not even a chink of sunlight came through. But it felt like day. Midday, quiet, too hot outside to even think of movement. That was what it was: no movement. A humid, drowsy day. And the room was dimly lit; wall lights turned low, and a shaded bedside lamp. But I'm way ahead of myself. At first I didn't see a damn thing, I only felt the pain in the back of my skull.

"Then, as I gradually came to, I heard voices speaking in Italian. I knew the language well enough to know they were talking about me . . . and Natasha. 'After the girl,' one voice said, 'then you can have him. But first, I want him to see and understand—the spoiled English *brat!* I would have had her myself a long time ago, except that might have been problematic. Even so, I was tempted. And if she'd been a little more willing . . . but I won't force any woman, it's too demeaning—to myself, I mean. Anyway, our colleagues in Moscow think highly, much too highly, of this bitch. And now this brat has spoiled her. Well for me, at least. I don't take anyone's leavings, Jean Daniel, so this is your lucky day; you get to do it for me. Let's face it, you've watched her often enough, and I'm sure you've fancied her just as frequently, eh? So, what better way to pay him back for what he did to you?'

" 'Fancied her?' the other voice said. 'Hey, I'm only human, Luigi! And this is . . . this is a lot . . . a lot of woman. . . .' "

As for Jake's own voice as he told or relived his story: it had sunk very low, become guttural, until at this point he was choking on his words, having difficulty getting them out. Trask saw this and said, "Jake, we can leave it there if you like."

But the other shook his head. "No," he said grimly. "No, I think I'd like to finish it. Maybe it's *good* for me to remember what went down. Because then I'll be sure I was right in what I did. Yes, and it also serves to remind me of what remains to be done. . . ." And after a moment:

"These voices," he went on, "were very distinctive. The one belonged to Castellano, as I was about to find out. It was very deep and powerful; like a rumble, a purring sound, even when he was speaking quietly. And the other, this Jean Daniel's voice, it had an obvious French accent in keeping with his name. But it also had something of a lisp, which explained itself as soon as I saw him.

"Anyway, I must have twitched, moved my head or something. Maybe I groaned, but suddenly they knew I was awake. Then shadows moved in that dim room.

"They came from behind me, one pausing to stand beside my chair, the other moving towards the bed, positioning itself in an easy chair on the other side of the lamp. They were men, of course, but to my blurred vision more like shadows. But as my eyes adjusted and my head stopped swimming, finally I saw Natasha, spreadeagled there on the four-poster. And because she'd lifted her head she could see me, too. Maybe that—that look on her face, expressing her relief that I'd finally come to—was how they knew I'd regained consciousness. But in any case, it was an expression that didn't last much longer.

"The one beside the bed spoke, and his deep purring voice told me that this was Luigi Castellano. 'Ah, Natasha, Natasha!' he rumbled, as she turned her pale, frightened face to look at him. 'First the injury and then the insult,' he said.

'To have spurned my friendship, my warmest offerings of affection, for this . . . this *Englishman's*. Perhaps you didn't understand that in the game we play it's always business first—no such thing as mixing business with pleasure, Natasha. And if there was we might reasonably expect you to take your pleasures with one of us, not some stupid outsider. Perhaps it's my fault; I allowed you too much leeway? But no, for I hate to blame myself.'

"I tried to look at the speaker but he was still a shadow, a dark silhouette hunched behind the cone of faint yellow radiance from the bedside lamp. And he went on speaking:

" 'But then again, what if this foreign playmate of yours wasn't so stupid after all but a member of one of those agencies we haven't yet got to, eh? You took too many chances, Natasha—took too *much* pleasure, I fancy—and now you must pay. Ah, but what price? Well, since you don't seem to care too much for the company of a business partner, I was obliged to find a punishment to fit your . . , your what, your crime? Ah, but no—too harsh by far—your error of judgement, then. A punishment to fit *both* participants, that is. Tit for tat, if you like. Or better far, *tits* for tat?' Castellano's tone was much harsher, harder now. 'Yes, and the rest of your more than ample charms in the bargain. . . .'

"He looked up and beckoned to Jean Daniel. My chair was a swivel. The man beside me spun it, and I went turning, turning, feeling sick as a dog as the room revolved around me. At least it gave me a chance to identify my tormentor, his cold, smiling face passing before me as the chair slowed down. It was Natasha's tail, of course, and Castellano's tall pale-faced watchdog.

"Finally he spoke to me in broken English through a broken mouth, which accounted for his lisp. I hadn't realized how hard I'd hit him. 'Bastard!' he said. 'Stupid, English, pig *bastard!* When I finish with her, then is your turn. We see who hit hardest, eh?' He made to move towards the bed.

" 'If you hit her,' I mumbled, 'if you strike her just once, I swear I'll—' But he turned, cut me off, said:

" 'Hit her? With fist?' For a moment he frowned, looked

puzzled. But then, grinning as best he could through split lips, he said, 'No, stupid, I not hit. I *fuck* her!'

"And he did. . . ." Jake's voice was a growl now, a sob, a low moan. "With that dog Castellano watching, and laughing. And me: I couldn't look away. I *had* to look! He ripped her underclothes right off her. The skinny bastard—he didn't pause to get undressed—he just . . . he just . . . And Natasha, she didn't even speak, didn't cry out. But she *did* cry. I heard her sobbing. . . ."

And Trask cut in. "I'll take it from here, Jake, okay?" And before the other could protest:

"You were found in an alley badly beaten. Four broken ribs, and your nose much as we see it now. The rest of your face was a mass of bruises. You'd been kicked, too—someone had really worked on you—so badly that for a day or two the French doctors couldn't be sure they'd be able to save . . . everything. But you still had your plastic, and paper money in your pockets, so it looked like the motive wasn't theft. In fact, they never discovered *what* the motive had been; even when you could talk you weren't telling anyone, said you didn't know. Now why was that, Jake?"

"I was going to handle it my own way," Jake answered, dispassionately now. "And I did, eventually."

"Yes, you did," Trask nodded. "But that came later. Do you want to pick the story up again?"

The other's face was white, drawn, but he nodded.

"I was three weeks in hospital," Jake eventually continued. "No word from Natasha; I didn't know what had happened to her, but I prayed it wasn't physical. Or rather, nothing more than she'd already suffered. As for what *I* had suffered . . . I think it was as much mental as physical, worrying about Natasha, I mean. But at last they turned me loose. By which time there'd been plenty of time to think things out. Now it was up to her. If she still wanted out—if she still dared—I was her man. *Huh!* That old motto of mine: 'Who Dares Wins.' Well, I dared for sure, because I loved her. See, I still hadn't learned my lesson. Then again, do fools in love ever learn?" He managed a wry grin. "How about that: Jake Cutter, philosopher!

"About Jean Daniel, which was the only name I ever knew him under: my initial intentions towards that bastard had been very bloody. At first . . . well, I admit that I'd equipped myself. And I had gone looking for *them*, too—the Mob, I mean—but carefully. And as I healed, so I had quit abusing myself with booze and maybe some other stuff. The army had trained us hard: 'body maintenance,' my section commander had used to call it. But now I found it really difficult to get back into the routine. Oh, I was still young, but as you've pointed out, Mr. Trask, that Jean Daniel had done a hell of a good job on me. Such a good job, it took me four long months to put the damage right.

"I completed my recuperation in England, went back to Marseille. But time was passing and I still hadn't heard from Natasha. I had given her both my English and French telephone numbers; if she couldn't speak to me, she should certainly be able to speak to friends of mine. Still I hadn't heard from her, and time seemed against me, seemed to be flying. But where Natasha was concerned, it was like some kind of paradox: the months passing like so many years! I couldn't forget her—I still wanted her—and the debt that the Mob owed us was slowly slipping out of memory and into the past.

"Earlier, however, not long after leaving the hospital, I had found Castellano's villa. I did it the easy way, by tailing the tail. I'd grown a designer beard, tinted my sideboards grey and changed my mode of dress, even developed a limp. Or rather, I had deliberately held onto the limp I'd been left with, legacy of Jean Daniel. In all I looked quite a lot older. And I was staying out of bars, places where people might have been warned to look out for me. But one lonely night— I don't know, maybe I was hoping against hope that Natasha would be there—I went back to the bar where I'd first met her.

"I suppose I was lucky I'd developed my disguise, for Jean Daniel was there. He was on his own, didn't notice me. But when he left I was waiting in my car, followed him to the villa. And having found the place, I sat back out of sight and watched it, watched its clientele . . . hard men, all of them! Then, for some few weeks, I followed them, too. Well and good—now I knew the places to avoid if ever Natasha came back to Marseille; I mean, I knew which routes *not* to take getting her out of there. And I knew to get her out fast.

"For despite all my earlier intentions, finally I was getting some sense. These people played rough, played for keeps. So maybe I'd be wise to forget the revenge thing, simply take Natasha and run for home. *If* she ever came back.

"And eventually she did.

"It was less than three years ago, in early November. I got a message from a friend, who gave me a Moscow telephone number. And when I called . . . I knew it could only be Natasha. She was scared. Castellano had done a job on her, ruined her reputation with the Moscow Mob. For a long time they'd left her alone, let her go to the dogs. She'd been unable to find work, and finally she'd become desperate. Then she'd begged a Mob boss to let her run drugs again. And now she was coming to Marseille. But Castellano knew she was coming and she was more afraid of him than ever.

"I asked her if she remembered our previous plans. She did, and was ready to do whatever I'd worked out for us. But her own idea was a lot more daring: to dump her drug consignment cheaply on a rival French gang, and then to run with the money! Even cheaply it would still be worth a quarter million sterling.

"At first I backed away from it. But the more I thought it over the more I liked it. Wouldn't it be as good, even better, than the somewhat more physical revenge that I'd once planned? And it would hit them all, not just Jean Daniel, who obviously had been my principal target.

"Natasha had already contacted her buyer; she was supposed to come by yacht but instead would fly into Marseille. That way she'd have time to dispose of her load and get out of France—with me, of course—before Castellano and his people even knew she was missing. My part of it would be simple: drive like hell for Lyon, Dijon, and Paris, finally the tunnel. I'd studied the routes, couldn't find any fault with the plan. We'd be on board a train and passing beneath the English Channel before the Marseille Mob even thought to backtrack Natasha's movements. So we reckoned, anyway.

"Maybe it would have been easier to fly. But that way would have meant leaving my car behind. I had a beauty, an almost new Peugeot. Also, if we'd flown the Mob would find it a lot easier to track us. Idiot that I must have been, I still hadn't fully appreciated just what kind of people I was fooling with. . . ."

Jake paused to look at Trask. "You compared the modern Mob to terrorist organizations. Well, I thought I had learned something about terrorism in the SAS. Maybe I had, but plainly not enough. And anyway, that was just classroom stuff. Whatever, I thought of the Mob a lot differently from you: as just a bunch of hoods, I suppose. But you were right and I was wrong.

"They were probably watching her all the way down the line. They'd probably always watched her . . . maybe they have watchers for all their couriers and dupes. Take Jean Daniel for example. That spindly bastard was just another watchdog. Not so hard to understand when you consider the street value of the merchandise . . .

"Natasha was wearing dark glasses, a wig and all when I met her off the plane. But I knew her immediately. And so did they. Then . . . it was like a repetitive nightmare, almost a repeat of last time. Except *this* time there were five of them at the villa, and the way they went at it . . .

". . . Oh God! Oh *God!*—I knew they wouldn't be taking prisoners this time."

Jake's face was ashen now. Earlier tonight he'd known more or less what to expect; even if he had only half believed in it, still he had been doing a job. But at the time of his collision with the Mob, Castellano's people—*that* kind of monster—he had been . . . what, naive? Well, no longer.

Ben Trask knew it was time to step in, but more forcefully now. "That's enough, Jake!" he said. "You don't need to go into any further details. Why upset yourself? We've all heard enough and we're on your side. As for 'justice'—the justice you received?—I might know a lot more about that than you do. So for now, let's skip that night at the villa." But:

"That long, long night," Jake husked, sweating and shivering at the same time, his skin almost visibly crawling. "All of them, and that bastard Castellano watching it from the shadows. God, I *still* don't know what he looks like! But afterwards, oh, I remembered the rest of them in minute detail, would never let myself forget them. And their laughter, like jackals. And their jokes. The way they went at her, leaving no marks, no signs . . ."

"Skip it, Jake!" Trask's grating voice, shaking him out of it.

Jake sat back and gulped at the air, gradually quit shuddering. Eventually a little colour returned to his face, and finally he was able to continue.

"I came to in the water. Underwater! My car's windows were half open and we were sinking like a brick. At first I was disoriented, didn't know what the hell was happening. I think I woke up because I couldn't breathe. Like when I was a kid: I'd come screaming awake thinking I was drowning, only to discover that my head was under the covers. But this time it was river water. And I was stupidly trying to push back the covers . . . I mean, I *felt* stupid, drugged—which of course I was! But then, as I remembered what had gone down, I looked for Natasha in the passenger seat. She wasn't there, and I thanked God—

"—Thanked Him, as I somehow managed to wind my window down and drifted out and up and free. But as the car went down and I floated up, buoyed up in an eruption of big bubbles, I saw Natasha in the back of the car! Her face . . . her hair floating . . . her eyes wide open . . . her mouth gaping. And her spread fingers flattened and white, the hands of a corpse—I hoped!—against the curved back window.

"But dead? I didn't know, I still don't know to this day if she was dead or alive. But I've got to keep telling myself that she *was* dead, because that's the only way I can bear it.

And in any case, I couldn't have done a thing about it. Weak as a kitten, I felt half dead myself! My lungs were bursting—my ears too—we were that deep. And I drifted up oh so slow, while the car went down, disappearing into the deeps. And this girl I had loved, still loved, Natasha disappearing with it . . ."

This time it was a while before Jake could go on. He was like a man apart from reality; he started and sat up straighter in his chair when the Old Lidesci coughed, and looked around for a moment as if wondering where he was.

"Are you okay, Jake?" Liz asked him.

A nod was his only answer, until he was able to continue.

"Don't ask me how I got back to Marseille," he finally went on. "I can't for the life of me remember. But I did, and I laid low with a trusted friend. By then my earlier plans for revenge were firmly back in place. Before that, however, I actually considered going to the police. Then I remembered what Natasha had told me about the police being in Castellano's pocket and decided against it. I would wait it out, see what happened.

"I didn't have long to wait. It was in the newspapers home and abroad. My car had been found in the Verdon River where it comes down from the Alps of Provence near Riez. Locals had been alerted by a hole in the wall of a stone bridge over a torrential gorge. Natasha was still in the car, along with a quantity of illicit micro-drugs and other evidence that she'd been a bad lot. As for me: well, with my past record I would have been a wanted man—her partner, obviously—except they assumed I was dead.

"But I wasn't dead. And now I had absolutely nothing left to lose. Also, I knew a few things about Castellano's people, where they hung out and who with, and I wasn't about to waste any more time.

"There was one thing I had been really good at during my couple of years with the SAS: sabotage. Sabotage, booby-traps, and demolition. And I still remember—and I *cherish* the memory—of the night I found Jean Daniel drinking alone in that discreet little bar that I knew so well. I was there, watching the place, when he arrived, and I was there when he left.

"It was a rainy night. As he got in his car in the alley, I stepped out of the shadows maybe twenty-five yards in front. I stood there with my legs spread like an inviting target, and I waved at him. And I started oh so slowly to walk towards him. He saw me; I saw him flinch, knew that he'd recognized me. Then he turned the key in the ignition, and I knew exactly what the bastard was thinking: that he would run me down.

"By then I'd turned my back and hit the deck just in case. But no, there wasn't much of a blast; what little there was of flying glass went over my head. So I got up, walked to his car and looked in through the shattered window. I knew pretty much what I'd see, for I'd been determined to make the best kind of job of it. And I had.

"I had taken a small hacksaw and cut halfway through the four spokes of his steering wheel close to the column. And I'd fitted a trembler to the high-explosive charge that I'd placed under the plastic casing where the column was jointed for adjustment. It was a hellishly sensitive mechanism, far too sensitive to ignore the vibrations of a revving engine.

"The blast had driven the steel core of the steering column through Jean Daniel's middle, stripping its plastic casing as it went. The core had broken his lower ribs and torn through his stomach, and done a lot more damage along the way. Yet somehow it had missed severing his spine. He sat there—alive but barely—pinned to his seat with this fat cylindrical rod right through him; sat blinking at me, the steering wheel still gripped in his spastic hands.

" 'This is a different kind of rape, Jean Daniel,' I told him, watching as blood filled his mouth, and his eyes began to dim, and his twitching gradually stilled. 'My own special version.' And then, just before the bastard died. 'So now you know who hits the hardest.' "

6
More of Jake's Story

BEN TRASK, IAN GOODLY, AND THE OLD LIDESCI were first away from the gutted, smouldering remains of the vampire enclave; Liz and Jake followed behind Trask's commandeered transport in their own vehicle. They would be taking it easy, so it shouldn't be a problem that they'd lost the windshield. If they kept well back from Trask, the dust thrown up by his Land Rover wouldn't bother them. And the cool night air would be a definite bonus.

Just as they rolled onto the ramp cut in the steep face of the bluff, Jake slowed almost to a halt and looked back.

Apart from the smoke there was very little to show for the earlier activity. Several members of the team, dressed in fresh combat clothing but no longer armed or gas-masked, were hammering sharp signposts into the stony earth. One such post carried a legend only just visible in moon- and starlight:

HEALTH HAZARD!
TOXIC WASTE! KEEP OUT!

E-Branch took no chances.

"What next?" Jake jerked his head to indicate the scene of recent devastation. "For this place, I mean?"

Liz shrugged. "The mine's sealed, there are no life signs. Tomorrow the sun will come up and scorch the bluff clean. Maybe they'll bulldoze the surface and dynamite the ramp, eventually. But there's no real hurry now. The main man was Bruce Trennier, as yet a lieutenant but a would-be Lord. If he had got away . . ." Again her shrug. "Tomorrow they'd be back to tracking him down again. As it is, the operation was a complete success."

"And this was the first time you've seen this kind of action?" Jake slipped the Rover into third, let gravity draw them down the dusty ramp. "How come you know so much more about this stuff than I do?"

Liz tossed her hair back. "I've had a little time to study what they do—the Branch, I mean—and I'm 'aware' of my own talent, which makes their talents so much more acceptable. Once you begin to realize that all the weird stuff is real, it's not so difficult to believe the weirdest stuff of all."

But Jake only wondered, *And that's a good thing?—to actually believe in all of this?* But still it was hard to deny his own five senses. Assuming they were his own, of course.

Down on the level, he turned onto the old road. A quarter mile ahead, Trask's taillights glowed red. "I still can't accept that we were simply thrown in at the deep end," Jake said.

"It was a test, as Trask told you," Liz answered. "I guess he knew that once we'd actually experienced it, gone up against the plague itself . . . well, that we really *would* accept it."

"So why don't I?" Jake wanted to know.

For a while she was silent, letting the wind blow her hair back, breathing the night air. Then she said, "Jake, about your story tonight, in the ops room. There are terrible experiences, and there are terrible experiences. There are monsters and monsters, and I don't know which ones are the worst. But your life has been one of extremes. Maybe if mine had been messed with as much as yours, I'd start to wonder what was real, too. But this talent of yours, that's *really* something else. I mean, what you did tonight was—"

"—Wasn't me!" he said sharply, cutting her off. And with a shake of his head: "I can't explain it any better than that."

"Try," she said. "If we are to be partners, surely you can try? Look, this isn't something I suggest lightly—the Branch has its own internal code of conduct for espers, telepaths, empaths, and such—but if you'll just let your thoughts flow free, I'll—"

"You'll what?" he looked at her. "Read my mind? See if I'm as messed up as you suspect? Well, I probably am. Probably have been ever since ... since Natasha died. The *way* she died." Then he sighed and relaxed a little. "On the other hand, you could be right. My life *has* been a mess, and fate seems bent on screwing me around more than my fair share. So is it any wonder I have a problem sorting out what's real from what's fantasy? And as for E-Branch," Jake shook his head wonderingly. "Gadgets and ghosts—yeah!"

"And they want you for one of their gadgets," she said.

"Huh!" he answered. "Maybe one of their ghosts, if things had gone wrong tonight!"

"You've changed the subject," Liz accused. "Look, back in the ops room you started to tell your story. A good start, but you didn't nearly tell it all. Now me, I'm a hell of a listener. And right now, right here, there's just the two of us."

"Oh, really?" he said. "A good listener—and bloodthirsty with it? Like one of those things we destroyed tonight?"

"That's not fair," Liz answered. "And that's not the part that interests me." She gave a little shudder. "I mean, I know you killed all of those men—"

"No, not all of them," Jake said, coldly. "Castellano and one other, they've still got it coming."

"—And that your methods were ... extreme, but that's not what I'm talking about. I've heard Ben Trask going on about the way you use what he calls the Möbius Route. That's your talent, right, Jake? It's how you moved us to safety back at the lair."

He nodded, growled, "And that's what I keep trying to tell you. It's *not* mine! It's like—I don't know—somebody else? Someone who gets into my head, anyway. Someone who's living in there like a bloody squatter. Trask keeps mentioning this Harry Keogh. Well who *is* this Keogh? Some kind of telepath? And if so, why is he so damned keen to mess with my mind? Why not pick on someone else, someone more receptive? No, I can't see it. Maybe it's a part of me that *this* me—I mean the *real* me—doesn't recognize. Like I'm a . . . a split personality or something? God, maybe I really am crazy!" He banged on the steering wheel with the flats of his hands, stamped his feet and set the Land Rover to swerving.

Liz gave him time to cool down, then said, "Jake, how can I get through to you? This isn't just for me, nor even for Ben Trask or his people; it's mainly for you. I wish you'd tell me about it: how you escaped from jail and all, and ended up with E-Branch. I know it happened, but not how it happened. So what do you say? Will you tell me?"

And he knew she wouldn't let it go until he did. . . .

"I got sloppy," Jake began. "When I killed the third and last but one of Castellano's men—of the men who had been present at the villa that night—it was a sloppy job. A case of familiarity breeding contempt?" Glancing at Liz, he shook his head. "I would really hate to think so; hate to admit that I was getting used to it. But who can say? Maybe I was at that.

"Anyway, he was an Italian and I killed him in Italy. And I got caught there, too. Maybe they were waiting for me. After all, I had been working down a list, like a serial killer, you know? Of course, Castellano must by then have made the connection—must have figured out that this wasn't just another gang war—and it's possible he had tipped off the authorities, the police. When I thought it out, it was even possible he'd sent that last victim out of France to put distance between himself and me! If so, then I'd actually managed to get to the bastard—I'd worried him considerably— which felt very good. But in any case:

"I was tried and convicted in Italy, and there was no hope of extradition. Having dual nationality—English and French—only made the legal side of it even more tangled, complicated, hopeless. And to put the cap on it, current European law made it imperative that I was tried 'in the country where the crime was committed for any serious offence against nationals of the said country.' Well, you can't get any more serious than murder, which was their term for what

I'd done, even if I called it an act of justice. And finally, if found guilty—which of course I was—I had to serve out my time in that same country.

"That's why I think it was Castellano who set the trap for me, and baited it with his own man. Castellano's a Sicilian, or an Italian if you like. And it's like Trask says: the gangs are highly organized now—computerized, integrated and all—and as always they have their fingers in every pie.

"So, why do you reckon this bastard thug wanted me in an Italian jail? Obviously, it was one of those pies in which he had a finger! Jake Cutter was a dead man. If not immediately, soon.

"But to me the hell of it was I'd never been able to get a sniff of Castellano himself. The villa in Marseille was always guarded to the hilt, and if he'd ever left it . . . well, I certainly didn't know about it. How could I? I still didn't—still *don't*—even know what he looks like. This is one secretive son of a bitch! But I will find him one day, and when I do—"

"But not while you're working for E-Branch," Liz broke in. "The one thing you mustn't do is compromise the Branch. They're your protection, Jake. And you've got to remember: Trask is the only thing standing between you and a return visit to that cell in . . . where?"

"In Torino," Jake answered. "Turin, where they're alleged to have found the Shroud, and where I was being fitted for one! I tell you, Liz, there were some hard men in that jail. It took me maybe—oh, twenty-four hours?—to figure out that I wasn't getting out in one piece. The looks, the nudges, the winks. But what I said earlier about the size of my . . . er, you know what, that wasn't true; could have been but wasn't. No one came sidling up to me offering their protection for a little buggery on the side; I guess because the word had gone out that I couldn't *be* protected, and that anyone who tried it might well need some protection himself.

"And there were a couple of narrow squeaks. Knife fights I wasn't involved in, that I somehow *got* involved in. And once in the prison hospital—I was in for abdominal bruising and a suspected fractured rib . . . yes, another one—someone tried to inject me with a hypodermic full of human shit.

"Anyway, I'd been in there for eleven weeks when this guy—just a guy, no one sinister, I thought, but someone who probably pitied me—got me on my own and told me that it was coming. And *when* it was coming. I had a week to live, he said. And no good going to the prison staff; they were in on it, and the governor was a man who knew which side his bread was buttered.

"Then a funny thing. This same little fellow said he was working in the machine shop. He gave me a rough key—just a strip of metal, really—showed me how to make an impression of the lock on my cell. This was an old, old prison, Liz. Not like the home away from home you'll find in a lot of modern English jails. Anyway: 'You take the impression,' he said, 'and I make finish the key.'

"So what was in it for him? He already had his own key, he said, and a plan. But he couldn't do it on his own. And he figured I might be just desperate enough to go along with him. Oh, he supposed I had seen those old prison movies—of the double double-cross kind—but hey, it was his life, too, wasn't it? Did I think he was suicidal or something? So maybe he was, but he'd got one thing right at least: I *was* desperate enough.

"Okay, my reasons for wanting to escape were plain enough: I wanted Castellano dead, and couldn't do it from inside where my own life seemed destined to be a pretty short one. But what about my new-found friend's reasons?

"Apparently it was for a woman. 'A dear old friend of mine, he fucking my Maria,' he told me, grinning emotionlessly. 'The last man who did that, he dead . . . is why I in here. This time I going fuck *both* of them, Maria, too. After that I not care.'

"Funny thing is, I understood him well enough. Just didn't realize how far he'd go to clear this little matter up, that's all.

"Came the night. We got out into the exercise yard way too easy and I felt it was all wrong, all fixed. But it was far too late to go back and lock myself in . . . and what if I was simply being paranoid? I mean, this was my one last chance. It was his one chance, too, this bald, scrawny little Italian murderer who made the keys.

"His plan was simple: he had a length of chain he'd welded hooks to. Between us and freedom there was a twelve foot wall, barb-wired at the top. He was a little guy; he would get on my back, use his chain like a grapnel to grab at the barbed wire. He'd tried it in the workshops and it worked. By God, it also worked out there in the exercise yard!

"So Paulo scrambled from my shoulders up the chain, took a prison blanket from around his neck and tossed it over the barbed wire, which his weight had pulled flat. He balanced himself up there with a leg over the wall, stretched out a hand for me. But when I was on the chain and as I was reaching for his hand . . . he withdrew it! And I saw his eyes, looking beyond me into the night. I glanced over my shoulder, saw them:

"Prison guards, armed and taking aim! I looked up at Paulo, his face staring down at me. 'I sorry, Jake,' he shrugged. 'But they promise me—' And then, cutting him short, the *crack!* of a rifle shot."

Jake paused, swerving to avoid a pothole, and Liz took the opportunity to ask, "Is that when it happened? When you . . . moved?"

He shook his head. "Not quite. But Liz, you know how they say you don't hear the one that kills you? Well, it's true. I know because I *heard* the bark of that first shot, but I didn't feel a thing. Paulo, on the other hand . . . His blood splashed me as his right eye turned black. Then he was falling, and taking me with him. It was only a few feet, but with him on top of me I hit the ground like a ton of bricks. Just as well because there was more shooting, shouting, the flash of bullets sparking where they spanged off the wall.

"That's when it happened. But exactly *what* happened, I don't know to this day. And something very weird: if you don't hear the one that kills you, how about seeing it? I mean, did you ever hear of anyone actually *seeing* a bullet in flight? Of course not; and please, no cracks about phoney stage magicians who catch them in their teeth!

"Yet I saw . . . something. A flash of fire from a ricochet? It could be. But it didn't look like fire. It was tiny, bright, and it came came right at me—at my head—and couldn't have missed me. If it had been a bullet, then I was dead . . .

". . . But it wasn't, couldn't have been, and I only thought I was dead."

Liz nodded, her mouth suddenly dry. Because for a moment, as Jake had finished speaking, she had received a vivid impression of something alien to all science and knowledge, something from outside. She'd "seen" his meeting—his confrontation?—with what he'd described. A transitory thing, it came and went, like a bright flash of fire reflecting from the surface of his mind . . . or still burning *in* his mind?

"That was when you did it," she said hoarsely, and cleared her throat. "That was when you moved, took the Möbius Route."

"There was an indescribable darkness," Jake told her. "More than darkness, a nothingness. It was death; I mean, I *thought* it was death, for what else could it be? But I was drawn into and through it, towards a point of light."

"A typical out-of-body experience," Liz said. "A near-death experience, as certain survivors are supposed to have known it. The Light, which you refused to enter."

But Jake shook his head. "Refused nothing; I had no choice; I was dragged right in! But suddenly there was gravity, weight, and I'd been struggling with the darkness—whatever it was—and was the wrong way up. I emerged upside down, fell, smacked my head against something . . . a desk, as it turned out. So you see, the second bout of darkness wasn't nearly so drastic. I was merely unconscious. Or about to be.

"Anyway, even as I passed out I remember there were alarms going off, someone hammering at a door, a voice shouting. Then nothing more."

"Not until you came to at E-Branch HQ in London," Liz said. "That's where your talent had taken you: to Harry's Room, sanctuary."

He shook his head in denial. "Not my talent. Oh, someone's, as it appears. Harry's, maybe? But not mine, Liz, not mine. . . ."

The radio crackled into life, Trask's voice saying: "All callsigns, but especially Hunter One, this is Zero One. Maybe five miles up the road from here, the chuck wagon. Base camp, where we eat, drink and debrief. Those with beds in the ops vehicle, use 'em. Tentage for the rest. Or should you prefer to stretch your legs you can put up your own tents and bivouacs. And Hunter One, I'll be wanting to speak to you. All acknowledge."

"Hunter One, roger," Liz answered into her handset. And in strict numerical order, coming through the hiss and crackle of static:

"Hunter Two, roger."

"Hunter Three, roger," and so on.

Jake shifted his position in the driver's seat, cranked his neck, and glanced back along the dark, winding road through the ancient river valley. Back there, stretched well out, a handful of headlights made a lantern string in the night. And from dragonfly shapes on high came the steady, near-distant *whup! whup! whup!* of powerful blades slicing the air, the occasional flickering beam of a searchlight.

"Five miles," Liz said. "Maybe seven or eight minutes. Will you tell me the rest of it while we still have time?"

"The rest of it?" Jake was reluctant again. "You still need convincing I'm crazy?"

"You're not crazy," she said. "Just troubled. Come on, Jake. You ran away, escaped again, this time from E-Branch. What happened? How did that come about? Was it any different?"

He sighed and said, "Once you stick your claws in you just don't let go, do you?"

"Or could it be that I'm simply fascinated?" she answered. And quickly added, "Er, with your story, I mean."

"Huh!" Jake snorted, but he also angled his face a little, turned it away from her. Liz could have sworn that he was

grinning and didn't want her to see. But that was a good thing.

"Okay," she said. "I'm fascinated, period. So now will you tell me the rest?"

"So you can report it to Trask, right? Well I've got news for you: your boss—our boss—has already had this from me, oh, at least a dozen times. Don't you get it? I can't tell you what isn't there."

"Then tell me what is," she said.

Again Jake's sigh, before he succumbed to the inevitable. "Okay, this is how it was. . . ."

"When—or rather where—I woke up, everyone was speaking English. I don't know what I thought. Oh, several things. A jangle of things, rattling around in my skull. Maybe, following injuries sustained in the failed jailbreak, I'd been extradited back to England after all. But what injuries? While it's true I was flat on my back with a sheet and blanket thrown over me, I didn't feel in any way injured. Also, I was in no way conscious of the passage of any real time; it felt like *snap!* . . . I had been in Turin and now was here. So logically, while this wasn't the prison, it had to be a place somewhere in or near Turin.

"As for the people, Trask and Co.—they weren't jailers or even physicians. So if this place was a hospital, well, it wasn't like any I'd ever heard of! And they kept asking me a lot of nonsense questions, the silliest with regard to my identity. 'Who are you?' they all wanted to know. Huh! Who were they kidding? If they didn't know who I was, who would? Who was *I*? But the question I kept asking myself was, who the hell were *they*?

"Then a real doctor arrived who checked me over, giving me a thorough physical before I was allowed up on my feet. I supposed I was lucky that I hadn't at first been able to talk even if I'd wanted to. The whole experience had struck me dumb. But then it dawned on me that they really didn't have any idea who I was. So why should I tell them?

"I kept quiet, told them nothing, didn't even speak.

"But Trask—he knew I wasn't on the level. Right from square one I could see that he was more than curious, positively suspicious about me. I suppose he had every right to be; I know now that the place I—er, *emerged* into? 'Harry's Room?'—is highly significant to the Branch. More than that, though, Trask knew I was lying. Even without me saying a word, he knew I wasn't telling the truth, knew I was hiding something.

"Well, of course I was! Wherever I'd 'escaped' to, anywhere had to better than the vermin-infested slaughterhouse in Turin that I'd escaped from! And yes, I had already made up my mind that as soon as this weird crowd gave me room to breathe, I'd likewise be escaping from here—wherever 'here' was!

"Finally, instead of asking me stuff and getting no satisfactory answers, no answers at all, Trask said, 'You're in the headquarters of a branch of government, a very off-limits establishment, Mr. . . . whoever you are. You shouldn't be here, and the penalty for trespass is a high one. But I'm really interested in you, in how you arrived—especially *where* you arrived—and I'd very much like you to start explaining. If you don't, I'll have to assume you're a common criminal and deal with you on that basis.'

"But then he got a certain look in his eye, like he'd suddenly stumbled across the truth—maybe a truth even I didn't know—and quickly went on, 'Or maybe an *un*common criminal? In which case we might just be getting somewhere.'

"Some of Trask's people had guns and there didn't seem too much point in trying to break out of there, not at present. So I just had to keep playing along.

"Finally, I was escorted to the HQ ops room." Jake glanced at Liz. "Do you know the place? I take it you've been there."

He waited for her nod, the one word that summed up her own feelings the first time she'd seen the ops room. "Awesome . . ."

"Yes, awesome," he agreed. "I don't know about ghosts, but E-Branch certainly has the gadgets! Anyway, as soon as we entered—before anyone could stop me—I stepped to a window and yanked the blinds. It was night but there were plenty of street lights. There could be no mistaking where I was; the very sight of it set me reeling. That skyline, that city. Impossible, but it was Westminster! London! The centre of bloody London!

"And grabbing me, looking at me with those all-seeing eyes of his, Trask said, 'Surprise, surprise! So where did you think you were, Mr. Nobody?'

"By then a lot of other people had arrived. They'd got the place up and running. It was the middle of the night after all, and my being there was just as big—maybe a bigger—shock to them as it was to me. But they must have a good emergency call-in; the place was fully operative in no time at all. And every man-jack and woman of them wide-eyed, whispering, curious . . . maybe even awestruck? But why? What was so special about me?

"Anyway, things were happening at a rapid pace.

" 'Prison clothing,' Trask said. 'At a guess, continental. Very well, get fingerprints, mug shots—do it now. Then get a link to Interpol, see if we can get a match. But let's *not* get carried away, not yet. Let's *not* think the unthinkable, or the incredible. Check the security system and see if it recorded a physical break-in. And let's have a check on all doors and windows, and the elevator. Then get me the duty officer. Didn't I hear him saying something about not being able to get into Harry's Room because the door was locked? Now why would Mr. Nobody here first *break* in, then *lock* himself in? And how could he do it anyway without a key . . . assuming he broke in at all?'

"Trask said all of these things, if not in the same words. And he probably said a lot more that I can't remember before he finished up with: 'Answers, people, I want all the answers. And I do mean tonight.'

"I had been fingerprinted and photographed by the time two new agents entered the ops room. Trask greeted them with, 'Current Affairs, and Tomorrow's Affairs. And not before time, you two.' "

Liz nodded, said, "Millicent Cleary and Ian Goodly. Millicent is a telepath, but she's also an expert in current affairs. She has that kind of memory. You want to know what's gone down in the last ten years, ask Millicent. And Ian Goodly—"

"—A precog," Jake said. "Yes, I know that now. But then—I couldn't make head nor tail of their conversation. Trask wanted to know why Goodly hadn't 'seen' anything, and he asked the woman if she was 'getting' anything. That was the way he talked to everyone around him. It all seemed pretty esoteric to me."

"Espers have an almost different tongue," Liz answered. "It takes some getting used to."

"Anyway, Ian Goodly was at a loss to explain his lapse. And the woman, Millicent Cleary? She stared hard at me, frowned and said there was a lot of confusion. Damn right there was!"

"The confusion was in you," Liz told him.

"Looking back on it, you're dead right," he said. And after a moment:

"By then all the wall screens were up and working—people processing my pictures and feeding them into machines, computer keyboards tap, tap, tapping away—but I was a little less the centre of attention. I saw my chance, snatched a gun from a man who was momentarily distracted, grabbed ahold of Goodly. I had the gun to his neck, his arm up behind his back.

"For a moment I thought Trask and the others might rush me. But then Goodly said, 'It's okay, Ben. Everything will be fine. Just let us go, and be sure we'll be back.'

"I told him, 'Do you want to bet?' But now . . . I'm glad he didn't! I'll cut a long story short. I got Goodly out of there and into the elevator. He used his card without argument. Then we were out in the street. Which was when he turned the tables on me. How? Well, I suppose he saw the future, knew I wouldn't shoot him. Or maybe he saw that I couldn't?

"Anyway, he just twisted round to face me, grabbed the gun and started wrestling me for it. I was so surprised . . . I just let go of the thing! And the fact was I couldn't have shot him anyway, not an innocent man. But I couldn't say the same thing for him, now could I? And there he was, crouching down, aiming the gun at me!"

The vehicle was nosing down a slight decline. As they came round a shallow bend, Jake saw campfires and started to brake. Then a man stepped out onto the crumbling tarmac and made signals, directing them into a makeshift roadside parking area.

As they slowed to a standstill, Liz sat motionless, said, "Finish it."

And Jake thought, *Why not? Except there's nothing left to tell!* Or if there was he couldn't possibly explain it. But he could at least try. "It's already finished," he said. "When I thought Goodly was going to shoot me, I made a dive for cover. I mean, I *knew* I was diving to safety . . . but that wasn't possible. How could there be any cover, any safety, out there in the middle of the street?"

"There couldn't be," she said.

"No," Jake answered huskily, pale in the flickering firelight. "There couldn't be. Not out there in the street. But it wasn't me who reacted to the perceived danger, Liz. Not me but someone in my head. Someone or something that reckoned I would be safer—that I'd be safer—"

But Liz, reading it clearly in his mind, came to his aid and finished it for him: "—That you'd be much safer back in Harry's Room, yes," she sighed.

He shook his head, frowned and said, "But safe from what? From Goodly, who didn't intend to harm me in the first place?"

She made no answer but thought: *No, just safe—period.* Maybe Ian Goodly's gun hadn't triggered the thing at all; maybe *it* simply hadn't wanted Jake out there on his own, on the streets. For whatever it was, this thing had been new to him at that time. Still very strong in him—and having only recently found him—it hadn't been about to let him escape. Not without first exploring him, and not until Jake had explored its possibilities, its potential.

Such were Liz's thoughts. But bringing them back to earth:

"We're there," said Jake. "So are we going to sit here all night? Me, I'd like a mug of coffee and a bite to eat."

7
More Gadgets and Ghosts

AS LIZ AND JAKE GOT OUT OF THEIR VEHICLE, Trask came over and checked it for damage: a few scratches to the paintwork, some small dents in the hood, and the missing windscreen of course. "Did you have this attended to?"

Liz knew what he was concerned about: not the damage itself but rather its origin, and any possible contamination that might have been left behind. She nodded. "Back at the Old Mine gas station. A squad sprayed her down, cleaned up the mess."

"I worry, that's all," Trask explained. "But having seen some of the measures the Travellers take on Sunside, I suppose that's only natural." He shrugged. "I don't know . . . maybe I'm too cautious." His reference to Sunside flew over Jake's head, but he was getting used to that kind of thing.

"I didn't see you taking too much care of yourself," Jake told him. "Back there, I mean. You and the old man, Lardis? It was as if you didn't give a damn between you! No nose plugs or combat gear. No gas masks. No precautions."

Trask looked at him. "Double standards? Is that what you're saying? Do as I say, not as I do? Not really. Maybe one day I'll tell you *my* story. But couldn't it simply be that some of us have less to lose?" And before he could be asked to elaborate:

"As for Lardis Lidesci, he's been doing his own thing all his life. Perhaps there's a partial immunity among the Szgany, I can't say. But even so I watch him, just as he keeps his eye on everyone else. And the day he gets rid of his silver bells, or starts shrinking from the sun . . ." He let it go at that.

"Maybe I haven't been listening very much," Jake said. "In fact I'm sure I haven't. There's been too much happening—not only *to* me but all around me—for my tiny brain to accept it all at once. But what if I start listening as of now? Am I asking too much that we sit down sometime so you can fill me in, put me fully in the picture about E-Branch? I mean, if I'm to work for you, isn't it only right I should know something of what's going on?"

"So you've finally decided you'll work for us?"

Jake pulled a wry face. "Actually, I thought you had!" And all three walked towards one of the campfires.

The rest of the vehicles were arriving and lining up on the road before being allocated parking areas. Making himself heard over the revving motors, Trask shouted a few instructions, then answered Jake. "Oh, I think there's work for you. But there are still a few things I need to clear up. If I'm to control you, I need to know what I'm controlling." He looked at the other, his gaze seeming to pierce the younger man through and through, and with a wry smile continued, "I've got to be sure you won't just cut and run—like maybe in a crisis, when you're most needed. After all, you do still have your own agenda."

"Don't you ever trust anybody?" Jake growled, knowing that indeed Trask had seen right through him.

But enigmatic as ever, Trask wasn't buying it. "In my time with the Branch," he said, "I've seen what trust can do . . . and what it's *done* to some of my favourite people."

They sat by the fire with one or two other agents, most of them keeping to themselves, lost in their own thoughts now that the night's work was done. It was a night they'd been building up to for some time. The Old Lidesci dished out food—steaks, steaming stew from a container on a military shallow-trench back-burner, and man-sized chunks of bread fresh from the burner's oven—but with the exception of Lardis himself no one was much interested in eating. Maybe it was the back-burner's roar, the way it sounded so much like a flamethrower. . . .

By the time the three had done eating, and washed it down with mugs of coffee, the big articulated truck was in situ and Ian Goodly had gone to check on incoming messages. By then too the rest of the agents had sat down to eat, and the atmosphere wasn't quite so heavy.

Liz had been yawning for some time, and though she swore she would never sleep, still she'd gone off to seek out a bivouac for herself. Watching her go, Jake put down his empty mug and said to Trask, "Me, I'm not tired either. In fact my mind is going every which way. So all misgivings aside, I'm asking you to tell me what I've got myself involved with, how it all began, and how you think I can fit in."

Trask stood up and for a moment looked as if he might say something. But just then Ian Goodly came striding from the direction of the ops vehicle. On top of the first trailer, in fact the mobile ops room, a cluster of antennae and radio dishes had poked up, locked into position, and aimed themselves at the sky . . . also at several communication satellites.

"Ben," Goodly called in his piping voice. "David Chung is on the wire from London. You can get him on-screen if you want. He got your message, and he appears to be rather excited." But as Trask headed for the ops truck, Goodly had second thoughts; at least he made it seem that way. "Oh, and Ben! Er, maybe you should take Jake with you? Introduce him to David . . . ?"

The two of them looked at each other in passing, and Jake could swear some sort of silent exchange took place. Then Trask called back to him, "Jake, if you'd still like to know how you might fit in, perhaps you should come along with me."

In the ops room, the duty officer and one other were on listening duty within the oval desk. The D.O. got out of the way when Trask lifted a flap in the desk, walked through and parked himself in the command chair. Jake followed and stood close behind him. Trask looked at the D.O. and said, "Chung?"

"London HQ, waiting," the other nodded. "Do you want him on-screen?"

"Put him up there," Trask said, indicating a screen on the wall. And the D.O. hit a switch.

As the other lights dimmed a little, the wall screen flickered into life and its picture quickly firmed up. This was the first time Jake had seen E-Branch's chief locator, David Chung. He was small, middle-aged, Asian as they come, and very serious looking. And he was quite obviously highly intelligent. It was in his eyes just as it was in Trask's; a light behind them, shining out. But it was also in the high dome of his head. Jake didn't need advising of the extraordinary brain that was housed within. Chung's raven-black hair was thinning; there might even be a few strands of grey here and there. But his skin was clear and unwrinkled and his posture was straight as a ramrod. He was sprightly, alert . . . and excited, yes. That, too, showed in his eyes.

"Hi, David," Trask greeted him with a smile—but in a moment got down to business. "How did it go?" he said.

"Ben," the other nodded, then immediately fixed his attention on Jake. And Jake could see that his curiosity was intense. But Trask had seen it, too.

"Save it," he told the locator, his tone of voice carrying something of a warning. "I suggest we deal with the other matter first." And turning to the D.O.: "Are we scrambled?"

"Yes," the D.O. nodded.

And Chung said, "All bad news, I'm afraid. It's as Greenpeace and the others suspected. In fact, it's worse then anyone suspected. The Russians are still doing it, but now it's *where* they're doing it. You know, if we'd had Anna Marie English in on this we could have cracked it without even leaving the HQ."

"I know," Trask answered, his shoulders slumping a little. "But we don't have her, and anyway she's happier where she is—God help us all! But is it really as bad as you make out? What, yet another treaty gone up in smoke—or nuclear pollution? I suppose you'd better put me in the picture, but not on-screen. Let me have a printout."

Chung spoke to someone off-screen, turned again to Trask. "It'll take a few minutes. And later, when I've done a little checking, I'll also be sending you, er, a weather report? Some unexpected smog? But I'd like to check it out first and see if it's still hanging around, you know? Meanwhile, what about the other business?" His gaze switched to Jake however momentarily, then back to Trask.

Understanding Chung's "coded" message, Trask gave a cursory nod and said, "Do you remember what happened at E-Branch HQ when Nathan arrived in Perchorsk? I mean you personally? Do you remember how you proved his identity, or his connection?"

Chung grinned, his excitement plainly in evidence. "Do I remember? How could I ever forget? I'm way ahead of you, Ben." And he held up a hairbrush, showing it to Trask and Jake.

"I wasn't sure you still had it," Trask sighed his relief. "It wasn't in Harry's Room; I had it searched immediately after Jake . . . came visiting. But I knew that if you had it, it would be secure with your special items at the HQ. That's why I asked you to go and dig it out as soon as you got finished with what you were doing."

Now the locator looked at Jake again and said, "I suppose this is Jake Cutter?" He nodded a greeting. "So why is he looking so—what, lost?"

Before Trask could answer, Jake leaned over him and said, "I look so 'what, lost,' as you put it—though personally I'd prefer 'stunned'—because no one has bothered to tell me what the *fuck* is going on! It's okay for E-Branch to put my life in jeopardy, set me in conflict with . . . I don't know— vampires? Mutated things? Alien invaders that live on the blood of human beings?—but totally out of the question to tell me what it's all in aid of. The human race, perhaps? Well, great! But since I'm a member, don't *I* have any fucking say in the matter?"

"Right first time," said Trask. "And on both counts. It's

in aid of the human race, and no you don't have any say in the matter."

Chung saw now why the head of E-Branch was so cautious: as yet Jake Cutter knew very little. But Chung was already certain that Jake would have to know it all eventually. And so he said, "That's fine for now, Ben. But if you're asking for my opinion, he'll have plenty of say in the not too distant future."

Trask quickly held up his hand. "We understand each other, and that's for the future—maybe. But don't say any more right now. Instead you can tell me about the brush."

"Oh, it's active," Chung said. "Very definitely. Why it's like a live thing in my hand even now!" He looked at the man's hairbrush—just a well-used wooden oval tufted with pig bristles, some of them coming loose—and smiled. But alive? From what Jake could make out the brush was about as dead as . . . as a piece of wood with pig bristles.

"So," said Trask, speaking to Chung. "Can I take it you're thinking that just like once before maybe something of— well, let's for now call him a *once*-friend of ours—has come back to us? But if so, come back from where? And in what form?"

"Absolutely," Chung answered—then stopped smiling as the meaning of Trask's words sank in and he began to understand the other's caution. And: "I think I see," he said. "So now we must ask ourselves whether or not it's beneficial. Is it here under the aegis of a friend, to help us, or is it here—"

"—For something else?" Trask cut the locator short. And after staring at him for a long moment, he said, "That's it for now, David. Stay there at the HQ. The chair's yours until we're all sorted out at this end. Okay?"

"Whatever you say," Chung answered, his face once more inscrutable. And the D.O. blanked the screen. . . .

"What was all that about?" Jake queried the Head of E-Branch on the way to his tent. Trask had a "room" in the ops vehicle but preferred a little more space. In keeping with his status, his tent was somewhat bigger than a bivouac.

"When we have a little light, I'll show you," Trask said. "Some of it, anyway. From which time on you'll need to be aware that you've signed the Official Secrets Act."

"But I haven't!" Jake said.

"But if you ever give me reason, I'll say you have." Trask grinned his cold grin. "And you'll have to anyway, eventually."

Jake snorted, said, "Could this mean you're actually going to let me in on some secret or other?"

"Sarcasm will get you nowhere," Trask said. "Except maybe in a whole lot of trouble."

The camp wasn't far from the edge of a watering hole. Several large Australian night insects were fluttering, occasionally buzzing, through the smoky, flickering firelight. There were clusters of knobbly, fat-boled trees of a type Jake didn't recognize; Trask's tent stood shaded by one of these, in comparative darkness.

Trask squeezed a rubber button on a cable hanging outside the tent, and as a light glowed within he drew aside the canvas flap and a fine-mesh gauze fly screen to invite Jake in. Inside, a folding table supported Trask's briefcase, a bottle of liquor, and two glasses. There were folding chairs and a camp bed, and in a screened-off corner a portable toilet. Comfortwise it was better than a bivouac, certainly, but scarcely luxurious.

Trask sat Jake down, opened up his crammed briefcase, fumbled out a flat machine the size of a box of typing paper, and flipped a switch. The device whirred softly, and a slot opened in one end. Feeding Chung's printout into the slot, Trask said, "It's enciphered, and this is a decoder."

"Gadgets and ghosts," said Jake.

"Yes," Trask answered, "I have to agree. This is certainly a gadget, and Chung's message is about ghosts—of a sort."

"Are you kidding me?" Jake couldn't any longer be sure of anything.

"I suppose I am," Trask suddenly looked tired, "though not necessarily. Don't you believe in ghosts, Jake?" And before the other could answer: "Well, *these* ghosts are sub-marines. They're dead Russian subs, yes—except they're still very much alive. A paradox? Not really. Just wait a minute and you'll see what you'll see. Meanwhile, why don't you pour us a drink? And consider yourself lucky. It's Wild Turkey."

Jake poured; the machine whirred; eventually two sheets of paper slid from the slot, pushed out and followed by the original. One of the decoded sheets was a large-scale map of Europe and the seas around, with numbered, circled pin-points of reference. The other was a list of grid references, numbered to correspond with those on the map. All of the grid references were oceanic: two pinpoints in the Black Sea off Varna in Bulgaria, another off Podisma in Turkey; two more in the Tyrrhenian midway between Naples and Sardinia; one in the Atlantic off Portugal's Algarve; and three more between Iceland and Norway south of the Arctic Circle. And there were others marked out by tiny question marks instead of dots. Looking at these little black marks on the map, and matching them with the grid references, Trask's expression was very bleak.

"Look there," he indicated the question marks. "As close to home as that: the Barents Sea, off Norway. Crazy!"

"Close to home?" Jake echoed him.

"Close to the former Soviet Union," Trask answered. "Odd, because the Russians are usually more careful than that. Chernobyl taught them that much of a lesson at least—taught them to look after their own, anyway. So maybe those two were accidental? Maybe they didn't intend for them to go down just there. Jesus, but whatever they intended, still it's a mess!"

"I'm not with you," said Jake, shaking his head.

"Then let me explain. Each of those pinpoints represents a hulk resting on the bottom. But what kind of hulk? The answer's almost unbelievable, but since I've already told you . . ."

"Submarines?"

Trask nodded. "Those innocuous little black dots? Each

one of them is a disaster just waiting to happen or already happening. They're allegedly 'decommissioned' *nuclear* subs we thought had been cleaned up, made safe, taken apart and stored with ten thousand tons of other radioactive rubbish years ago. Relics of Russia's penniless, outmoded, unwanted cold war navy, yes. But the Russian military was lying to us—which is nothing new—and this is the truth."

"And it's a bad thing?" Jake still didn't see it. "I mean, that these things have been sent to the bottom, miles deep, out of harm's way?"

"Out of harm's way? God, what an infant!" Trask shook his head. And before Jake could get upset again:

"Look, most of these subs have twin atomic engines. There are two possible meltdowns in each hulk. *Barely* possible, mind you, but possible. We don't know if they've been shut down properly, or even if they could be. But the very means of disposal tells us they're less than safe! Why else would the Russian military dump them on someone else's doorstep? What's more—since they're capable of this—how do we know they didn't load them to the gills with other high-level waste before scuttling them? What? They might have even left their leaking missile payloads aboard. These were ships of war, Jake! And sooner or later the bastard things will start spilling their guts!"

"What—in ten, twenty, fifty years? And a mile or so deep?" Jake still wasn't too impressed. "And anyway, what has this to do with you and E-Branch?"

Trask scowled at him, actually clenched a fist and thumped the table. "If Anna Marie English were here right now . . . she'd knock you arse over breakfast!"

Astonished, Jake drew back. "Anna Marie English? Isn't she someone who Chung mentioned?"

"She worked for us," Trask snapped. "An ecopath, she gave warning of Earth's decline—I mean personally. She was 'ecologically aware,' or as she herself would put it, she was 'as one with the earth.' It was her talent—or her curse. Funny, isn't it, Jake? But there are very few in E-Branch who are happy with their talents. They would much prefer to be ordinary. But since they can't be, they're E-Branch."

Jake wasn't sure of Trask's meaning. "So how did this help you? Her talent, I mean? How did it work?"

Trask shook his head. "None of us can tell you how our talents work, only that they do. In Anna Marie's case:

"As water tables declined and deserts expanded, so her skin dried out, became desiccated. When acid rains burned the Scandinavian forests, her dandruff fell like snow. In her dreams she heard whale species singing of their decline and inevitable extinction, and she knew from her aching bones when the Japanese were slaughtering the dolphins. She was like a human lodestone; she tracked illicit nuclear waste, monitored pollution, shrank from holes in the ozone layer. Anna Marie was an ecopath, Jake: she felt for the Earth and suffered all its sicknesses, because she knew that she was dying from them, too. . . ."

Trask was eloquent, Jake would grant him that much. "You're saying she's dead, then?"

"No," Trask answered. "I'm saying she's somewhere else. But by now . . . she might well have started to suffer again, yes." He sighed and sat up straighter, seemed on the brink of coming to a decision, finally continued:

"Me, I believe in ghosts, Jake. I really do, for I've seen a few in my time. And they weren't always of the moaning, chain-rattling and mainly harmless variety. But I also believe in listening to my colleagues. Now it seems a ghost has come among us, possibly a beneficial one. Well, according to Chung and Goodly, anyway. Unfortunately it's come at a very bad time. The coincidence is just too great—that this should happen *now,* just as we find ourselves in conflict with the Wamphyri and the plague they've brought with them out of Starside—for me to take any chances. That's what holds me back from telling you everything: the thought that perhaps *you* are an agent, albeit an unwitting agent, of the Wamphyri!"

"Me?" Jake's surprise couldn't have been more genuine. And Trask, a human lie detector, knew it more certainly than any other man ever could. Ah, but he remembered other times, when Harry Keogh had fooled him, too! And Jake went on, "How in hell could I be anyone's agent? And I'm certainly no ghost!"

"No," Trask agreed, "but what's in you might be."

"What's in me?"

"Don't play the fool, Jake!" Trask snapped. "We're talking about what's in your head. This talent you've suddenly come by, which brought you to E-Branch and then *returned* you there when you tried to run off. But is it the ghost of Harry Keogh—or is it something that merely *tastes* like him? Should I take you into my confidence, or shoot you dead right here and now?"

Jake started to his feet and upset the table. His face was a snarl, his hands reaching for Trask. "I've had it up to here with your threats and your bullying. You're an old man, Trask, and as far as I'm concerned you're an old fraud . . . too!?"

But by then he'd seen the gun that Trask had been holding under the table; it was aimed right at him. And he understood the other's apparent fumbling when he'd taken the decoder from his briefcase. But what he didn't understand was the way Trask stared at him, the urgent, burning question in his penetrating gaze.

"What would you have done?" Trask snapped. "What would you have done to me?"

"Done?" Jake looked at the gun, then at Trask. "Nothing. I . . . I might have shaken you, or tried to shake some sense into you. Or maybe I'd have tried shaking a little *out* of you! God, can't you see you've got me going in circles?"

And Trask actually smiled as he slowly lowered his gun and put it away. "Yes, I can see that," he nodded. With which Jake got the idea.

"What? Another bloody test?"

"To push you hard," Trask told him, "and see what answered. You . . . or something else."

"Well, if I were you," Jake said, "I would have supposed it was something else!"

"But you're not me," Trask told him. "And you passed. That leaves just one more test to go."

"Then let's get it over with."

"Not now, no."

"When, then?"

"Tomorrow morning. I'm having a man flown in from Carnarvon on the coast. An expatriate Brit, and the best in his field."

"What, yet another great 'talent'?" Jake was still angry.

"Not the way you mean," Trask shook his head. "But he has talent enough, yes. Oh, and by the way: that's some temper *you* have, Jake. You said you might have shaken me? Well, you shook me all right. I thought you might actually attack me!"

Jake relaxed a little, grinned. "I scared you?"

"I was scared I might have to *shoot* you, yes."

But before that could start Jake off again, a voice called from outside the tent. "Mr. Trask? Phillips here. We have a bit of a problem." A male figure stood silhouetted behind the gauze fly screen.

Trask let him in, said: "Shouldn't you be on your way to Carnarvon?"

"Would be," said the other, "if not for this problem. Its name is Peter Miller, and it won't get its ugly arse out of my chopper!" The speaker was small and young, and looked very hot, sticky, and agitated in his flyer's gear.

"Miller's in your machine?" Trask raised an eyebrow, then nodded decisively. "So he wants out of here. And once away, he intends to take his story to the authorities, or worse to some newspaper or other. Well, it can't be allowed. Yes, I want rid of him. No, I don't want the trouble he'll bring. Only a handful of people in the very highest places know what we're doing, and if we're compromised it will make them look bad. As for the man in the street . . . well, it's simply out of the question. The world's insecure enough as it is."

He turned to Jake. "Go and find Lardis Lidesci, will you?

Bring him to the chopper park in the clearing on the far side of the road." And speaking again to Phillips. "You and me . . . let's go and have a word with Mr. Miller."

"Just what *is* that fat jerk doing here anyway?" Jake wanted to know.

"He was supposed to give us some legitimacy," Trask answered. "He's liaison, a go-between, that's all. But he took his job too seriously, discovered the location of our original base camp near Lake Disappointment, which is after all his province, and since then he's insisted on staying aboard. Well, *with* us is one thing, but against us is another. Now, after seeing far too much of what we're about, he's all too eager to leave. I can't very well stop him, but I really should warn him against doing anything stupid. Now go and get Lardis, will you?"

And Trask and Phillips went off through the night. . . .

The Old Lidesci was in a fold-away chair, dozing by the guttering campfire. But as Jake approached he gave a start and looked up. "Eh, what is it?"

"Trask wants you," Jake told him. "At the helicopter park. Some trouble with Mrs. Miller."

"Mrs.? Eh?" Lardis frowned at first, then burst out laughing. "Oh! *Ha-ha-ha!* But you know, the truth is I've been thinking much the same thing: how that poor excuse for a man reminds me of a chattering old woman. A week on Sunside would sort that one out, I fancy. But no, no . . . the poor bastard wouldn't last but a day."

Jake assisted him to his feet and the Old Lidesci stamped his left foot a little. "Cramp," he said. "I'm getting past it. We call it the Crippler where I'm from. But it's rheum—er, rheuma—er . . ."

"Rheumatism," Jake said.

"Damn right!" said Lardis. "It's rheumatism here. Ah, but it's a *sod* in any world."

And with the old man leaning a little on Jake's arm, they made for the road and the helicopter park.

8
"Mr." Miller and the Trouble with Dreams

IN THE HELICOPTER PARK, VOICES WERE RAISED in anger. One was a rasp: Ben Trask's. And the other was high-pitched, shrill, and threatening. In short, blustering; but the mind behind it held threatening knowledge, certainly. .

"Try to see sense, man!" Trask was growling, as Jake and Lardis Lidesci approached the well-lit area where a handful of Branch agents and chopper ground staff stood in a clearing and watched the show.

"Sense? Sense?" Miller was in one of the two helicopters, belted into a passenger seat near the section of aluminum frame that formed both cabin wall-panelling and steps. At present the steps were "down" and Miller was seated opposite the open door, from where he looked down on Trask outside the aircraft. "What? Are you telling me my attitude is nonsensical? But I know what I saw tonight, and it wasn't of this Earth. It was intelligent, and alien . . . oh, and it was ugly, yes. But I also saw the devastating force that your thugs used against it, which was even *more* inhuman! So who the hell are you, Mr. Trask? Some kind of monster yourself? You and your people: you're not the military, not even Australian. It's obvious to me that you've duped somebody somewhere. As for those poor aliens: whoever they are and wherever they're from, they deserved a lot better welcome than you gave them. This is Earth Year—dedicated to the ecological survival of the planet—and you might well have condemned our world to interplanetary isolation. Worse, we may even find ourselves at war!"

The precog Ian Goodly stepped out of the shadows and spoke to Jake and Lardis. "This idiot obviously has some kind of bee in his bonnet. 'The flying saucers have landed,' and all that rot. He seems to think we've been murdering aliens—visitors from another world, that is—out of hand!"

"Haven't we?" Jake looked at him.

"No," Goodly answered. "We killed invaders. Visitors don't arrive uninvited, stay, and kill off or enslave the occupiers. But invaders frequently do . . . and the Wamphyri *always* do! Not knowing everything, Miller sees our action tonight as an unprovoked assault, a preemptive strike against 'beings' whose intentions hadn't been fully determined. We, on the other hand—knowing the entire story, having been here, or there, before—see it differently. We see tonight's action for what it really was: the only cure for a nightmarish plague that submits to no other antidote."

And meanwhile:

"Miller, come down out of there." Trask was insistent. "The airplane you're sitting in has been serviced and fuelled for an important mission. You're cutting into a tight schedule."

"That's *Mr.* Miller to you!" the other snapped. "And I'm delighted to be disrupting your vile schedule! What, am I preventing another massacre like the one you organized tonight? Good! My God! How many of these poor people have landed, then?"

"You see?" Goodly muttered. "They're 'poor people' now. I mean, is Miller unbalanced or what? He had a ringside seat for tonight's show, yet he's *still* not convinced!"

Lardis had seen and heard more than enough. Freeing himself from Jake's helping hand, he moved up alongside Trask and in a lowered tone, said, "Why don't you just drag his arse out of there?"

"I was trying to be diplomatic," Trask answered under his breath.

"It didn't work," said Lardis.

Trask nodded and said, "That's why I sent for you." Then, turning away, he said, "Get him out of there. And bring him to the big ops truck. Maybe his own authorities can convince him, for I certainly can't. Jake, help Lardis after he's got Miller down from there."

"Why don't I just do it for him?" Jake was surprised. "The old boy, well . . . he's old."

Trask agreed. "He's full of old ways, too. So don't worry, he'll manage okay, and probably scare Miller half to death into the bargain. Serve the bastard right!" And without another word he went on his way, and Ian Goodly went with him.

Meanwhile Lardis had climbed the steps, leaned inside the chopper's open door, and was showing Miller his machete. "Sharp as a razor," he said. "You could shave with this—except you'd get tired holding it up to your face. See these notches in the grip? Twenty-seven of 'em. Twenty-seven exec—er, excecu—er, *killings,* yes. And all of them were these 'people' you seem so fond of. D'you know why I killed 'em?"

"Bloodthirsty old lunatic!" Miller hissed. "Well, I don't know where *you* come from, but where I'm from we're educated and civilized. Don't try to threaten me. I don't give a *fuck* for your big knife!" Which was more bluster, for anyone in his right mind would certainly give a fuck about Lardis's machete. And Miller's language was slipping, too.

In any case it was as if Lardis hadn't even heard him. "I killed 'em 'cause they eat fat little girls like you," he said. " 'Cause they're a contam—er, a contamin—er . . ."

"Contamination," said Jake from the foot of the steps.

"Damn right!" Lardis nodded. He put the point of his machete up to Miller's neck inside the nylon seat belt, and continued, "Now Ben Trask wants you to come down out of there. He was asking you nicely, because he believes in being diplomatic. But me, I don't."

Miller tried to cringe away from the glittering blade, but his seat belt trapped him in position. "Are you . . . do you *dare* to threaten me?" he gasped.

"Dare to threaten you?" said Lardis, his dark eyes narrowing to slits. "Hell, no, 'Mr.' Miller! This isn't a threat but a promise. If you don't move your arse out of there, I'm going to cut your fucking ears off!" And he made, a sudden slicing motion with his machete.

Miller screamed aloud, and for a moment Jake thought that Lardis really had cut him. But no, he'd sliced upwards and outwards, and his fine-honed blade had passed with scarcely a hiss through Miller's seat belt above the shoulder. Miller had been straining away from the Old Lidesci; freed from the safety harness, he jerked from his seat in that direction and fell to his hands and knees on the helicopter's floor. Lardis stepped over him, and while the little fat man was still off-balance grabbed him by the scruff of the neck and the seat of his pants to send him bouncing down the steps. It didn't take too much effort.

Miller's blubber saved him from any real hurt, but still he yelped as he hit the dirt; yelped yet again as Jake hoisted him to his feet—only to put him in an arm lock. "Mr. Trask is waiting for you," Jake told the babbling fat man, as he frogmarched him in the direction of the operations truck. . . .

In ops, Trask stood inside the oval control desk, speaking earnestly into a telephone. "Yes, I appreciate the lateness of the hour. . . . I understand perfectly, sir, and I agree entirely. But in this case I'm sure that only the highest authority will suffice. . . . You may believe me when I tell you that this really is as important as your Minister for Internal Security has reported, a matter of the gravest security. I certainly wouldn't have had you brought from your bed for anything less. . . . He's called Peter Miller, sir—that's 'Mr.' Miller— our so-called 'local liaison.' Not very helpful, sir, no. Indeed, completely hysterical, as I've said. . . . That's what I would suggest, yes, absolutely. . . . Until we're finished here, yes. That is, of course, if you're in agreement . . . ? Confinement. I'm afraid so, yes. Oh, we have the means. But Miller—*Mr.* Miller—is an Australian citizen, sir, and we're not. Which is why I need your . . . ?"

Trask looked up, saw Miller's face throbbing with rage and 'righteous' indignation where Jake's hand was clamped over his mouth. The sight of the man, in no way pacified, seemed to convince Trask of the course he must take. And:

"Perhaps you'd like to have a word with him in person?" he continued into the phone. "See for yourself, as it were?" With a nod and a grimace he passed the phone to Miller, at the same time indicating that Jake should release him.

Miller shook himself, reeled, and said, "Eh? What?" Intent on freeing himself from Jake's grasp, he'd taken in very little of Trask's conversation with the unknown other.

But now Trask said, "It's for you . . . someone who wants to know how you're keeping."

"Bloody crazy pommy bastards!" Miller raved. "And who the hell is this, the Prime-bloody-Minister?" He snatched the telephone from Trask's hand, yelled, "Whoever you are, the man you were speaking to is not a reasonable human being. He's fucking British, a fucking murderer, and I'm a God-fearing, completely innocent fucking Australian! This is my goddamned country, for Christ's sake, and I demand to speak to the police, to the military, to someone in authority, to—"

"—To the Prime-bloody-Minister, perhaps?" said Ben Trask, coolly examining his fingernails. And under his breath, to the others in the trailer: "Lance Blackmore, whose platform slogan, if I remember correctly, was 'sanity, sobriety, and common decency in speech and spirit.' Oh, and something else: he's decidedly pro-British!"

Miller's round face was suddenly wobbling, its colour visibly changing, paling. "Eh?" he gulped. "Do I what? Your voice? Do I recognize it?" Well, maybe he did . . . and maybe not. With his pig-eyes narrowing, he stared suspiciously at the phone—then at Trask—and spat, "Some lousy fucking pommy con man *you* are! And this is supposed to be Lance bloody Blackmore, right? Oh, *really*? What, at two o'clock in the morning? After what I've seen and been through tonight, you expect me to believe that my own Prime Minister, the *Australian* Prime-bloody-Minister, would condone—"

But the telephone was making loud noises in Miller's ear, and suddenly his face was floppily mobile again. For this time the owner of the now angry voice was fully awake and the voice itself unmistakable. As Miller's flabby mouth fell open, Trask took back the telephone and spoke into it. "There you have it, Prime Minister. Now you know what we're up against." And a moment later: "Yes, certainly, I shall see to it myself. Physical restraint—house arrest, shall we say?— until we're through here? Thank you. And there will be a copy of my report on this phase of the operations on your desk by noon, yes. So far it's looking good. My pleasure, sir. Thank you once again. And goodnight." He put the phone down.

"It *was* him!" Miller gasped, his mouth opening and closing like a stranded fish. "It really was Lance Blackmore!" Clenching his pudgy fists, he glowered at Trask: "You duped him! You even duped the Prime Minister! Who the fuck are you people?"

Trask shook his head in disgust. "Once your mind's made up it really is made up, isn't it, Miller?"

"That's *Mr.* Miller—"

"Oh, shut the fuck up!" Trask was mad now. He reached over the desk, grabbed the fat man by the front of his sweaty shirt, bunched a fist and drew it back . . . then thought better of it. Instead he gave him a shove, sent him reeling back into Jake's arms. And before Miller could start up again, "You're under arrest. If you protest too loudly I'll have you gagged. If you come on all physical I'll have you bound. If you attempt any interference with the work going on around you, I'll put you under constant surveillance by Lardis Lidesci. And if you're stupid enough to make another run for it, then you'd better be aware I'll deal with you . . . far more severely. Have I made myself clear?"

"Why you . . . *you!*" Miller mouthed, his furious expression speaking volumes more than all of his frothing bluster.

"When I turn you over to your Internal Security people in Perth tomorrow," Trask went on, "they'll read you the riot act, demand that you sign an Oath of Silence, give you to understand how very much in error you are, and generally threaten you with all sorts of dire things if you so much as mention anything you witnessed as our regional liaison person during this operation. And believe me, Miller, even if they can't make it stick I can. Don't for a moment think I'm going to forget the trouble you've put me to. And something else you should remember: in this modern world of ours distance isn't a problem. I'll be back in the U.K. shortly—I hope—but I have the longest arms in the world. And if I ever suspect that you're out there somewhere flapping those soft self-righteous lips of yours—"

Trask paused for breath, and Lardis Lidesci said, "—Then he'll send me to *stop* you flapping them—perhaps permanently!"

The Old Lidesci stood in the narrow doorway holding his machete to his chest, thumbing its blade and turning it in his hand to make it reflect the ops room's lights into the fat man's eyes. "Twenty-seven notches, remember, Miller? But in your case, I'd just love to make it twenty-eight."

Miller flinched a little but his expression didn't change. And again he blurted, "You . . . you . . . *you!*"

"Obviously I haven't made myself clear," Trask sighed. And to Jake: "See if there's a spare bunk back there, will you? And lock this fuckhead safely inside it!"

And that was that, for the moment.

Finally, they could all get some sleep. To some, a blessing. . . .

But Jake Cutter didn't much care for sleep. For some time now, in fact since his weird escape almost a week ago, sleeping had been a problem. Oh, he could do it, and he could do *with* it—indeed, his eyes felt heavy from the lack of it—but he didn't want to do it. Because when he went to sleep, that was when the Other woke up. That bloody Other, that one who was there in the back of his mind. And when Jake slept . . . why, then he couldn't be sure that his dreams were his at all.

He hadn't told Ben Trask about it, mainly because he suspected that Trask would be interested. It was the relationship that was developing between them: just as the head of E-Branch continued to hold things back, so did Jake Cutter. In his book trust was something that could only work if it was mutual.

And so he was left to face it on his own, and sleep was a necessity he avoided as best he could while yet recognizing, of course, that it *was* a necessity. It wouldn't be so bad—or so he told himself—if only he could remember what these troubled dreams of his were about afterwards, when he was awake; or then again maybe it would. And maybe that was why he couldn't remember them: because he didn't want to. . . .

Lardis Lidesci sat with Jake awhile, heaped a little wood on the dying fire, opened a can of sausages and beans in tomato sauce and ate them cold. The Old Lidesci smacked his lips appreciatively. "Some of the things in this world . . ." he said, then started again, "—Hell no, *most* of 'em!—I could do without. But a can opener and a can of beans . . ." he grinned, smacked his lips again, and shook his head. "Well, these beans and the meat in these sausage things, they're a sight easier on these gnarly old tusks of mine than roasted shad, I can tell you!"

"Shad's a fish," Jake said, tiredly.

"In this world, sure," Lardis nodded. "But the first time I see a fish pull a caravan . . . I'll quit drinking plum brandy, and that's a vow!" He held the empty can in one hand, the can opener in the other, looked at each in turn admiringly, burped, and uttered a sigh. "But since my people don't have cans, what good's a can opener?"

"You and Trask could drive a man mad," Jake told him without looking up. "You come up with this weird stuff right out of the blue, as if I'm supposed to know what the hell you're talking about! I mean, I've seen enough now to know this isn't some gigantic leg-pull, so what the hell is it?"

"Hell's just about right," Lardis grunted, creaking to his feet. He laid a hand on Jake's shoulder. "But son, take my word for it: Ben's not trying to drive you mad, and neither am I. It could be we say these things hoping you'll recognize something, hoping you'll perhaps remember."

There was something in Lardis's gruff old voice that

caused Jake finally to look at him. "But remember what?" he said.

And it was as if they stared deep into each other's souls. So that for a moment—just for a moment—it seemed that they had known each other, oh, for quite some time. Then Lardis nodded, and as though he had read Jake's mind said: "Other times, maybe? Other places?"

"Times and places?" Though Jake tried hard to understand, still it was beyond him. "Make sense, can't you?" There was no anger now, just a need to know.

"A time on Starside, perhaps," Lardis said, still staring hard at Jake, "when a man and his changeling son laid waste to the aeries of the Wamphyri? Or a time when the same man lay in the arms of a wonderful woman, whose name was Nana Kiklu. Or a time when we met—met for the last time, that man and I—in the ruins of The Dweller's garden, when it was already far too late for him. . . ."

Lardis's words conjured pictures that came and went. They meant something—Jake knew that much at least—but they were monochrome things; they flickered like the frames of some ancient silent movie . . . jerky scenes and twitching puppet figures. And despite that Jake thought he recognized some of them, still it was as if he saw them through someone else's eyes:

He looked down on a plain of boulders, lit silver-grey beneath a tumbling moon, where distant spires climbed to a sky of ice-chip stars. And that alien sky was alive with flying beasts whose weird shapes . . . ! God, those shapes! *Designs not of Nature but of Nightmare!*

As quickly as it had come the scene was gone, disappeared, and another took its place.

*A garden—*The garden?*—where a younger Lardis stood by a wall and gazed upon a scene of desolation. A windmill's crumpled vanes slumped all lopsided atop a skeletal, tottering timber tower; some of the roofs of low stone dwellings had fallen in; the trout pools were green with algae, and the greenhouses were tangles of shattered frames, leaning or* *fallen flat, with clumps of bolted vegetation sprouting through their torn plastic sheeting.*

The pictures continued to flicker and blur, and the oddly young Lardis turned jerkily to stare at Jake . . . or at the one gazing back at him through Jake's eyes.

But in this not-so-Old Lidesci's eyes there was fear, and in his hands a shotgun that came swinging, frame by flickering frame—click, clickety-click—in Jake's direction. And the look in Lardis's eyes was no longer fear, or not entirely, but fear combined with deadly intent!

Abruptly, the scene changed:

To the straining face of a handsome woman. Handsome, yes, but by no means beautiful—yet beautiful, too, in her way. Her body was beautiful, certainly. And hands (Jake's hands?) on her breasts where they lolled in his face. And her breath like fire in his (or some other's?) flared nostrils, and the sweat of her passion as slippery and hot on his hands as the wet core of her womanhood where it sheathed his jerking flesh.

Nana?

"Nana!" Jake exclaimed, as the scene slipped from memory—but *his* memory?—and he found himself seated by the campfire, his hands before his face, perhaps to fondle (who? What was her name?) the handsome woman's breasts, or perhaps to ward off Lardis Lidesci's shotgun. Well, there was the old man, sure enough, but now more surely the "Old" Lidesci as Jake knew him; and he had no shotgun but a strange satisfied look on his face.

"And it's Nana, is it?" Lardis said, with a knowing nod, as Jake's mind swam back into focus and he slowly lowered his trembling hands. "Took you back a ways, didn't I, my young friend?"

"What . . . what did you *do* to me?" Jake whispered, the words sighing out of him.

"I have an ancestor's seer's blood in me," Lardis answered. "It smells things out. And I think that it has smelled you out, too, Jake Cutter. For just as this art of my forebears has been passed down to me, so something has been passed to you. It's *in* you, man! Not in your blood, as it was in Nestor's and Nathan's blood, but buried in your mind and your soul for sure!" And now the look on the Gypsy's face was one of awe as much as anything else.

"It's in me, yes," Jake agreed, knowing it was so. And then coming very close to desperation, "But what is it, Lardis? What *is* it?"

The other shook his head. "No, no. Ben wouldn't want me to say any more. Indeed, He'd nag that I've already said too much! It will have to take its own good time, that's all. But what's in will out, of that you can be sure. And now, goodnight to you, Jake Cutter." With which he backed off, and like the wild thing he was faded into the night. . . .

Maybe Jake had been too tired to dream, or perhaps he had managed to fight it off this time. Whichever, he had slept deeply, soundly, and dreamlessly, and remembered coming awake only once, when he'd thought to hear a vehicle's engine starting up. Then he'd eased his cramped body off the chair, zipped himself into a sleeping bag, and curled up right at the edge of the fire's cooling embers—

—And now came starting awake as the toe of a boot nudged him and Trask's voice rasped, "Jake, get up. Have you seen anything of Miller? Obviously not. Well, the fat bastard's run out on us, and in *your* bloody vehicle! Damn, I thought for a moment you'd gone with him!"

Throwing back the mosquito net from his face, Jake unzipped the bag and struggled out of it. Now he remembered the engine starting up, dipped headlamps swinging faint beams out onto the road, and the cautious crunch of tires on dirt and pebbles. He had thought at the time that someone was being very careful not to awaken the camp . . . and he'd been only too right!

"My vehicle?" he mumbled, but Trask had already moved on.

The entire camp was coming awake, and overhead the shrill, pulsing whistle of a jet-copter cutting its thrusters; the *whup whup whup* of its vanes lowering it down from a sky in which the stars were only just beginning to fade. And the first faint nimbus of dawn silhouetting the treetops and shining on rising, writhing wisps of mist.

"Hell's teeth!" Lardis Lidesci groaned where he came stumbling from the direction of the big articulated ops vehicle. As he came, his trembling right hand gingerly explored a blackened patch of bloodied, matted hair on the left side of his head. It looked ugly, and was made to look worse by a flow of blood that had run down and congealed around his ear. "Damn the bloody man to hell!" he said.

Meeting him halfway, Trask grunted: "Miller?"

"Wouldn't you just know it?" Lardis nodded, then groaned and held his head again. "I bedded down under the steps at the back of ops. And I heard something in the dead of night, something breaking. But these damned short nights of yours . . . my system's all out of kilter with them . . . I'm used to *sleeping,* not these forty winks that you people take!"

"You didn't wake up till too late," Trask grunted.

"I'm not a damned watchdog!" Lardis snapped.

Trask shook his head. "I'm not blaming you, Lardis. Hell, I didn't think the crazy bastard had enough guts to make a run for it! So if it's anyone's fault it's mine. I should have posted a guard on him."

Ian Goodly came loping, looking more than a little angry with himself. "The camp's awake," he said, sourly.

Trask looked at him and growled, "You too? It seems we're each and every one of us blaming himself."

"But I'm the precog," Goodly chewed on his top lip.

"Right," Trask agreed, "but one man can't foresee it all. And let's face it, if you could anticipate everything that was coming . . ."

". . . Then I would probably have killed myself a long time ago, yes," Goodly nodded. "But damn it, I *did* see this one!"

"You what?" Jake was wide awake now. "So why didn't you do something?"

"I saw it in my sleep," the precog answered. "Saw it as a dream. *Huh!* When is a dream not a dream? When it's a glimpse of the future! But even if I'd known what it was, how would I have woken myself up? When you're asleep you're asleep. And the future guards its secrets well."

"And I thought I was the only one who was having problems with his dreams!" Jake said. At which Trask looked at him very curiously . . . but only for a moment. There was too much to do.

"Okay," Trask said, "let's forget it. I'm to blame, Lardis is to blame, Ian is to blame, and so is Jake—"

"Me?" Jake raised an eyebrow.

"For leaving the keys in your Rover," Trask nodded. "Anyway, no one is really to blame. The problem is we've grown too used to dealing with the weird, the abnormal, the monstrous. I mean, if it's mundane we tend to let it slide. And you couldn't ask for anything more mundane than Mr. bloody Miller!"

"I beg to differ," said Goodly.

"Eh?" Trask looked at him.

"Can I put you fully in the picture now?" the precog said. And when Trask nodded: "Miller's a strange one," Goodly continued. "When finally I woke up I was worried about my dream. So I went to see if everything was okay. I missed Lardis where Miller must have pushed him back out of sight behind the trailer's steps, but I found the duty officer. He's going to be okay, but he, too, had been bashed on the head. He was lying in the corridor outside Miller's bunk with the door on top of him. They're pretty flimsy, those doors. The hinges had been worked loose.

"I wasn't sure how long the D.O.'d lain there, so I checked that he was okay then went to see if the ops room was safe. The place was working as normal . . . incoming, that is. Several messages, waiting for answers, and situation reports coiling up on the floor. There was some Cosmic Secret stuff that the D.O. must have been processing when Miller attracted his attention. Quite a bit of it had been decoded. Then I remembered how you'd asked for background information on Miller. That was there, too, coming out of the printer even as I got there. But there was stuff that *should* have been there and wasn't . . . like a lot of Cosmic Secret stuff from HQ?

The printouts had been ripped through and some of the serials were missing. We'll need to get them duplicated, find out what was on them.

"Anyway, I grabbed the stuff on Miller, then began to wake people up. Now they're all awake, though I don't see what they can do to help. Oh yes, and here's all the background information on Miller. . . ." He thrust some sheets of printout at Trask.

But before Trask could even begin reading, Goodly went on. "Miller isn't as mundane as you think, Ben. But he *is* an obsessive nut, and the black sheep of the family. His uncle was big in Western Australian politics, got him work as a minor official in a job where he didn't have a lot to do but could indulge his thirst for power—in however small a way. Why else do you suppose he's the guardian of a million square miles of nothing? To keep him out of the way, that's why. Good grief, and we had to get lumbered with him! Come to think of it, it's likely that that, too, came about as a result of his uncle's influence.

"Okay, his obsessions. Anything! I mean it: this fellow can get hooked on literally anything! An obsessive personality, it's as simple—or not as simple—as that. But guess what? Back in the late 1970s, early '80s, he saw *Close Encounters* and *E.T.*—well, who didn't? But this is Peter Miller we're talking about. He joined a wacky UFO group, of which he's still a member, and wrote two 'Friendly Aliens Are Here' books that didn't get published. Need I say more? No way you could have convinced this bloke that we were in the right last night, Ben. No way at all."

"I see," said Trask. And, after he had given it a moment's thought, "Do we have any idea how long he's been gone?"

"Judging by the D.O.'s signatures in the message log, maybe three, three and a half hours," Goodly answered.

Trask nodded. "Then he could be anywhere by now. Two hundred and more miles away, for all we know! So no good our trying to chase him. Very well, here are the priorities. I want Lardis and the D.O. taken care of as best possible. And I want a ,man—you, Ian—in the ops chair sending out wanted notices to all the police authorities in a two hundred miles radius . . . better make it three hundred miles . . . or better still, all of Western Australia!" But on second thought: "No wait, send out just one, to the Internal Security people in Perth. He's their man, after all, so let them go after him. Oh, and check that they have his profile, too, which ought to scotch any 'wild stories' that Miller may be circulating. And finally, I want to know what was on those missing printouts."

Trask paused, shrugged, and eventually continued. "Anyway, there's one good thing come out of all this: I won't be wasting half a day handing Miller over to the I.S. people in Perth. And as for right now . . . I'm hungry." He headed for the trench with the back-burner, which someone had fired up. "I'm going to have breakfast."

By which time an agent was tending to Lardis, and all over the camp sleepy-looking people were on the move. The jet-copter had landed, and Phillips the pilot was leading a tall, grizzled stranger—strange to Jake, anyway—through the grey predawn light between the trees into the camp's clearing. Trask spotted them as they came striding through thinning ground mist; waving to attract their attention, he diverted his steps in their direction. Jake followed on behind him.

"Grahame." Trask smiled a greeting. "If it's no the laird himself. It's been quite a few years now." But while Jake might wonder at Trask's assumed accent, the stranger's seemed perfectly in keeping and went well with the swing of his kilt:

"Aye, that it has," he rumbled through the full grey beard that gave him his grizzled aspect, grinning to display a bar of strong, square teeth. "What, twelve years? How goes it with you, Benjamin? You and yere bleddy gadgets!"

They shook hands . . . but in the next moment the stranger's searching eyes, those oh so dark eyes of his, transferred their gaze to Jake. "And this'll be the subject, is it no?"

"It is," Trask nodded. "As for the gadgets—like the one

that flew you here in a matter of hours—well, they're improving all the time, if that in itself can be considered an improvement. But to be truthful, which I always am, I find it harder and harder to keep up. Future shock or something. Anyway, it's not that side of the equation that concerns us, not this time."

"Then if it's no the gadgets, it must be the ghosts," said the other, still staring at Jake.

And Trask nodded. "One ghost, anyway," he said.

Part Two
The Why of It

9
Regression

AS THEY SEATED THEMSELVES AT A FOLDING
table, to a breakfast of black coffee in plastic mugs, and
bacon and eggs on paper plates, Trask made belated introductions. "Jake Cutter, mah guid friend here is Grahame
McGilchrist, Laird o' Kinlochry. . . ." But then he ahemmed
his embarrassment, and went on, "Who, despite my atro-
ciously false and corny accent, is the genuine article."

Shaking hands with the big Scotsman across the table,
Jake said, "A Scottish laird, living on the other side of the
world? There has to be something of a story in that."

"No much o' a one," the other rumbled. "It's simply a
matter o' choice. See, the McGilchrist estate went broke all
o' a hundred years ago. Oh, ah had mah crumblin' old castle,
but in truth Ah wiz a figurehead in the local community, and
that wiz a'. But Ah still had mah pride. So, when a cousin
o' mine pegged it out here in Oz and left me his wee place
in Carnarvon, Ah came out and took over. That was some
nine years ago."

"That 'wee place' Grahame's talking about," Trask cut in,
"is two and a half thousand acres of well watered farmland
east of Carnarvon. If he wanted to sell up he could go back
home and be a proper laird again."

"But Ah willnae do it," McGilchrist said. "Ah have lads
tae tend mah land and animals, while Ah have mah own
interests."

"He has a practice in Carnarvon," Trask explained. "His
own special slant on psychiatry."

"Aye, and there ye have the other reason why Ah made
mahsel scarce frae they so-called 'British' Isles." McGilchrist

cocked his head, frowned at Trask, and winked at Jake. "Tae escape frae these bleddy E-Branch types!"

"He worked for us awhile," Trask said.

But Jake had been quick to latch onto something else. "Psychiatry?" he said, suspiciously. "And I'm the subject?"

Liz Merrick appeared out of nowhere, looking great in black slacks, cowboy boots, and a frilly white blouse. Seating herself beside Jake, she said, "And a suitable subject at that!"

"Thanks," Jake told her sourly, while he waited for Trask's or McGilchrist's explanation. And:

"Hypnotic regression," Trask said without further preamble. "That's Grahame's speciality. It's not a 'talent' as recognized by E-Branch—that is, it isn't some strange parapsychological ability, though the way it works for Grahame it might well be—but it does come in useful in cases like yours."

"Cases like mine?" Again Jake waited.

"Where the subject has subconsciously deleted some part of his memory," Trask said. "Or something else has blocked it—"

"—Or he has simply forgotten it," McGilchrist finished it for him. "Ye're no a nut case, if that's what's bothering ye."

"You don't know him yet," said Liz, and Jake scowled.

McGilchrist grinned at Liz across the table and said, "Will one o' ye kind gentleman no introduce me tae this beautiful wee thing? Oh, Ah ken Ah'm a mite late—a mite too old, maybe?—but still Ah'd like tae be in wi' a chance!"

"Too late?" Liz blushed at his words. But McGilchrist simply looked at Jake, smiled, and went on eating. . . .

Jake had been studying the Scotsman, and despite his apprehension he discovered that he liked him. McGilchrist seemed as open as a book. The hypnotist was tall, yes, but with his huge chest and massive girth looked almost stocky. Jake could well picture him tossing a caber, and for that matter he could probably toss big men around as well. Except, Jake reckoned, that wouldn't be in his nature. He was the salt of Scottish soil, the hard flint of wooded mountains, however far removed; but there was a kindness—an understanding of nature, human nature, especially—in those dark eyes of his, however deeply they might probe.

It was frequently the same with men of rare ability. Even in Jake's few days with E-Branch he had been aware of it in Ben Trask's espers, the ones he'd met, and of course in the head of E-Branch himself. The big Scotsman might not be as parapsychologically endowed as a true esper, but still there was that special something about him; in those eyes, mainly—those hypnotic eyes, and the way they studied a man. . . .

Jake suddenly realized that they'd been studying him, reading him much as he had been reading the other. Perhaps reading him more, or more cleverly. And breakfast was over now.

"So when's it tae be?" McGilchrist stood up, stretched, and yawned. "God, but ye got me up early, Ben Trask! Ah wiz barely in bed . . . then up again, when yere chopper landed in mah backyard. Ah wiz expectin' yere man, aye, but no at that hour."

"I'm sorry about that," Trask said, "but we never know how long we'll be in any one place. And in fact we could be moving on at any time. I'm just waiting on some information from London, and then we'll be out of here."

He got to his feet; Jake and Liz, too, and she said, "Can I come in on this? Jake's my partner, after all."

"He might *yet* be your partner," Trask answered immediately. "We won't know that until we know."

And Jake, as fidgety as ever, burst out, "Then for Christ's sake let's get *on* with it! For whatever it is, it seems my future's hanging on it."

"Yere future?" said Grahame McGilchrist, as Trask led them towards his tent. "Ah, no. Ye'd be better off askin' the precog about that. And ye'll find that even he isnae that sure. But as for the past: well, that's different. What's been has been, and it cannae be changed. But even if it's been well and truly buried—buried in or by the mind, that is—we can usually dig it up again, aye. And as for me: Ah'm one hell o' an archeologist!" He turned his attention to Trask.

"So then, but this is a verra different E-Branch to the one Ah used tae know. They pilots, talkin' over there: Australians, aye? And a couple more fiddlin' wi' those vehicles there? Seems ye're recruitin' far afield these days, Benjamin."

"No, not really," Trask answered. "Not even if it was just our espers you were talking about. See, in E-Branch we've never much cared about colours, creeds, or nationalities. In that respect you could even say that we've always recruited far afield. For example: David Chung is of Chinese stock, you are Scottish, and poor Darcy Clarke's forebears were French. As for Zek Föener, Zek . . ." Trask's voice faltered and his face clouded over.

"Aye, Ah ken, and Ah'm sorry." McGilchrist took his arm.

They had arrived at Trask's tent. Freeing himself from the Scotsman's grip, his well-meant but inopportune commiseration, Trask turned his face away, occupied himself in fastening back the entrance flap to let in the predawn light. And in a while:

"Currently the team consists of a small nucleus of agents, mainly from London HQ," he went on. "But the backup squads are Australian military, and likewise all their gear. It's not likely that anyone would know that, because the tac signs have been removed from the vehicles and choppers, and of course the men themselves aren't wearing their standard uniforms. But the discipline is the same. And you're quite right, Grahame, there have been several changes in E-Branch. For one, we're no longer the shoestring outfit that we used to be. Financially we're pretty stable now; when you can pay your own way, it gives you that much more clout.

"Five years ago, through our dealings with Gustav Turchin, the Russian Premier, we got ourselves accepted and well established. We could afford to come out of hiding—emerge, as it were, from the esoteric closet—but never too far. For let's face it, an organization like E-Branch can't remain secret if everyone knows about it.

"As for these Australians: obviously they're all subject to their own version of the Official Secrets Act, and they've all been hand-picked for their loyalty, their unswerving devotion to duty and their country. Isn't that just exactly how it should be? Who better to do . . . well, what I'm calling on them to do, than loyal subjects of the country under threat?"

"Under threat?" Suddenly McGilchrist's tone was sharp as he took his seat at Trask's small table.

Trask nodded gravely. "Perhaps the entire world," he said. "Except the world doesn't know it yet, and it mustn't."

"A secret invasion?" McGilchrist looked from face to face, trying to fathom their expressions. "As bad as a' that, is it? Than ye can only be talkin' about one thing. Oh, Ah dinnae need tae ken it a', but is it . . . Them?" An ex-member of the Branch, he'd had access to the files on their long-term war against the Wamphyri; indeed those files had long been required reading for all Branch operatives and senior affiliates.

"Grahame, you weren't part of the Sunside/Starside thing," Trask told him, "and from past experience I know how dangerous it could be to put you in the picture now. So please let it be. But yes, it is . . . Them. And now perhaps you'll forgive me for getting you out of bed in the middle of the night? As for Jake Cutter here, he could be very important to us—but *very* important—in the work we've still to do."

The big Scot had heard enough and was suitably impressed. "Then we'd best be at it," he said. "But tell me, just what am Ah supposed tae be lookin' for? Can ye no offer a wee clue?"

Trask looked torn two ways. He glanced first at Jake, then turned back to McGilchrist. "I can, but that would mean telling Jake, too."

"What's that? But doesnae he have a right to know?" McGilchrist frowned. And Jake said:

"*Huh!* My point exactly."

"But," Trask countered, "If he does have such a right, why doesn't he *already* know? If he's been denied access, it must be for a reason. In which case, what right have I to give him access now?"

McGilchrist shook his head, frowned again. "Well, doubt-less ye ken well enough what ye're on about, but Ah'm as much in the dark as Jake here! Can ye no gi' me a startin' point?"

"Oh, yes," Trask answered. "That I can do. Just a week ago Jake was in jail in Italy, Turin, when—"

"Undercover?" The hypnotist cut in.

"Er, no," said Trask, and the big Scot sat back and scratched at his beard musingly. "Anyway," Trask went on, "Jake escaped from the prison, barely. But it's the *way* he escaped that interests us. And it's where he escaped to . . ."

"Eh?" said McGilchrist. "Escaped to . . . ?"

"To Harry's Room, Grahame," Trask told him. "You'll remember Harry's Room, at E-Branch HQ?"

"Ah!" The other stopped scratching on the instant, stared hard at Trask, and harder still at Jake. "He *escaped* there, ye say?"

"Arrived there," said Trask. "But the question is, was he brought there, or did he come of his own volition . . . or was he sent? And if the latter, by whom was he sent?" And again:

"*Ahhh!*" said McGilchrist. "Verra well, then that'll be our startin' point: the prison, the escape." He unbuttoned a tartan shirt pocket, took out a small vial and uncorked it, gave it to Jake and said, "Sit down here and swally that."

Jake sat, looked at the colourless liquid in the vial suspi-ciously. "Do what?" he said.

"It's only a wee drug." McGilchrist was completely matter-of-fact about it. "We've had truth drugs a long time now, stuff ye had tae inject. But we've come a ways since then. This isnae a truth drug, but it does open the mind . . . it lets ye see more clearly intae yere own past. Aye, and it lets ye *talk* about it! Oh, and one other thing: it enhances mah power over ye."

"Your power over me?" Jake didn't like the sound of that, especially since he'd already poured the draft down his gul-let.

"It simply means that unless there's a verra strong post-hypnotic block on yere mind, ye'll gi' me all the assistance Ah require. Ye willnae hold anythin' back."

"And if there is a post-hypnotic block? Will that mean I've been hypnotized before?"

"Well, if no hypnotized, ye'll have been got at, certainly."

"And you'll be able to clear it?"

"Man, Ah cannae make ye that kind o' promise." McGilchrist was honest about it. "As Ben here will tell ye, there's hypnotists . . . and then there's hypnotists. And if what he fears has been here first . . ." He shrugged.

"I understand," said Jake, though in fact he didn't.

"Now, that's a fast actin' drug that's in ye," McGilchrist continued, "so Ah'd best be tellin' ye one or two things. Ye're tae sit verra still and upright in yere chair; oh, dinnae fret, Ah wouldnae let ye topple over. And ye're tae look at me, at mah eyes. Verra big and black, mah eyes, are they no?"

They were *very* big and black, and Jake's head was beginning to spin oh-so-slowly, languidly at first, but gradually getting faster; as if he were drunk, flat on his back on a bed, and the room spinning around him but without the sick feeling.

"And here's me bringin' mah eyes closer, lookin' at ye, and lookin *intae* ye." McGilchrist's voice was so very low now, like the growl of a great wolf. So low, so dark, and so close. "Ah'm lookin' intae ye, and yere lookin' intae mah eyes, or is it mah eye? For see, there's only one o' they now! The two have merged intae one, like a wee swirly black hole in mah face. Or maybe a big black hole? And it's suckin' at ye, Jake, suckin' at ye . . ."

It was indeed. That blackest of black holes, spinning faster and faster. And Jake felt its lure, its attraction. God, if he could back out of this now he would! But he couldn't. And:

"Dinnae fight it, laddie," said a voice that burned in his head. "Just let it go, and come to me. Open up to Grahame." And then:

The black hole had him! He was sucked in and whirled

like a bug down a plug hole. It was as quick as thought; it happened before he could even cry out, if he had been able to. . . .

Paulo has slid a length of rubber tubing over the links of the chain to deaden its clanking. Now he looks at me, gives me the nod, and I cup my hands for him. He steps into my hands, and I can smell his groin . . . he smells of fear, and I imagine I do, too. Thank God there's no moon!

He's up on my shoulders now, swinging the chain. I hear it swish through the dark night air . . . hear it clatter, too, just the once but enough to make me grit my teeth. And now there's a scraping sound as Paulo hauls on the chain, flattening the roll of barbed wire to the top of the wall. But he's done it! Paulo is on his way up the chain!

I look up; his head and shoulders are silhouetted against the black horizon of the wall. He clings to the chain with his right hand, takes the blanket from around his neck and lobs it up and over. The wire is covered. Damn! The man's a genius!

Now he's balanced up there with one leg over the wall, and he's reaching down for me. My heart is thudding, hammering away in my chest, but at last I'm on the chain. Up I go, and I reach for Paulo's hand. But what? What? He withdraws it!

I don't believe it! (But I do, I do! I just knew it was too bloody easy!) And I cling to the chain and look up at him, look into his eyes, that are looking down into mine. Except now they look beyond me, into the night.

And dangling there, I glance over my shoulder and see them: prison guards, armed and taking aim across the exercise yard. I look up at Paulo, and his sweat falls on me like rain. He gives a shrug, says: "I sorry, Jake, but they promise me . . ." And then he jerks as I hear the shot. And now Paulo's blood splashes me as his right eye turns black.

He's falling, taking me with him . . . we hit the ground like a ton of bricks! Paulo's body is on top of me, which is just as well, because I can feel it jerking, shuddering to the sound of more gunshots. I struggle under his dead weight, somehow manage to throw him off and rise into a crouch. But God, I'm a dead man—I have to be! Fat white sparks light the night like angry fireflies where bullets ricochet off the wall and spit concrete splinters at me. But now—

—Now there's a spark that . . . that isn't a spark! I don't understand it, haven't the time to understand it. But it hovers there like a golden dart, level with my eyes, only twelve inches away, seeming to follow my movements as I dodge bullets. And now it moves, too. And I know that it has to be a bullet after all, because it smacks me right between the eyes!

And I fall face-first, but I can't feel it when I hit the ground. Of course I can't feel it, because you don't feel anything when you're dead.

Dead and weightless and rushing somewhere, rushing out of my body I suppose. Rushing to heaven or hell, if I believed. I wish I had believed now . . . and I'll bet I'm not the first man who thought that! But Jesus, I'm not going out without a fight . . . not Jake Cutter! I struggle and twist and tumble. But this can't be right, because I can feel myself. I'm not dead yet!

And now I see a light in the darkness. I rush towards it, fall into it . . . no, I fall out of the darkness!

My head! God, I'm sick, dizzy, and my head . . . !

But I'm not dead yet.

I'm not dead yet.

Not dead yet.

Not dead.

Not.

No.

!

"It's been an hour," said McGilchrist's voice. "Ye ought tae be comin' out o' it now, Jake mah lad."

Jake remembered where he was and would have jerked erect, but since he was already erect—sitting upright in his chair, just as the "doctor" had ordered—instead he became aware of incredible cramps in all his limbs, whose pain was physical and of course far worse than the imagined thump on the head that he had "experienced" for the second time around just a few moments ago.

He opened his eyes, tried to reach up and touch his head, maybe cradle it in his trembling hands, but even the slightest movement caused violent shooting pains in his arms and shoulders, freezing him in position.

"G-God Almighty!" he groaned, his throat dry as kindling.

McGilchrist dropped two white pills into a glass of water, swirled them, and watched them dissolve. "These'll do ye a power o' good," he said.

"And I . . . I should believe you?" said Jake, blinking rapidly as his eyes grew accustomed to the full dawn light.

"Eh? But they're only wee aspirins, man!" McGilchrist told him. "For yere headache, ye ken? Which is a side-effect o' that draft o' mine. What, d'ye really think Ah'd poison ye?"

Slowly, Jake allowed himself to slump in his chair. And as his blood began to circulate and pins and needles took over from the true pain, so he took the glass and drank. And then he remembered not only what had gone before, but also something of his regression.

Again he straightened up, but much more carefully now, and said, "That dart. A golden dart or splinter. I seem to remember it . . . it entered my head?"

"Just like you told me," Liz Merrick sighed from where she sat close to him. "Except you didn't call it a dart."

Jake carefully turned to squint at her through the tent's luminous air. And Ben Trask said, "I think that's all we needed to know. It makes any further questions I might have academic, conjectural, meaningless. For the time being, anyway." He, too, was seated—looked like he needed to be— and his voice was trembling to match Jake's limbs.

"Great," said Jake, unsteadily. "Fine. So now that all of *your* questions are answered, how about mine?"

"Yours?" said Trask, stopped dead in his tracks. And: "Ah, well! We'll deal with those shortly, yes. And Jake, I'm really,

really very sorry about that—I mean, that I had to be so secretive. I'm sure you'll understand when you know it all."

"But for the next few minutes," said McGilchrist, with his massive hand on Jake's shoulder, "ye're tae take it easy, until ye're back on yere feet. And then ye should stop worryin' about what's happened tae ye. Ye're in the verra best o' hands, after a'."

The stiffness was draining from Jake's limbs and his headache was in recession. "Did I do okay?" he said, looking at Ben Trask. "Did you get all you wanted? It was that dart, right? It was that dart that I thought was a bullet. What in hell was the thing?"

But while Jake was beginning to feel okay, Trask was still shaken. "It's not so much what it *was*," he replied, "as what it *is*, but definitely. And what that makes you."

"Makes me?" Sensing something of Trask's quandary, perhaps his reluctance to accept whatever he was having to accept, Jake had stopped feeling okay on the instant. Now, frowning, he said. "How do you mean, what it makes me? What I am is plain: a fugitive from so-called justice, hiding out under the protection of E-Branch. Unless you've changed your mind, that is. Is that it? Did you learn something that makes you want to throw me back to the wolves? Am I in fact the sick, psychotic killer that people have been made to believe I am?"

And perhaps Trask would have started to tell him there and then, but at that moment Ian Goodly's piping, excited voice was heard from across the clearing:

"Ben, Ben!" the precog was calling. "Those serials. I know which ones are missing. And I think we're in a lot of trouble!"

"Think?" Trask called from the open door of his tent.

"I *know* we are." Goodly was closer now, and his voice commensurately less strident. "I've seen it coming, Ben," he said, heading towards Trask's tent at a fast, agitated lope. "Trouble with a capital *T*, yes. So whatever it is you're doing, put it aside for now. This is just as important—maybe more so—and I think you need to hear me out."

As Trask ducked out under the tent's awning, Liz took hold of Jake's hand and said, "No one thinks badly of you, Jake. What you told us when you were under only serves to corroborate what Ben Trask has been hoping all along. But that's for him to tell you, not me. And as for throwing you to the wolves . . . *au contraire,* Jake Cutter: on the contrary. But it could be his intention to throw you *at* them. . . ."

Ten minutes later, Trask had called his small nucleus of Branch people to him. And at the last moment he'd invited Liz and Jake into the briefing. Everyone was crowded into his tent.

Wasting no time, when all of his people had arrived, Trask said, "I won't make a meal of this and as soon as we're through here I want you to start packing up. I'd like to be out of here A.S.A.P. Ops truck and vehicles: strip them of everything important to us because we're leaving them behind. Our next target is too far away to simply drive to. It was possible we might have stayed just as we are now, but something has come up. Our Aussie friends will have to follow on behind us, but as the brains behind the brawn, as it were, time is a luxury we've just run out of. So . . . what's the big hurry, eh?

"Well, you all know about our Mr. Miller. But you don't know *all* about him. To recap: Miller's some kind of nut who believes in friendly aliens, and despite having seen the enemy pretty close up he thinks that *we* are the butchers. He thinks the work we did last night was a totally unjustified preemptive strike against a landing party of explorers from outer space, and that they only turned nasty in order to survive. He has even written books on the etiquette of first contact. So obviously, in Miller's warped perceptions, we're sadly lacking in manners.

"It doesn't matter that our 'aliens' are stinking, murderous vampires from a parallel world; Miller's mania would never accept that. He doesn't believe a word I've said to him— probably doesn't even believe they're vampires—but he does think he can talk to them.

"Well, that in itself wouldn't be a problem. His own people can look after him, lock him up or do whatever they deem necessary to make him look like an idiot—which he is—if Miller should start babbling his 'crazy stories' about our work to the press or other sensationalist outlets. So when I found out that he'd made a run for it, in a way I was pleased. At least he was out of *my* hair. Yes, but that was before I discovered what he'd taken with him.

"People, last night our locators at London HQ, headed up by David Chung, found us a new target: they detected a hitherto unsuspected patch of mindsmog on the other side of the Australian continent. It was only there for a moment—someone's mental shield slipped, shall we say?—but it was the real thing, the unmistakable signature of a Lord of the Wamphyri. I'm talking about a Lord, yes. And what we have to remember is that the Thing we went up against last night, Bruce Trennier, *that* was a mere lieutenant—someone in thrall to a Lord—left behind by his maker and master for whatever reason.

"Okay, this mindsmog: it was detected at the same time—I mean *precisely* the same time—that we were dealing with Trennier. Now, we know that many of the Wamphyri had the power of telepathic contact with their thralls even over great distances, so it's possible, indeed probable, that Trennier's unknown master 'felt' his lieutenant's death, and it so surprised or startled him that he let his guard down, if only for a moment. He might even have done it deliberately, tried to establish better contact with Trennier to find out what was happening. As for our people in London, they were lucky; someone happened to be looking in the right place at the right time, and that's when they detected the evil 'aura' of a Great Vampire.

"Of course Chung forwarded this information to me, only to have it intercepted by Peter bloody Miller! And now I couldn't give a damn about him speaking to the media or anyone else for that matter. But I do care that he might be on his way to deliver a warning to one of the worst threats our world has ever faced.

"A warning that *we* are on our way to destroy it!"

10
The Vampire File

WHEN EVERYONE WITH THE EXCEPTION OF JAKE
and Liz was clear of his tent, Trask opened his briefcase and
plumped a thin file down on the table.

"Read it," he told Jake. "It will give you something to do
for a while, for we may be here a little longer than I anticipated. I was forgetting that we'd have to fly Grahame back
home again. Even though he's on his way now, it will still
be three to three and a half hours before the chopper gets
back. But on the other hand, and since I'd like E-Branch to
move as a unit, that's probably just as well; it gives us more
time to get our act together—our thoughts, too—for which
I'm grateful. I hate starting something without being able to
think it through first."

He looked pointedly at Jake. "That file is your chance to
think things through, too. You see, I don't want anyone in
the Branch who doesn't fit or doesn't want to be here. However, in the event you do decide to move on, you needn't
worry about my handing you over to the law. That's not my
way. I would simply wash my hands of you. But if you stay,
then you're with us *all* the way. I have no time for quitters,
and in that case I would assist the law in any way possible."

"Huh!" Jake answered. "And just when I thought you'd
begun to appreciate me. Okay, do you want my answer right
now?"

"Read the file first," said Trask curtly, "then ask Lardis to
tell you about Sunside/Starside. After that I'll fill you in on
some of our history, bring you up to date on the current
situation, and how we got here, and generally try to explain
where you fit in the grand scheme of things. Oh, you'll find
it lots of fun, Jake, I can guarantee that." But despite his

guarantee. Trask's words were dry as dust; he was deadly serious, his face utterly devoid of humour.

"Oh, good" said the other, just as drily and seemingly unimpressed. "I can't wait."

"God, why him?" Trask asked under his breath, of no one in particular, as he went stamping from the tent. It was a question he would be asking himself for quite some time to come. . . .

"So why are *you* still here?" Jake asked Liz.

"Because I'm good company," she answered testily. "Or maybe I'm maintaining some kind of balance: my good and pleasant aura versus your miserable, messed-up, self-pitying—"

"—I don't pity myself," Jake cut in, scowling.

"Then have pity on me and leave it out!" she told him. And abruptly, angrily starting to her feet: "Very well, do it your way. Who needs you, anyway?"

"Wait," Jake said. "Sit down. I may need *you*—to help me with this." He waved a dismissive hand at Trask's file.

Liz took a very deep breath, but despite her annoyance she sat down, folded her arms, said nothing.

And after a while Jake said, "You know why I'm pissy, even with you?"

That "even" told Liz something at least . . . mainly that she was special, different in his perception. But she remained cool towards him and simply said, "Go on."

"Ben Trask, Goodly, Lardis," he said, "especially Lardis!— he can give you bad dreams, that one—it's as if they were all waiting for something to happen." And he thumbed himself in the chest. "To happen to me!"

"Or waiting for you to do something," she said.

"Exactly," Jake narrowed his eyes at her. "And you, too?"

"Well, and weren't we justified in that?" she countered. "I mean, we've seen one of the things you can do. The way you move . . . without moving."

"But I thought that was agreed." His frustration was mounting. "I've already told you that's not me!"

"Maybe it's *trying* to be you," she said—and at once bit her lip.

Jake nodded, and his voice was harder when he accused: "So you are in on it."

"Jake," Liz told him, "if you were to learn everything all in one go, it might be too much for you. I can understand that even if you can't. Ben Trask and the other espers, they've recognized a germ in you. But maybe it's more than a germ. Especially after last night, and again this morning with McGilchrist. Anyway, they would like it to grow; they don't want to kill it off with the shock of sudden awareness. That's why they'll let you in on it slowly, gradually. That way, when it all becomes clear to you, you'll be ready for it."

Jake looked at her and saw only truth in her eyes. Then he looked at the file again. "So reading this stuff is like Trask said: just another step in my gradual education, right?"

"I think so, yes," she answered.

"*Huh!*" And muttering darkly to himself, Jake picked up the file. It had a yellow plastic jacket with a red diagonal stripe stamped with the word COSMIC. A once-white, well-thumbed label gummed in the top right-hand corner bore a scrawled legend in india ink: VAMPIRES AND THE WAMPHYRI—BASIC.

But as Jake Cutter was about to discover, there was little or nothing basic about them. . . .

Jake had, of course, been briefed prior to last night's foray: a very sparse—even a *brief* briefing—before being "thrown in at the deep end," as he had had it. He'd seen a jerky old black and white film from a place called Perchorsk in the Ural Mountains, which at first he'd thought was a clip from some old horror movie that a sensitive twentieth century film censor had refused to pass for general viewing. It was just too graphic, too real, too horrific. And its special effects had been . . . well, something else.

But the rest of the footage (of the underground Perchorsk Complex, which was obviously real, and of an incredible, nightmarish flying creature that two USAF fighters had sent to hell over the Hudson Bay all of thirty years ago, coupled with Ben Trask's matter-of-fact, voice-over commentary) had finally served to convince Jake of its authenticity . . . well, almost. But still not quite with it, and at that time not really wanting to be, he had allowed himself to arrive at his own incorrect conclusion:

That all those years ago Soviet scientists had been breeding something—probably biologically engineered soldiers—in subterranean laboratories in the Urals, and that an unspecified number of genetically mutated monsters, not to mention several "altered" human beings, had somehow escaped . . . which even now seemed a far more acceptable explanation than the fantastic story he was beginning to piece together from the notes in Trask's file.

"WAMPHYRI," (Jake read the heading again): "The following notes result from Harry and Nathan Keogh debriefs. The Keoghs, father and son(s), were mainly responsible for the destruction of the Wamphyri. This file should be read in conjunction with 278, HARRY KEOGH, 279, NECROSCOPE, and 311, NATHAN."

And then he started on the text:

The Wamphyri are the original vampires of "myth" and legend. For the last two thousand years vampires have been periodically "banished" from their own world into ours. Prior to that time it seems possible that several of them found their own way to Earth via a "wormhole" situated in Starside, having its exit in a subterranean cave under the foothills of the *Carpatii Meridionali*, the Transylvanian Alps. This is obviously the reason why, even to this day, that region is associated with vampires and vampirism. It is the source of the so-called "myth."

But the Wamphyri are not a myth. They are the inhabitants of an Earth-*type* world lying parallel to Earth in a "universe" on "the other side" of our familiar space-time continuum; and but for the fact that the wormhole enters our world deep underground on a watercourse subject to flash flooding, it is quite feasible that by now the human race would have been conquered, converted, and enslaved by vampires.

However, and whatever *might* have been Mankind's fate, one thing is certain: there will be no more vampires in this world. The only means of entry have been closed. In 2007, the Russian premier, Gustav Turchin, diverted hydroelectric dam waters from the Urals Pass into the subterranean complex at Perchorsk, thus drowning the singularity or "Gate" in the heart of the complex. This action served to preserve the integrity of both worlds and guaranteed the future safety of at least one of them, ours. For further reading see 262, PERCHORSK, and 297, THE REFUGE.

STAGES OF VAMPIRISM—*the Vampire Life-Cycle (in large part speculative):*

In the east and west of Sunside/Starside lie swamps which are always gloomy under rolling banks of fog. In a time immemorial to Sunside's Szgany (nomadic humans), the first vampires came out of these swamps.

The morphology or evolution of the Wamphyri would make for a fascinating study in its own right. *(But we must consider any clinical, laboratory, or experimental study of* ANY PHASE *of vampires and vampirism far too dangerous.)* Cyclical, it frequently involves forms other than human. Vampire DNA is unique in being mutative within a single life-cycle without the benefit of generation. Like any disease, but almost sentiently aggressive, it invades non-vampire tissues to infect them. But instead of destroying the contaminated body it passes on its mutant DNA causing the host to adapt—and indeed to mutate—within its own span. Since longevity is invariably a result of vampirism, and barring accidental death or fatal diseases, the lifespan of the victim, then a vampire in his own right, might easily extend to many hundreds and perhaps even thousands of years.

First Phase:

In the vampire swamps of Sunside/Starside, the first (or final) phase of the cycle may be found. It is a black mushroom that ripens to give off red spores. SPECULATIVE: The spores are the genesis of vampiric life and carry the as yet "blank" form of vampire DNA. Breathed in, the spores attach to animal lungs and commence leaking their "poison" into the bloodstream along with oxygen. Then the mutation quickens, the victim falls ill, and following a period of some three days emerges as a vampire in his own right. In Transylvania, the illness would occasionally appear fatal and the victim dead. Hence the legend of the vampire rising from his grave after three days in the earth.

The spores do not discriminate; they infect who or whatever breathes them in. An infected fox or dog would have vampire instincts. But the true vampire has instincts of its own.

Second Phase (in part, speculative):
Within an infected host, certain special strands join up to take on a separate, parasitic identity. This may take a few years, decades, or even centuries; the reason for these variations are as yet undetermined. But the symbiotic creature that results is the *true* vampire: a semi-protoplasmic leech clinging to the spine of the host and extending its own nervous and sensory systems into his brain, literally possessing his mind. It is him, and he is it. And the parasite or symbiont's appetite is for blood. It feeds on the source of life itself: the blood of its host's future victims. Indeed, "the blood *is* the life."

The symbiont is not necessarily "faithful" to an original host; in Sunside, should a dog or fox host come in contact with a human being, a wholesale transfer of leech from the animal to the human is possible, especially if the animal is stricken and dying. In other words the leech will seek a continued existence—or even better, a higher life-form—in its new host. Among the Szgany of Sunside, the tenacity of the leech is a legend in its own right.

Third Phase—Wamphyri:
Not only has the symbiont become an integral part of its host's body, but the host's being—even his thought processes, his personality, and of course his DNA—have been altered forever. Just as strands of that DNA have mutated into the leech, so the host's flesh has become in itself mutative. His flesh is now metamorphic: he can within certain

limits bring about physical alterations in his shape and form. He *is* Wamphyri.

Fourth Phase—Back to the Origin (speculative):

In the event of death the symbiont leech (and even the host's "dead" flesh) may attempt a secondary existence by way of reconstitution. Essential fats and amino acids—the building blocks of life—may seek to escape into the earth, there to develop into mushroom spawn that lies dormant until a time of maximum opportunity. How the "vampire essence" or mushroom germs recognize this one opportune moment remains unknown. In Transylvanian legends as in those of Sunside, certain vampire Lords store native soil and sleep upon it—clear evidence of the instinct for survival. And once again, immemorial Sunside myths have it that the Drakuls—an especially infamous line of Lords—kept loam from Starside's swamps for the same purpose, against just such an eventuality.

Final Phase—The True Death:

Decapitated, a vampire dies. (There is no brain for the leech to control to its own ends—but the symbiont itself may still attempt to escape its host's termination). However, the bulk of a symbiont is located mainly on the left or heart side of its host's spine, and a stake driven through the heart will usually suffice to pin the creature there for a time at least. A stake soaked in garlic will certainly do the job, for garlic like silver is a quick-acting poison to vampire flesh. But the only sure way to kill a vampire is to burn it to ashes. Wherefore Sunside's Szgany stake, decapitate, *and* burn all vampire manifestations wherever possible. Only then can they be certain that the vampire has died the "True Death."

There exists one other phase in the vampire life-cycle (see "Egg-son" or "-daughter" in the next section following).

VAMPIRISM: *Infection, Deliberate and Accidental.*

By a bite. The virulence of a vampire's bite, which is usually delivered in the act of feeding, would seem to differ from vampire to vampire. But a Lord of the Wamphyri's bite is especially infectious. It can cause delirium and death, though not necessarily the True Death. When a Lord (or Lady) seeks to "recruit" a vampire thrall or servitor, the bite isn't usually deep and little blood is taken. In this case the bite has been used to transmit vampire DNA, but only in an amount sufficient to bring about the first phase of the change. It may then take years for a leech to develop and the servitor—or, later, the "lieutenant"—to "ascend" and become Wamphyri.

But when a Lord or Lady's bite is excessive and too much plasma is taken—and a commensurate amount of vampire essence transfused—then the result may be "death" of a sort, lasting the specified three days. Then, too, when the victim ascends it will be with the germ of a leech established and growing within him.

"Accidental" infection may occur when an infected animal (such as a dog, fox, or wolf), fighting to avoid entrapment and/or execution, bites a human being. In such a case it is possible for a person bitten in this manner to develop the characteristics of the original host beast. This is the proven source of the werewolf legend; it seems feasible that in Earth's past there were even ("genuine") vampire bats other than *Desmodus* and *Diphylla*.

Accidental infection may also occur when vampire blood is spilled, such as in Sunside executions of suspect vampires by the Szgany. In common with AIDS and similar contagious diseases, open wounds and mucous membranes are especially susceptible. Even healthy, whole skin splashed with a vampire's blood or urine should be treated immediately. (Oil of garlic applied with a silver scraper is the best remedy, though no guarantees may be given.)

The most definite, and definitely the most effective form of vampiric infection is obtained when a Lord or Lady wishes to create an "egg-son" or "-daughter." Apart from one rare exception (see "Mother," below) a symbiont leech is capable of producing only one cryptogenetic "egg" during its lifespan. In this the parasite relies on the judgement of its usually human host to provide a superior vessel for habitation. The egg—a flexible ciliolate spheroid half an inch in diameter—is "willed" into being by the vampire host and passed on mouth to mouth, or by sexual intercourse, or by simple spillage when it must find its own way.

A spilled egg, being protoplasmic, will seep through the skin of a designated host or other acceptable vessel, interacting with him to cause speedy infection and transformation. Any such changeling is considered to have ascended and *is* Wamphyri.

Not all exchanges of bodily fluids between vampires (the Wamphyri) and human beings are necessarily infectious. The vampire has a degree of control over his parasite, and also over his blood and other plasma fluids. A Lady of the Wamphyri may consort with a human lover without converting him. She simply avoids taking his blood, and following intercourse "wills" her vampire essence to destroy his sperm. Likewise a Lord may will his sperm free of vampiric influence to keep a concubine pristine.

This cannot in any way be taken as indicative of love or even affection; it is simply that the Wamphyri do not casually "create" other Wamphyri. Egg-and blood-sons and daughters are chosen with infinite care, and among the reasons are these:

A powerful egg-son may one day usurp the father; knowing and even accepting this, the nature of the man, the prospective host, must first be explored to the full. And egg-daughters—as all Wamphyri Ladies—are treated with great care not only by their sires but also other Lords, because while the occurrence is rare, nevertheless the occasional Lady will prove to be a "Mother" or breeder of vampires. The exception that *dis*proves the general rule, a Mother's parasite has the ability to spawn a great many more than the usual single egg.

THE NATURE OF VAMPIRES—A Possible Explanation of the Wamphyri Lifestyle:

The Wamphyri are aggressive, tenacious, territorial, egotistical, ruthless, and proceed in each mode or mood with passions exaggerated to a degree quite beyond human understanding.

It appears that the symbiont leeches are directly responsible for their hosts' invariably antagonistic natures: unless the host is made strong, the parasite cannot be certain of its own longevity. Lacking aggression the host would be seen to be weak, easy prey to his contemporaries. And without tenacity or the will to survive, he must fail. If territory exists for the taking, a vampire will take it; extending his boundaries makes a Lord safer within his own sphere of jurisdiction. And as for ruthlessness: since the driving instinct of the leech is survival, the question of law and order—and especially justice—never arises. Might is the only right. The "evil" of the Great Vampire springs naturally from all of his other vices.

As for the vampire's ego: that becomes glaringly evident in the *pride* he takes in his violence. According to Szgany legends the first of the Wamphyri was Shaitan, in our world Satan. And pride (or ego, as we understand it) was his downfall, too.

It will have been noticed that the above vices are identical with Man's, forming in the main *our* definition of "evil." In that respect it should also be pointed out that the vampire has no recognition of evil. *Regret, shame* and *guilt* are in all probability words that he does not accept, or emotions which—if experienced at all—are held in abeyance by his parasite.

As for any comparison with Man's "evil": the scale of difference—the enormity of the gap between ours and the vampire's capacity for evil—simply does not allow for comparison.

DISEASES AND VULNERABILITIES:

The Wamphyri shrug off most diseases common to man; their leeches produce antibodies to order. There is one ailment, however, whose morbid encroachment may only be delayed by the symbiont's healing powers and the host's protoplasmic DNA. Leprosy, "the bane of vampires," disfigures and kills them no less than it kills wholly human beings, but the disease's progression is usually far slower in the Wamphyri. The symbiont is itself susceptible to the disease, and once the infection breaks through a vampire's resistance and reaches the leech the process becomes irreversible and the True Death results.

Silver is a poison to the Wamphyri. The mythical "silver cross" may well turn aside or stay a vampire's hand, but not by virtue of any mysterious religious power in the cross. The silver itself is the deterrent and may not be considered a "supernatural" element in this regard but simply a poison to the Wamphyri, much as mercury, lead, and plutonium are poisons to humans. But it does more nearly compare with plutonium in this respect, as it is quite deadly when used correctly. (NOTE: In E-Branch, while the supernatural is never scorned, neither is it accepted until scientific explanations have been ruled out.)

Silver will sear the vampire's flesh. Wounded with a silver knife, the wound will take longer to heal and leave a permanent scar. Injected internally, as by a shotgun using silver shot, or a gun firing silver bullets, it will cripple and even kill. Vampire flesh damaged by silver in this way must be shed and new flesh manufactured by a protoplasmic process.

Garlic is also a poison. And once again, no supernatural reason is attached; garlic is simply poisonous to the vampire, even as various fungi, poison ivy, and many fruits and vegetables are poisonous to man. The smell of garlic, offensive to many humans, is emetic to the vampire; its oil will sting him, causing his flesh to slough; taken internally, if it does not kill him it will certainly damage organs and make it difficult for the symbiont to effect repairs. The Szgany of Sunside make extensive use of garlic, not only in their cooking but also as a poison with which to daub their crossbow bolts.

"Nevertheless—and despite the fact that silver is by no means rare and garlic is plentiful on Sunside—still the Wamphyri have been a scourge among the Szgany from time immemorial to the most recent of times.

THE SZGANY—*How They Relate to the Vampire:*

The Szgany (Travellers, Romers, or Romany) are so called because they are kept on the move by Wamphyri raiders who come nightly into Sunside to hunt. The Szgany are their prey, their livelihood, their sole means of survival and continuity. Without the Szgany there would be no Wamphyri, for the leech would never have had access to humanity and the means to rise above the intelligence level of, say, a dog or wolf.

The Szgany provide sport, women for the Lords of the Wamphyri, and men for their Ladies. Szgany blood is the staple diet of Starside's vampires; their flesh feeds vampire beasts; even their skin, bones, and hair are fashioned into furniture or decorations for the manses of their persecutors. The Szgany are to the Wamphyri of Starside as the coconut to the twentieth-century South Sea Islanders: useful in every part, with little or nothing going to waste.

But when the Szgany are no longer of use as lieutenants, concubines, or thralls, then they are drained of their blood and butchered, and all unappetizing parts ground down for "the provisioning," as meal for the flying creatures and warrior beasts of their masters.

Wamphyri ESP, And Other "Supernatural" Skills:

Most Lords and Ladies of the Wamphyri are to some extent telepathic. In addition to being physically stronger than entirely human beings (in an approximate ratio of four or more to one) their sensory skills have also been enhanced—including several "sixth" or higher senses as defined by E-Branch. It is therefore fortunate that their intelligence has *not* been enhanced; their symbionts can only make use of what native intelligence was there to begin with, and ruthlessness and deviousness must compensate for the untutored peasant mind, a lack of learning which, ironically, has come about as a direct result of centuries of Wamphyri predation.

On the other hand, in response to Wamphyri ESP—and apparently as a process of natural selection—the Szgany are adept at disguising their thoughts; mentally they are equipped to "hide" from the telepathic probes of their hunters. But the "supernatural" abilities of the Wamphyri almost always tip the balance their way, and our science is hard-pressed to find an answer to certain of the Great Vampire's skills.

Metamorphosis:
The entire life-cycle of the Wamphyri could be said to be a series of metamorphoses; a constant ongoing mutation is apparent even in the individual specimen. But in certain circumstances the vampire's *spontaneous* metamorphosis is theoretically improbable, scientifically baffling, and physically awesome. It is, too, a reality. In battle, the "normal" or "usual" morphology of a Lord of the Wamphyri (the basic structure of his anthropological form) becomes something else entirely when whatever aspect he has assumed is put aside in favour of his parasite's best protective armour and weaponry.

His flesh stretches, tears, and refashions itself; hands become talons, while jaws elongate fantastically to accommodate teeth or tusks worthy of a sabretooth or wild boar. His usually pale aspect turns grey to leaden as his skin thickens to hide; the wild, feral yellow of his eyes turns from flame to red (as in infrared perhaps?) especially at night, possibly enhancing his already incredible night-sightedness. And in the fullness of his change, the very sight of him is as a weapon in itself. The closest approximation in Man would be the rage of the berserker—*without* the berserker's disregard for his own safety. For over and above all else, survival is uppermost in the vampire's symbiont-controlled mind.

Survival: the basic instinct that quite literally lends a vampire wings. For in certain extremes many of the Wamphyri can so change their shape as to flatten their bodies, lengthen their arms, sprout webbing like the membranes of a bat or flying squirrel, and form aerofoils to support their weight or at least allow for gliding. And the most adept of all are capable of controlled flight and aerial manoeuvers. In this respect it seems reasonable to suspect that there is something of the bat about them. There are giant bats in Starside—they are often the watchdogs of the Wamphyri—and if an infected bat with a spore grown to a leech were to bite and pass on its characteristics to a man . . . ?

This theory might well account for the sensitive, convolute snout to be found in a great many Lords and Ladies of the

Wamphyri; also their night vision and of course their tendency to flight. But what theory or accident of evolution could possibly account for their mist-making? Or is this "simply" another facet of the vampire's powers of metamorphosis?

For when the Great Vampire is in danger—or conversely, when he sets out to creep up on prey or a foe—he can "create" or "call up" a mist to cover his movements. And vampire mist is not the often humid and softly lapping vapour we know but slimy and cold as a cold sweat. And the vampire Lord's enhanced senses—the normal five along with his telepathic probes—are carried in his mist like electricity in a wire but faster than the speed of light, at the speed of thought.

As for the mist itself:

It issues from the vampire's pores, as sweat issues from ours. But the process is brought about through his will. There is a theory, however fanciful, concerning the way in which the earth itself is caused to release its moisture: That the vampire mist is some kind of catalyst, as when dry ice is released over a cloud to excite precipitation. But this scarcely explains the *volume* of such mists as are generated by the Wamphyri.

For HYPNOSIS, ONEIROMANCY, AND OTHER POWERS OF THE WAMPHYRI, see also the Appended Notes to 176, E-BRANCH AND OTHER TALENTS. . . .

This brought Jake to the end of a paragraph a third of the way down a page that was two-thirds blank. Turning the page, he read: "A more comprehensive file is in preparation."

Then nothing more, except perhaps the feeling that he was floating at the centre of a weird sphere of inexplicable understanding. . . .

11
The Lidesci's Story

SILENTLY CLOSING THE FILE, JAKE STARTED AS Liz's voice reached him through the vacuum of concentration—a zone exclusive to his mind and the words that the file had left mirrored upon it—which had somehow settled about him. "Well?" she said.

And surprising himself, frowning he answered, "Where have I read this before? I mean, do I know these things?" Too late, for the vacuum was dissolving, the familiarity fading. "No, of course I don't." And shaking his head, perhaps to clear it, he looked at her.

"No questions?" she said, staring hard at him.

"Should there be?"

Liz shrugged, but not casually. "You tell me, Jake. All I can tell you is that for the last half hour you've been sitting there like a man in a dream, totally engrossed."

Learning? he wondered. *Or remembering?* But aloud he only said, "Well, a couple of questions, maybe."

"Like what?"

"Oh, one or two ambiguities. Anyway, I think I've already worked out some of the answers."

"Go on."

"Well," he said, "this file cover, for one thing. It has a few dents in it . . . it's obviously not new. In fact, it's got to be years old. As for this label on the cover, it's been thumbed to death! But these pages, I mean the paper itself, is new, and the text has at least one glaring ambiguity."

"Oh?"

He nodded. "It talks about an underground exit in the Carpathian foothills—*one* underground exit, that is. But it also mentions Gustav Turchin, and how he flooded a Gate in Perchorsk in the Urals." He frowned again and continued, "Funny, but when I was reading this stuff it seemed to make sense. I don't know, I seemed to understand. But now I only remember the text."

"Like . . . eureka!" Liz said. "That word on the tip of your tongue. That abrupt but transient flash of insight. It's there, and it's gone. Right?"

Jake knew she was fishing—albeit for something he wasn't able to give her, not yet—and said, "Weren't we talking about Gates?"

"There are two," she answered. "The one under the *Carpatii Meridionali* is the original; it occurred naturally and has been there for—well, no one knows how long. It's like a black hole, or perhaps a grey hole, and its other end comes out in Starside in a vampire world. A long time ago, warrior Lords would throw their conquered enemies into it. It's how vampires got here in the first place."

Jake accepted that; it felt real, he *knew* it was so. "And the other?"

"Is man-made," Liz told him. And settling back, she said, "This is how the story goes:

"Thirty years ago the Americans put one over on the Soviets. A *big* one, that is. And good for them—for us, the whole world—too, because since World War II the Russians had been bluffing the West right out of its pants. Kennedy was the first U.S. President to call that bluff, over Cuba. Later, Ronald Reagan and Maggie Thatcher would have their say. They just said no. Thatcher was good at that."

"Said no to what?" Jake was no historian.

"To the Russian military build-up," she answered. "To trying to keep up with all of that expenditure on ships, aircraft, bombs, the space race. And so President Reagan or his advisors invented SDI, the Space Defense Initiative."

" 'Star Wars?' " He remembered that much at least.

"Right," Liz said. "A fantasy scenario if ever there was one. And the Soviets fell for it. Now the boot was on the other foot and eventually *their* expenditure went over the top. It was probably the beginning of the end for Russian communism. But in the early eighties, while they were still financially stable, their top boffins and physicists were tasked to dream up an answer to the USA's SDI—a program that didn't exist except on paper, and very thin paper at that.

"Well, that's what Perchorsk was all about. They built a dam across a powerful watercourse in a ravine to give them the hydroelectric power they needed, also to give them some camouflage against the West's spy satellites—which was something else that didn't work—and carved out a subterranean complex from the bedrock. They put in an atomic pile to boost the project's energy requirements, and bingo, they were in business. But they very quickly went out of business.

"The idea was . . . I don't know, some kind of radar? A fan of energy raking the sky, covering all the northwestern territories of the then Soviet Union. It was an experiment, but if it had worked they'd have built more complexes just like it as 'defensive' measures against incoming missiles or bombers. Hitting that fan would be like running into a brick wall; nothing was going to be able to get through. In effect, a force-screen. Huh! Talk about an 'Iron Curtain.' And what price SDI then, eh? Except of course, there was no SDI. . . .

". . . And no force-screen, either. During the first test it backfired, the pile imploded, and a new kind of energy—or perhaps a different and extremely primal kind of energy, a different kind of heat—was discovered. And where the pile had been, right at the core of the Perchorsk Complex, there was this . . . well, this hole. This hole that went right through the wall of our universe.

"In Starside the new singularity appeared in close proximity to the original, the 'natural' one. So—"

"—So," Jake took it up, "when Turchin flooded the Perchorsk complex he drowned *both* Gates on Starside, making any sort of travel through them impossible."

She smiled at him. "For someone who hasn't read the files, you figured that out pretty quickly!" Which gave him pause, because he'd been thinking much the same thing; and again he knew that what she'd told him was so.

But Liz was already going on: "Well, there you have it, the answer to at least one of your ambiguities. Now, what about the others?"

"Just one other," Jake told her, "but a difficult one. In a way it makes no sense, while in another—in the light of our involvement—it makes too much sense. The file talks about how the Gates were closed, 'drowned' by Gustav Turchin, which 'guaranteed' Earth's safety. Similarly, it talks about Harry and Nathan Keogh, father and son, men who it credits with 'destroying' the Wamphyri. But if the world is safe and the danger past, why is all of this information laid out in present tense? Also, how can it possibly fit with what we saw and did last night?"

Liz nodded. "This is the bit you already have the answers for, right? It's self-explanatory. Well, you're correct. Those inserts in the file are brand new, hastily prepared, and incomplete. Makeshift replacements for the old text that *used to be* past tense, which is now present because—"

"Because that's the nature of the problem," Jake finished it for her. "As we saw last night, it's here and now. Not left for dead in another world's past, but alive and well and horribly real in our world's present. Fine, or not so fine, whichever—but it still doesn't answer *my* questions, doesn't tell me where *I* fit in."

Liz tossed her head. "I, I, *bloody* I!" she said. "Is that all you exist for, Jake? You?" But he could get just as irritated, and:

"No," he rasped. "I exist for something else. Something I haven't finished, that I still have to do and that all of this is pushing to one side!"

"Jake?" came a gruff query from out in the morning. "Jake Cutter? Is that you in there, huffing and puffing again?" Lardis Lidesci, his shadow falling across the tent's doorway.

"Right on cue," Liz snapped. "And very welcome. If anyone can answer your questions, Lardis can. He'll certainly be able to add to your knowledge, anyway. And if nothing else comes of it at least I'll get a break from your moaning, and find something better to do with all of the valuable time I'm currently wasting on you!"

E-Branch staff and espers were busy all around the camp, stripping personal and Branch kit and equipment from the vehicles. A lot of the "gadgetry"—the hardware in the ops vehicle—was in reality common or garden stuff, computers and communications equipment on loan from the Australian army along with the truck itself. Mobility would be the key word in any future war—the mobility of ops centres, that is, and war meaning any "conventional" war between nations, not species—and all of the WACs, the Western Alliance Countries, used compatible equipment. But the software and such belonged to E-Branch. And just as Trask's people had been thorough in cleaning up last night's mess, now they were thorough removing every last trace of their work and presence here. For as Trask had pointed out, covert organizations such as E-Branch couldn't remain secret if too many people knew about them. And in the sort of war that *he* envisaged, the Branch's secrecy would be of the utmost importance—indeed, Cosmic.

"On Sunside," Lardis said, "oh, not all that long ago, the Szgany fought the Wamphyri with whatever weapons were to hand. Here your weapons are far super—er, *superior!* And not only your guns, grenades, and flamethrowers. No, for it seems to me that you're using their own tactics against them, too."

"Eh?" Jake queried, walking beside him.

"Disguises, smokescreens, visual lies—like that vehicle there. Beer? No such thing. A deadly weapons system! Or if not a weapon itself, a system capable of directing and controlling weapons. Ben has told me that in Earth's past the vampires had a saying: longevity is synon—er, *synonymous,* yes?—with anon—er, anonym—er . . ."

"Anonymity," said Jake, and knew it for a certainty, without knowing how he knew.

"Yes!" Lardis nodded his grizzled, bandaged head. "And in E-Branch they have another saying: secrecy is synonymous—*hah!*—with survival. Pretty much the same, wouldn't you say?"

"Pretty much," said Jake. "But vampires are one thing and I'm another. And frankly, I've had it with all the secrecy. If I'm so important to the Branch, why can't I be told about it?"

"At first it was because you might be less—or other—than you seemed," Lardis told him. "Now it's because you might be more. And also because you mightn't like what you are—*if* you are. Confusing? Well, not alone for you, believe me! Anyway, regardless of what Liz says, it's not my job to tell you about you but about me and mine and the way things were, and the way they could be again by now, on Sunside/Starside."

Around the camp, goodbyes were being said, hands shaken, the Australian contingent making ready to move out. Soon there would be just the ops truck, with its array of worldwide communications devices, one jet-copter, and another on its way back from Carnarvon. The two choppers were transport for Branch personnel and SAS commanders; the ops truck would stay until they were airborne, when it too would move out. In their next location, Trask's team of espers and support staff would be on their own until their Aussie backup teams caught up with them. Thus these farewells were temporary; the same parties would soon be meeting up again, next time on the far side of the continent.

This was something that puzzled Jake. "How come we don't move as a complete unit? Trask has all the contacts; why can't he order up one of those big military transport choppers? Better still, why doesn't he just call on ahead and arrange for a new fighting force to be waiting for us?"

"He could probably do any or all of those things," Lardis answered, "but how would it look if we all arrived together at our next camp? Wouldn't you consider that indis—er, indisc—er, *indiscrete*, Jake? Remember, it's no easy thing for a man or men to hide their intentions from the Wamphyri. Any event unusual enough to arouse the interest of ordinary citizens is bound to arouse theirs, too."

"Like a sudden influx of specialist troops?" said Jake.

"Indeed," said Lardis, with a nod. "And as for starting out fresh with a brand new platoon of soldiers, doesn't that go against the very first rule? The fewer people who know about us—"

"The longer we survive," said Jake.

"*Hah!*" said Lardis. "Finally we make progress. And the problem with Mrs. Miller becomes that much clearer, too."

The first vehicles were pulling out now, and the Old Lidesci grunted his approval. "This I like," he said. "It's what the Traveller is all about: constant movement between one place and the next. On Sunside, we Szgany became Travellers to stay ahead of the Wamphyri; we rarely stood still for very long in any one place. But here? Here *we* are the hunters. We move to track *them* down, and then we kill the bastards! Oh, *yes,* I like it a lot!" He smacked his lips.

The pair had arrived at the place of last night's campfire. The back-burner, stoves, and oven were gone, but a steaming pot of coffee and a few paper cups had been left beside the trench. And as these very different men from entirely different worlds sat down on the last of the folding chairs, Jake said, "Lardis, why don't you tell me about Sunside/Starside. I mean, *all* about Sunside/Starside, or as much as I can take in. For since that's where all this seems to have started, maybe it's my best starting place, too."

And Lardis said, "As you will. But I may as well tell you now, it still won't answer your one big question."

"I had a feeling it wouldn't," Jake grunted. "But tell me anyway."

And in a low growly voice, in words that strove valiantly to accommodate Jake's language—and when they failed reverted to Lardis's native Szgany, which the listener took in as best he could—the Old Lidesci complied.

"As its name suggests, though in more senses than one, Sunside/Starside is a divided world. On Sunside, a slow and benevolent sun spins out days to more than four times the length of Earth days. But it sits low in the sky and casts long shadows—the shadows of the barrier mountains—on Starside. And the gloom and the long nights of Starside must have been the greatest of aids in the evol—er, the *evolution*, yes, of the Wamphyri.

"We don't know how it started; it happened in a time lost to memory except in myths and legends, campfire stories carried down—and altered, of course—by word of mouth. But before the Wamphyri there *was* something of a young civilization, in a world much like this world, with oceans and mountains, islands and continents, and even seasons. And its peoples were setting out to explore it just as your first sailors explored yours.

"Then, an accident. Not of Man but of nature. A white sun fell from the sky. Ben Trask will tell you it was some kind of 'singularity'—but that is science, of which I know very little. Anyway, it bounced over the world like a flat stone skipping on water, and came to rest on the barren boulder plains of Starside. But its coming was such that it ravaged the world.

"Once a benign planet, our world became a place of nightmarish ferocity. Great storms lashed from year to year, oceans stood on end, and entire races were wiped out, gone forever in the tumult of earth and fire, wind and water. The seasons were no more, while far to the north, beyond the barrier mountains, the pitiless Icelands shone dark blue under writhing auroras. It was as if a hell had descended from the sky, and a handful of Szgany survivors were its mazed denizens.

"But they weren't its only denizens. . . .

"Time passed—oh, years and centuries and even millennia—and as the planet settled down the Szgany prospered awhile. Then came the Great Vampires, the Wamphyri! Don't ask me how, or from where, for I can only shake my head. Anyway, what does it matter? However it was, they came, and made their aeries in the rearing stacks of Starside beyond the mountains, where the sunlight never fell except upon the topmost ramparts of those accursed crags.

"Legend has it that Shaitan was the first; he changed men

into vampires in Sunside, and thus left his curse upon all the tribes of the Szgany—and even upon all men—for all time to come.

"Aye, for there's that of Shaitan in all of us, and I think in all of your people, too, especially the espers, though mercifully it amounts to very little. Watered down by time and blood, we see it only in such rare talents as Ben Trask gathers to use against the forces of evil. In him it's his ability to see the truth, and therefore to recognize falseness; in Goodly it's his visions of the future, and in me it's my seer's blood, warning me of dangers whose scent is blown on the air, felt in running waters, and glimpsed in the leaping flames of fires or patterns in the dust. When all is not well, I *feel* it. And in you—

"In you it is something else. . . .

"But do not let me stray.

"The vampires prospered; they raided on Sunside for blood and plunder. And the Szgany suffered every conceivable torment. They could move from place to place during the mercifully long days, gathering their food and learning the forest ways, but at night they could only hide themselves away—and pray to their stars not to be found. And when the sun went down the vampires would come on their flyers over the barrier mountains from Starside to hunt and 'play' in Sunside's darkened woods. And everything that the Szgany are today is built out of the incredible, the despicable depredations of the Wamphyri.

"The Szgany learned to hide, not only their trembling bodies but their very thoughts. Why, eventually they even learned how to fight back! But that was a long time in the coming. And as evolution taught the Szgany its lessons of survival, so the vampire—by nature lazy—found it increasingly difficult to take his prey. And then, from time to time, vampire would turn upon vampire, and all Starside would become a battle zone.

"The wars of the Wamphyri, their bloodwars, were endless, and except where truces were called they were times of rejoicing for the Szgany clans. But gutted aeries would always need replenishing, and deplenished larders filling, and fallen flyers and broken warrior creatures refashioning in their morbid masters' vats of metamorphosis. And however long it took, the Wamphyri would return to Sunside, its pleasures and plunders.

"It was during one such war that the rest of the vampire Lords rose up against Shaitan and banished him to the Icelands. And so he was gone a thousand years and more. . . . a pity it wasn't for good. And a greater pity that he left behind the spawn of his loins and tainted blood.

"But let me get on. . . .

"Now we move to modern times. How many years are flown? I do not know, I cannot say. But I was the chief of my tribe, the Szgany Lidesci, when Harry Keogh's Earth-born son, who was known to the Szgany as The Dweller, came among us; and later Zekintha—Zek Föener, to you— and later still that fighter of fighters, Jazz Simmons, whose name I gave to my own poor son, Jason, to honour him. Jason, aye, lost to the bloodlust of vampires. . . .

"And then, finally, there was Harry himself—Harry Hell-lander, called Dwellersire—he, too, came among us.

"But Harry and his sons—The Dweller and Nathan Keogh—they moved much as you move, Jake, *between* the spaces used by common men, along a route invisible! Nathan does so still, but in Sunside, in *my* world, on the far side of space-time; or one of its far sides, anyway. Which is Trask's voice speaking, you understand. Myself? *Hah!* I can't even say where space-time is!

"Anyway, I was chief when Harry and his son fought their battle in The Dweller's garden—their grand battle with the Wamphyri—and won! I couldn't be there with them, more's the pity, couldn't stand alongside Zek, and Jazz Simmons, and the Lady Karen, too; no, for I had problems of my own and arrived too late. But I saw what they had done: how they had used the science of another world, these Hell-lands, and weird talents from . . . well, from beyond *any* lands of the living, to defeat the vampire Lords and kick their backsides into the Icelands. Even the one known as Shaithis, spawn of

Shaitan, finally broken, defeated and thrown out.

"We thought that was the end of it—most of the Szgany thought so, anyway. But I have a seer's blood in me and didn't believe that the Wamphyri were no more. It simply didn't *smell* right, it didn't *feel* right, and I couldn't settle but watched and waited and held my breath. And I would climb high into the barrier mountains from time to time, to gaze out over Starside and think on things . . . and to worry.

"And not without good reason. . . .

"One time when I went there, Harry came. But he was . . . a changed man. Don't ask my meaning; he simply wasn't the man I'd known, but I believe he was still my friend. And the Necroscope had chosen a most opportune time to return to my world, for my seer's blood had told me no lie: the Wamphyri were back in Sunside/Starside! Not only the last of them, but also the first.

"Shaitan the Unborn himself, no longer a myth or legend but a terrible reality. Shaitan—brought back from the Icelands by his descendant Shaithis—come back to batten on the Travellers as of old, like a plague that can never die . . . !"

12
The Rest of Lardis's Story

LARDIS HAD PAUSED FOR SEVERAL LONG MOments, pondering the best way to finish his tale. Finally he went on:

"This must be a lot for you to take in all at one gulp. So best, I think, to cut a long story short. And to tell the truth what's left of it saddens me. I . . . lost some good friends that time. Not least The Dweller—who I *think* was my friend—and certainly his father, Harry Keogh.

"Aye, for they were beaten in the end, cruelly put down

by Shaitan, and by his descendant, Shaithis, who had returned from the Icelands. And I was privileged—if that is the right word, but horrified might do just as well—to witness the end of it, which came as the Great Vampires celebrated their victory close to that dome of dazzling brilliance called the Hell-lands Gate: in fact the fallen white sun of legend, or Ben Trask's 'singularity,' where it sits in the lee of the mountains on Starside.

"As to what happened:

"That Harry Keogh engineered it, I have no doubt. How is a different matter. But the Wamphyri, Lords Shaitan and Shaithis, had crucified and burned the Necroscope down there by the light of the Gate, and what followed was, I am sure, his revenge. For that was ever his way: an eye for an eye. Or, on this occasion, their lives and all their creatures with them, for Harry's one invaluable life.

"It came in a flash of light, a *crack!* of doom, a fireball and mushroom cloud. It was the Voice and the Breath of Hell itself, and it blew away those vampire Lords as if they had never been. We were there—myself and a handful of my Szgany faithful—safely distanced, high in the crags watching it all happen. We *saw* it happen, yet still we could scarcely believe it.

"Ben has told me what it was. A 'tactical weapon,' he says—which I'm told means a small one of its kind—had been fired through the Gate from the underground complex at Perchorsk. And would you believe it, he pretends not to understand why I still think of your world as the Hell-lands!?

"So, we didn't know it was a weapon, and since its deadly cloud swept north we didn't suffer its effects on Sunside. But when it was all over and done the Gate shone as bright as ever, and Starside looked no different, except now beyond the Gate a softly glowing plume lay fallen on the earth, forever pointing north in the direction of the Icelands. And no matter the rainstorms and howling winds, that plume was there for many a year, only very gradually fading.

"Then for a while we blessed the Gate, because it had issued that awful Breath of Hell that destroyed the first and last of the Wamphyri. So we thought for long and long. And this time I admit that I believed it, too. For with all we had learned of the tenacity of the vampire, we had not yet learned the lessons of history.

"Shaitan and Shaithis were indeed destroyed, aye—but the *last* of the Wamphyri?

"No, not yet, and not by a long shot . . ."

Again Lardis paused, and when he continued his voice was filled with emotion, throaty with the knowledge of a great debt.

"The next time: we couldn't possibly have survived without Ben Trask, Zekintha, Chung, Goodly, and Anna Marie English. Oh, and Harry Keogh's son, Nathan, of course—called Nathan Kiklu, in my world. And called Necroscope in both worlds.

"I won't delve into it too deeply: suffice to say that the Szgany came under threat from the east, from a place beyond the Great Red Waste, called Turgosheim. A place we'd never known to exist, because those regions were unexplored. But renegade vampire Lords and a Lady—the Lady Wratha, their leader—were on the run from Lord Vormulac Unsleep and his undead army, fleeing for their monstrous lives from sins against their own kind that we may only imagine. And Lord Vormulac and his creatures in hot pursuit. Ah, but his army was a horde!

"Wratha and her renegades were whelmed under, trapped and destroyed where they took refuge in the last great aerie of the Wamphyri, which had stood empty for so many years. But Vormulac, too, had been killed, 'deposed' by the Lady Devetaki Skullguise. And now, commanding his great army, Devetaki turned her attention on Sunside. For of course she must now replenish her forces and provision the last aerie. Provision it, aye, with flesh and blood out of Sunside.

"Which was when Nathan came into his own.

"Returning out of your world, this world, to Sunside, he brought back with him Ben Trask, Chung, Goodly, and Zek: sweet Zekintha, *ah!* And other good people, and weapons from the Hell-lands, or 'Earth,' as I must learn to think of this place. And at last we could take the bloodwar back to Devetaki Skullguise on Starside!

"And we did. But Nathan: it seems he had his father's powers and then some. Or perhaps it was the talents of all of that brave band, for certainly they were all in on it at the end. It was five years ago, Jake, but I remember it like yesterday. Who could forget such a thing?

"Nathan and the others had walked into a trap at the Starside Gate. He'd been trying to send his companions safely home again, back through the Gate to Perchorsk and out of the thick of the fighting. But vampire lieutenants stood in the way, and no room for manoeuvering. Nathan and his colleagues must stand and fight. They had Earth weapons, aye, but were low on ammunition; eventually they must be taken. And if Nathan were taken, what then of Sunside? But here I'm being selfish and perhaps I should ask: what then for your Earth? For Devetaki had learned the secret of the Gate; she knew that it was the entrance to a new world, ripe for conquest.

"Now, don't ask me how it was done, for I'm a simple man. But Nathan and the others, linking hands, they pitted themselves against the Starside Gate itself. The Gate is immovable—even that incredible 'tactical weapon' that destroyed Shaithis and Shaitan had not moved it nor even marred its surface—and sitting there on the boulder plains it seemed anchored in position, perhaps by its own enormous gravity. Wherefore, in order to move the Gate, a man or men must move the world!

"And they did. With all their weird talents together, acting in unison they *willed* the Gate to move south. South towards the rising sun, which had never once shone on Starside since an age long forgotten. And the Gate—and the world—moved! The world turned, all Sunside/Starside, turning like a great wheel, and the sun rising ever faster over the barrier mountains. And the Wamphyri, their lieutenants, creatures and all were seared in a moment. . . .

* * *

"And now, surely it must be over? Why, with the turning of the world even the last aerie had fallen like a felled giant, toppling onto the boulder plains! All that remained of that great and monstrous tower was its stump, like a flat-topped mound—or perhaps one of Ben Trask's 'buttes'?—glooming on the horizon, while its vile body sprawled like a corpse, crumbling in the new-found light of Starside.

"In the far east and west, as far as men were yet to journey, the vampire swamps were drying out, cracking open in their beds, cleansed by the sun. And in all the length and breadth of Sunside/Starside, no vampires existed—at least as far as men knew. But that didn't mean that men wouldn't keep watching, not while I lived, anyway!

"Nor was the transformation confined to the swamps. Water, presumably released from the Icelands, had brought great rains to the scrubland savannas, and showers even to the furnace deserts south of Sunside's fertile belt, until the land there was green. All of which processes of an altered nature, and others, would continue a while yet—

"—But not for long enough.

"As for the Starside Gate: that was scarcely the ominous place it had been. For now it was the centre of a lake, a constantly moving body of water diverted from its source in your world, in *this* world, Jake, and driven by its own weight into Starside. And the wormholes around the Gate—or 'energy channels,' as Ben Trask calls them, which wound through solid rock to the first or 'primal Gate,' the white sun deep in the belly of the crater—they had become whirlpool sinkholes, diverting the waters of the lake a second time and returning them to the Refuge at Radujevac in this world, Earth, and on into the Danube. Thus nothing was lost, and nothing gained.

"But what a wonder! That fountain of light, reaching up a hundred feet into the Starside night, lit up by the Gate glowing in its core, and raining its soft white waters on the land and into the lake! Moreover, it had closed off both routes out of and into Sunside/Starside, which preserved the integrity of *both* worlds. . . .

"And so things stood, for one and a half of your years—Earth years, that is—and seventy of my days, for the sun rose much higher now and the days were longer yet. Well, at least in the new beginning. But it wasn't destined to stay that way.

"Man can't master nature, Jake. Or if he does his reign is short. What Nathan and the men of E-Branch had done was against nature . . . what? To move a world? And slow but sure the lure of the white sun, its strange gravity, began to turn us northwards again. The days grew shorter, the sun sank ever lower, and Starside's shadows lengthened as before. The rains retreated, seasons we had known but briefly merged into one, the savannas wilted away to their usual russets and yellows. Nightly the rim of the barrier mountains showed more stars, flowing back into position from the north, and once again the grim Northstar, which had always shone on Karenstack, rode high in the Starside sky.

"But were the Szgany dismayed? Not a bit of it! For we had *enjoyed* our permanence of climate; what need had we of seasons, when the trees were always in fruit? But with the world turned, even the foliage—the *flora*—had suffered. Too much sun in the one season, a surfeit of rains in the next, and colder air in the third.

"And now back to normal, except there was no more scourge, no more vampires, no more Wamphyri! They'd been erased forever out of our world and the Szgany could sleep easy in their beds and not fear for their lives and the blood of their loved ones. Why, we might even begin to explore those lands and territories previously forbidden to us—Starside itself, perhaps! And the great lakes or oceans that lay north of the boulder plains. And those unknown lands to east and west of the no longer 'barrier' mountains, beyond the dried-out swamps and the Great Red Waste. How perfect it all seemed!

"Grand schemes and grander dreams, eh?

"Ah, Jake, but my seer's blood told me it wouldn't be so. And I fretted while I waited . . .

* * *

"There are myths and there are legends. A myth is a story come down the ages, so changed by its retelling over and over that we may no longer say if it is true or *simply* a story. One such myth was Shaitan the Unborn—until he became reality. A legend, on the other hand, is something much closer in time. A legend is not so old that it has lost its authenticity.

"Here in your world, Jake, you have a saying: 'he's a living legend.' Do you see what I mean? A thing—usually a man or woman—that attains legendary status even in its, his, or her own lifetime. But legends are generally older than that, if not as old as myths. In Sunside, our days being so long, the Szgany use them as a measure much as you use years. And we have a legend that dates back twenty-five thousand sunups. Not as long as your history, no, but still five hundred years. Oh, yes, I have learned your numbering system. I pride myself that I've learned many things, even though I've no use for them on Sunside.

"But five hundred years ago in my world, there were three Great Vampires unlike any others before or since. And they *were* legends. Two of them were Lords (for now, the time being, let's say that they *were* Lords, past tense) and the other a so-called 'Lady.' But Vavara, believing her name potent enough in its own right, a warning enough in itself, scorned all titles and cognomens. The name itself would suffice, and she was simply Vavara. And perhaps she was right. For see, even as I speak that name—*Vavaaara*—so I shudder. *Ugh!*

"Not that she was ugly. On the contrary, she was incredibly beautiful—irresistibly so. And that was Vavara's menace: she was a beguiler, a spellbinder. It was a kind of hypnotism, Jake but by no means the same as Grahame McGilchrist's. Grahame uses a drug to enhance the authority of his eyes and voice; his is a skill as opposed to a true Power. There again, who can say? Perhaps Vavara's hypnotism was just such a skill, but one enhanced out of all proportion by her vampire leech, as all human senses are enhanced by vampirism.

"Trask's science has it that not only humans but all creatures possess lures other than the purely physical attractions of face and form. But *in* humans the voice and the eyes are especially important in defining a person's—what, charisma? *Hah!* But that is also a Szgany word for personality. Ben talks about pheromones, and chemistry and such. But all I know of chemistry is how to mix a decent gunpowder. And it's a damn hard thing to beguile a rocket, or silver shot from double barrels!

Anyway, and whatever this attraction is, Vavara had it. And again, perhaps Ben's right. For the spell she cast over men was stronger than her power over women, and usually fatal. Any man who took her fancy—whether a simple Sunsider or even on occasion a Lord of the Wamphyri—he was a goner. To resist Vavara was a wasted effort.

"So much for the witch, and now the wizards:

"The other two were Lords, as I have said. Lord Szwart was one, for he had taken his Szgany name, by which the Szgany knew him: Szwart, pronounced like the German *schwartz*, which means black. And black he was, blacker than night, black as the black heart of the leech that empowered him . . . but with what strange powers? I've said he was blacker than night: a totally inadequate description. Lord Szwart *was* the night!

"Now, all of the Wamphyri are children of the night. Certainly they are, for they cannot bear the sunlight. And because night is their element—because they are awake at night, and see and revel and hunt at night—it is like a cloak they wear, disguising them even from the most keen-sighted of men. On Sunside when vampires were abroad in the forest, the Szgany would lie still in their hiding places and watch them pass. And sometimes when they passed a clinging mist would spring out of the earth, by which you would know they were there; or perhaps the stars would blink as a shape flowed across them, but you would not see whose shape it was, just a darkness in the lesser dark. And sometimes—oh, sometimes—the mist and the shape would come close, closer, and sniff . . . *and laugh!*

"But you must excuse me, Jake, the things of which I speak are not pleasant things. I may *not* speak of them without remembering. . . .

"Anyway, Lord Szwart's command over the night was so much greater than any other's that when the sun was down he was simply invisible. He made no mists, blotted no stars, and cast no shadows. Yet he *was* seen, but only once, by a man of the Szgany—seen in a storm, in a flash of lightning— and then no more. But the man who saw him was a madman until his dying day, which wasn't long in coming. For he went into the woods to dig a hole to hide in, but never stopped digging! And when finally the pit fell in on him, he didn't cry out in his horror at being buried alive but only his lunatic joy . . . for at last he was safe, and Lord Szwart could never get him now.

"I do not know what Lord Szwart was. Only that he was Wamphyri.

"Which leaves one other, and perhaps the most dangerous of all. Lord Nephran Malinari—called Malinari the Mind, or simply The Mind—was a mentalist, a thought-thief, a mind-reader without peer. None of the stripling telepaths in Ben Trask's E-Branch today would have stood a chance against Lord Malinari in any battle of minds, nor all of them together. Let me tell you how it was with him:

"Among the Szgany, even more so than in your people, there were weird talents. My own sixth sense—my seer's blood—is but one example. But we had mentalists, too, and oneiromancers, and even men like Ian Goodly, aye, despite that their precognition was a dubious art at best. For it's as I've said, there's a trace of the Wamphyri in all men of Sunside; their taint lingers on, and I fancy it has carried over even into this world. But Malinari . . . was special. His *evil* was special! Why, among the Wamphyri themselves, Lord Nephran Malinari had no friends. But don't let me mislead you, Jake: it's not that the Wamphyri were given to forming lasting relationships. They weren't, but some of them did form alliances; well, occasionally. But rarely with Malinari the Mind. How may a man trust, or remain on good terms, with a creature who knows his every thought, who is one step ahead of his every move? The Wamphyri are devious, secretive . . . but how to keep secrets from such as Malinari?

"Let him but touch a man, a mere touch of the fingertips, and it was as though the other's thoughts flowed like water— or like blood?—out of their owner and into the mind of Malinari. Ah, a vampire with a difference: he slaked two kinds of thirst, the one for blood and the other for knowledge! No idle curiosity, Jake, but the lust for knowledge itself. And once a thing was learned, Nephran Malinari never forgot it.

"But of course in Sunside/Starside, just as in this world, there were those who could not be read. Be it strength of will, or simply their nature, there was a wall in their minds no ordinary mentalist could ever breach. Ah, but Lord Malinari was no ordinary mentalist. I have said his touch opened the way. So it did, like opening a dam in a pent river. But if the soft brush of fingertips would not suffice . . . there was another way.

"Fingertips . . . and the incredible strength of the Wamphyri . . . Trask says it's their metamorphism that allows them to punch stiffened fingers into a man's chest to nip his heart. I think so, too, for it certainly wasn't brute force with Malinari. His fingers were fluid, like liquid, allowing the exploration of a man's inner ear, or the sockets behind his eyes, or the brain itself. And whenever The Mind stole a man's thoughts out of his very brain . . . then he left nothing behind. No, not even the will to live. . . .

"We're almost done. What will remain is not for me to tell but for Ben himself—in his own time, that is.

"Just one more thing. I spoke of Vavara, Lord Szwart, and Malinari the Mind in the past tense. For that's how I heard of them, around campfires when I was a boy, as part of Sunside's legends. The final part of the legend had it that four hundred years ago the rest of Starside's Lords and Ladies got together to be rid of them, and it took all of their strength and their fighting forces together to do it, to banish them into the Icelands.

"But five years ago—when Nathan and Ben Trask's espers turned Sunside/Starside towards the sun—it appears that some of the ice melted. And if Vavara, Szwart, and Nephran Malinari were locked in the ice, waiting out the long cold years . . . ?

"That's Ben Trask's explanation, anyway.

"And now we're done, for that's all I know of it, all I'm willing to say for now . . . except for one final thing that I'm certain you've worked out for yourself: the fact that they are *back*, Jake. All three of those monsters, they're back.

"And that is the nature of Ben's mission. It's what he and his espers are pledged to do. For once again there are vampires on the loose—

"—And no longer confined to Sunside/Starside!"

13
Trask's Story

WHEN JAKE LOOKED UP HE WAS ALONE. Perhaps he'd been asleep by the end of Lardis's story, but he didn't think so. It had gone in, all of it, and perhaps a lot more than Lardis had actually said. Weird, but that's how it had felt during the telling: as if Jake had been there on Sunside/Starside; as if he had known all or most of these things—the sights and sounds and smells of Lardis's world—and had only needed the old Gypsy's corroboration.

But that was during the telling, and now it was all receding; the scenes that Lardis had painted so inadequately, which Jake's own mind had coloured, and into which he'd inserted the finishing touches, were just words instead of feelings, sensations . . . emotions? And all that was left was a legend in its own right. Half of a legend, anyway.

"You didn't tell me everything. . . ." Jake accused, before he fully realized that he was alone. Then, looking all around and feeling foolish, he stood up, tossed aside the dregs of coffee gone cold in his cup, stretched the stiffness out of his limbs. It would be good to get some real sleep sometime.

Suddenly the silence, the emptiness, the loneliness of the place had become oppressive, weighing on him . . . until he spied movement in the clump of pale, stumpy trees between himself and the big ops truck. It was Ben Trask, dappled grey and green and gold in the partial shade of the trees, heading his way.

"Jake?" Trask called ahead. He wasn't shouting, but in the clear morning air—the silence of the near-deserted camp-site—sound carried a long way. And drawing closer, Trask asked, "Did I hear you talking to someone?"

"Talking to myself," Jake answered, rubbing at the stubble on his chin. "Or maybe to one of your ghosts—Lardis? That old man has this strange effect on me. He doesn't just tell a story but takes me with him! Says his piece and leaves me there, then vanishes."

"Sunside/Starside?"

Jake nodded. "But he left a lot out."

"He was told to," Trask said. "But that's okay . . . you can have the rest of it from me. Most of it, anyway. And if there's stuff *I* leave out, you'll just have to believe me that there's a good reason. Let's go to the ops truck. It's going to get hot out here in the next hour or so, by which time the chopper will be back and we can get on our way. Meanwhile, the ops truck has air-conditioning."

As they walked back towards the articulated vehicle, Jake said, "The stuff Lardis left out, I mean apart from the tech-nical stuff, or 'science,' as he calls it, was mainly to do with people. Harry Keogh, of course, the mysterious Necroscope? But also his sons: The Dweller and Nathan. *Huh!* I learned more about Vavara, Malinari, and Szwart than about these human figures."

Trask looked at him but said nothing, and so Jake went on: "That term, Necroscope. It comes up time and time again.

173

Now I know what a telescope is. *Tele* is from the Greek, right? Far, as in far away? Likewise *micro* in microscope, which obviously means very small. But Necroscope? An instrument for seeing corpses?"

"Something like that," Trask told him.

"And that makes sense to you?"

"And to you, eventually," Trask answered. "I hope."

Jake shook his head. "So it's your belief that this Harry Keogh, this Necroscope who sees dead folks, is in my head? Now, I know I've tried asking this before, but what the hell *is* this guy? Some kind of telepath?"

Trask nodded. "He was that, too, towards the end."

"Was?" Jake frowned. "Towards the end?" Then he snapped his fingers. "Oh, yes, and that's the other thing. Lardis mentioned a bomb—a nuke?—that came through the Gate into Starside. And I somehow got the impression that Harry and The Dweller?—that they were there at the time."

They were approaching the steps at the rear of the big ops vehicle. Trask paused in his striding to take Jake's arm. "They *were* there," he said, his voice hoarse now. "And before you ask me: no, Harry didn't escape."

"What?" Jake said.

Trask climbed the steps and made to enter, then turned and looked back. "Harry Keogh, Necroscope—the original Necroscope—is dead and gone, Jake," he said. "In one way an incredible waste, and in another a merciful release, and probably a blessing, too."

"Dead?" Jake said, and was suddenly cold in the full glare of the sun. "Then how can—"

"Harry's gone," Trask cut him short. "He's just another one of E-Branch's ghosts. But dead and gone or alive and living in you, he has never been more important to us than he is right now. . . ."

Inside the vehicle's ops section, the duty officer and the precog Ian Goodly were seated within the central control area. Liz was standing outside the desk, her elbows on its no longer cluttered surface, her chin cupped in her hands. Apart from minimum services—the permanent telephone array, one small radio crackling with static, and a dimly luminescent wall screen—ops had been more or less unplugged and decommissioned, however temporarily.

The muted conversation tailed off awkwardly as Trask and Jake entered, but the Head of E-Branch held up a hand and said, "It's okay, I want all of you to stay. I have to speak to Jake, and I can't see any reason to leave anyone out. Ian, if I slip up and forget some important detail, you'll be here to correct me. And Liz, there may be the odd tidbit of information that's new to you, too."

He hitched himself up onto the desk, and Jake let down one of the wall seats and sat opposite. Then without further pause, Trask told his part of the story.

"Jake, Lardis Lidesci has told you something about his world, a parallel world called Sunside/Starside by its inhabitants. He's told you about Vavara, Szwart, and Malinari, too. So by now you know that these aren't just legendary or mythical figures but a very real threat to everyone in *our* world. They're here, biding their time, hiding out somewhere on Earth. Now please take that for granted and *believe* that it's so, for last night was a mere lesson—a primer, a single leaf—out of the great textbook of the enormous threat posed by the Wamphyri.

"So let's deal with it step by step. How they got here has to be the first question, that's obvious.

"Five years ago the Gate in Perchorsk was closed. That was in large part Gustav Turchin's doing, for which our thanks. But Turchin is only one man, and Russia is a big place; the expansionist element hasn't gone away; there are still plenty of powerful people in the former USSR who hanker after the 'good old days' when their satellite subordinates paid tribute to Mother Russia. So while communism may have been wounded, its scars are quickly healing and the scene is set for a resurgence. The Russians are rather well known for their capacity for the odd revolution now and then, and their armed forces are now political factors in their own right. Well, the fact is they always have been, but never more so than now.

"In E-Branch we all remember how Turkur Tzonov, then head of the Opposition—our term for the USSR's answer to E-Branch—planned to take his partly nationalistic but mainly egomaniac schemes, along with a dedicated, crack military unit, into Sunside/Starside to conquer it for Russia. But Turchin had his own ideas about Tzonov's real motives, and so did we. Sunside/Starside is rich in gold, far richer than the Yukon's Klondike in its heyday. And it's not some kind of localized motherlode: gold is common in the vampire world, it can be found literally anywhere. Working with Turchin, we tried to keep that a secret, too, for obvious reasons. Or maybe they're not so obvious, so I'd better clarify:

"Russia is broke. Her army, navy, and air force are destitute, or so close it makes no difference. They can't even afford to decommission their clapped-out nuclear submarines and leaking missiles but have to dump them in someone else's backyard! But Russia's generals, her admirals and air-marshals are still very powerful. When that lunatic Turkur Tzonov went into Starside to get himself killed, he left many of his men behind, trapped in Perchorsk by Gustav Turchin's security forces. Tzonov had promised his men gold, and we all know what gold does to men. Gold *is* power, power corrupts, and ultimate power . . . ?

"So then, Sunside/Starside was literally one big gold mine, and the only sure access was through Perchorsk in Russia's Ural Mountains. Oh, it was blocked, flooded, that's true. But if you can turn a tap on, you can also turn it off.

"Okay, the rest of this can't be guaranteed as pure fact, but we're E-Branch and we do what we do, and we're not usually very far wrong. We keep our eyes and our ears—oh, and a lot of other equipment—open, and try to keep up to date. And we also have what Nathan Keogh told us. So it's a patchwork quilt of sorts, but pretty accurate, we think. . . .

"Where was I? Oh, yes: the Perchorsk Gate was closed, but somebody wanted it open. Enter Russian Internal Security, a militarized, updated KGB lookalike headed by General

Mikhail Suvorov. They stepped in and did just that: diverted the Perchorsk dam waters back into the ravine and let the Gate drain the complex dry. Then they had to decide who was going to explore Sunside/Starside, though 'exploit' might be a better word for it. But in any case, it didn't quite come to that.

"More than eighteen months had passed since Turchin closed the Gate, since when he'd had a hard time fighting off Suvorov, who of course wanted it opened up because he had heard rumours about the gold. And Suvorov eventually won the fight, because Turchin was over a barrel. Russia was in the red and Suvorov—who was *very* Red—had the answer: a huge gold mine in a primitive world at the other end of an interdimensional tunnel whose only accessible entrance lay deep in the earth and deeper still inside Mother Russia.

"Thus Turchin had very little choice: he could step aside and let Suvorov get on with what he'd promised would be a 'limited' exploration, or Suvorov would tell all the hungry Russian people about the unlimited wealth that their premier was striving to deny them. Well, we all know what that would have meant. . . . Only think back on the Klondike and you'll see what I mean. Everyone would want a piece of the action. And remember, Gustav Turchin knew something about the horrors of the vampire world—knew as much if not more than we do about what happened at Perchorsk in its early days. Certainly he realized that the fewer people who entered the Gate, the smaller the odds they'd bring something back with them out of Starside. Something other than gold, that is. . . .

"And in all that time—some eighteen months—we'd had no word from Nathan Keogh, who of course had made his home in Sunside. But how could we have heard from him, since the Gates had been closed? Ah, but Nathan had his own route to Earth, through the Möbius Continuum! That's the place where you go, Jake—er, between going places?—it's the darkness between leaving one place and arriving at the next.

"Okay, I know that's not good enough, but more later.

"Anyway, Nathan probably had his own reasons for breaking contact with us, but it wasn't as if we felt let down; indeed, without him we'd have been in a hell of a mess, 'we' being our entire world. It's bad enough that we have three of these monsters here, but without Nathan we'd have had an army. Come to think of it, Ian and I wouldn't even be here right now to talk about these things, and none of you would be here to hear what I'm saying. Oh, you would probably still *be* here—somewhere in the world—but not the way you are now. And damn few other people, not as you know them.

"Very well, Nathan's reasons for breaking contact:

"In turning his world and working out a means of preserving its integrity—for it had been Nathan's idea to flood Perchorsk, not the Russian premier's; Turchin was acting mainly on Nathan's suggestion—he'd also secured a measure of isolation for Sunside/Starside. Maybe he thought that if he left us alone we would leave him and his alone. He knew how far ahead we were technologically speaking . . . I don't know, perhaps he preferred to keep his people out of the rat race? Also, he wouldn't have forgotten that there were some people who would continue to see his world as a threat despite all precautions, and he knew they had the means to destroy it. And finally . . . there was all that gold, useless to the Travellers except as a maleable metal, but valuable beyond measure on Earth. An irresistible lure for the Helllanders?—meaning you, me, us—probably.

"Well, enough of that . . . he simply didn't contact us for whatever reasons. And during that same period of time Nathan's world was swinging back again, the shadows lengthening on Starside, and the sun settling back into its old, accustomed orbit. And far beyond the boulder plains, under the flutter and weave of strange auroras, a lot of the northern ice had melted.

"Enter Szwart, Vavara, and Nephran Malinari. The only possible explanation is that they had been locked in the ice—or they had locked *themselves* in the ice, preserving themselves in suspended animation—when they'd been thrown out of Starside. Wamphyri, they could do it; they *must* have done it, deep-frozen themselves, a handful of thralls, and however many flying creatures they'd required to bear them into the Icelands when they were banished from the aeries of the Wamphyri. The natural, or unnatural, tenacity of the vampire.

"And meanwhile, here on this world, our world, we weren't even aware that Mikhail Suvorov and a party of scientists, geologists, and prospectors—not to mention a platoon of heavily armed Russian soldiers—had entered Starside through the Gate in Perchorsk. Perhaps Turchin had been warned not to inform us; I like to think so. Or maybe he didn't want to, for that would have been to admit his own impotence in the matter. And he must have been just as ignorant as we were of the return of the Wamphyri. No way he could have known they were back in Starside.

"Nathan knew, though, and so did Lardis Lidesci. They knew because of the new spate of raids on Sunside. Ah, but this time the Wamphyri didn't have it all their own way, not by any means. Nathan had equipped his people with some devastating Earth-type weaponry, and because of his knowledge of our technology, Traveller 'science' was likewise leaping ahead. So that as quickly as Vavara and Lords Szwart and Malinari were recruiting, building up their vampire forces in the hollow stumps of the fallen aeries of the Wamphyri, Nathan and his Traveller fighting men were cutting them down to size again. But while this resulted in some kind of stalemate, still Szgany lives were being lost, especially in the farthest corners of Sunside, in tribal territories that lay far beyond the Lidesci sphere of influence.

"Despite Nathan's ESP, those amazing powers that he'd inherited from his father, he couldn't possibly be everywhere at once. And even in Sunside/Starside, charity begins at home. Of course his main concern was for the Szgany Lidesci, and he had his work cut out protecting them. Part of that work, which was of the utmost importance to Nathan, was to get the Old Lidesci and his wife, Lissa, safely out of there. For it's a fact that Lardis *is* an old man now—older than his years—as a direct result of living most of his life in the shadow of the Wamphyri. In his youth, life on Sunside was no bowl of cherries. Now Nathan would take over from him . . . just as soon as he'd taken him out of harm's way.

"So let Lardis complain all he wanted—and I'm told he complained quite a bit—Nathan gave him no choice but simply brought him and his wife to the supposed safety of our world. That's how he got here, and why Lissa is in the care of our people in London. Nathan would have protected his own wife, Misha, in the same way, but Misha wasn't having it. She'd lost him twice before; if Nathan was going to be fighting the Wamphyri yet again, she was going to be at his side. It's the same story for our own Anna Marie English: Anna had married a Traveller called Andrei Romani, and made a life for herself caring for orphans of the bloodwars. She wasn't going to leave Andrei or the children behind without one hell of a fight. And so she stayed.

"Very well, but just weeks before Nathan, er, *transported* Lardis and Lissa to Earth, there was a curious lull in vampire attacks on Sunside. When they started up again, the three principal survivors of four or five hundred years of frozen banishment were no longer in command of their lieutenants, thralls, and warrior creatures—or rather, they no longer accompanied them in their raids on Sunside. In order to find out what was happening, Nathan and his Szgany fighting men trapped a lieutenant, bound him to a cross with silver wire, and offered him the usual choice: he could talk and die a clean death with a crossbow bolt in his heart, or he could say nothing and be lowered facedown, undead and kicking, into a fire pit. He talked, died quickly, and *then* burned. There is no other way for a vampire.

"As for what he said:

"Vavara and the others had intercepted strangers entering Starside from the Gate on the boulder plains. There was a short, unequal battle—very short, for Suvorov's troops weren't prepared for this; but then, who would have been?—and Lord Malinari was now 'questioning' the handful of survivors before they were sent to the provisioning . . . that is, before they were used and drained by lieutenants and thralls, and their corpses turned to fodder for the beasts. For of course, following Malinari's kind of interrogation, they wouldn't be very much good for anything else . . ."

Apparently stalled by something in his story, Trask had paused. His face was drawn and grey now, his eyes sunken; he looked far "older than his years," much as he'd described the Old Lidesci.

The precog Ian Goodly knew what was wrong, and said, "Ben, I'll take it from here if you like."

"No," Trask husked. "When Jake was under pressure, he told his own story. So it's only right I tell mine. Hell, I've lived with it for almost three years now. . . ." But still he took a few seconds to straighten out his thoughts. Then:

"Call it coincidence," he continued, "or maybe synchronicity, but Nathan arrived at E-Branch, in Harry's room, yes, just a little too late. He had Lardis and Lissa with him, and a list of stuff he wanted to take back with him. But it was the middle of the night and there was only a skeleton staff; and I . . . was already on my way in, driving like hell through the empty, cold night streets. God only knows how many red lights I'd crashed.

"Why was I in such a hurry? Because of a dream—a bloody nightmare—a feeling that something was wrong. No, it was much more than just a feeling: the *sure knowledge* that something was definitely wrong. My espers: how often had I heard it from them that their talents were a curse? Mine, too, I supposed, when I had to sit and listen to rapists, pedophiles, and murderers trying to talk their way out of jail, sit there reading their lies and *knowing* that in fact they were cold-blooded killers, molesters, and defilers. But not once, until that night, had I really considered my talent a curse. And I can well understand how you felt, Ian, seeing the future in a dream, but not knowing it was *more* than a dream!

"For that's how it had been with me: just a dream, but oh so much more than a dream. And I . . . it had been 'a hard day at the office' . . . I'd just lain there, tossing and turning, reading the *truth* of the damned thing but unable to wake up, until she told me to. *God . . . !*" And again he paused.

But this time, before Goodly could speak up again: "It was Zek, my wife!" Trask blurted it out. "She was at the Refuge in Romania, where for a fortnight the outflow from the underground river had been almost at a standstill. The regular crew at Radujevac couldn't understand it, but since it coincided with low winter rainfall patterns right across Europe, that's what they put it down to.

"Anyway, that's not why she was there. Zek is—she was—a telepath of the highest order. But she was more than that. No one who ever met her could fail to be impressed by my beautiful Zek. Harry Keogh himself, Jazz Simmons, Lardis Lidesci . . . even the Lady Karen, they'd all been won over by Zek. And those poor Romanian kids at the Refuge, some grown into men now, but still suffering from deep psychological traumas dating back to Ceaucescu's time; of course she must try to help them. She could get inside their minds, track down their problems, even try to cancel them out. Sometimes it worked, other times she cried.

"And she was crying in my dream, crying out to me, to her husband, who knew he was only nightmaring yet at the same time knew he wasn't, but in any case couldn't do a damn thing about it. And despite what was happening to her, or about to happen, Zek was getting through to me in the only way left to her.

"It wasn't the first time. Once before she'd contacted me telepathically. That was in May, 2006, when she was with Nathan in the Mediterranean, more specifically the Ionian. They'd gone to Zante—or Zakynthos, the island of Zek's birth, from which she'd taken her name—so that she could, well, pay her respects to Jazz Simmons who was buried there. Jazz had been Zek's first husband . . . he was dead of natural causes. But Turkur Tzonov's people were tracking Nathan to kill him. And since Zek was with him they'd kill her, too. It was while they were trying to kill her that she'd contacted me, and for a moment I had experienced all that she was feeling. I had known what it was like to die. But she hadn't died, because that's when Nathan discovered the Möbius Continuum and used it to bring her back to E-Branch.

"In my nightmare, it was the same again, Zek in her—God, her extreme of terror!—knowing it was over, yet trying to get through to me, to let me know what was happening. In one way it was a cry for help, which she must have known I couldn't possibly answer, and in another it was this incredibly brave woman, passing on everything she knew about, about . . .

"It came thick and fast; telepathy is like that, conveying a lot more than mere words. What's that old saw about a picture being worth a thousand words? Well it's true enough; I saw half of it in pictures and half in thoughts, mind to mind. All of it while I tossed and turned and—damn my dreams forever—while I slept on!

"One of the Refuge's maintenance men, a New Zealander called Bruce Trennier, was down in the sump—the subterranean river's exit or resurgence—examining the system of hydroelectric barriers and the turbine that powered the Refuge during the Romanian rainy season. His being down there was partly in connection with the fall-off in the outflow, and partly because his instrumentation indicated that something wasn't right down there. The system hadn't been entirely reliable since the time when CMI—Combined Military Intelligence, disbanded now, thank goodness—made their biggest ever mistake and blew it up!

"Anyway, Trennier was in contact by landline with the Refuge's night staff, and he'd told them he was opening a dry inspection duct to go into the actual cave of the resurgence. He'd thought that perhaps something was clogging the works in there. And something was—a dead vampire lieutenant, his body rammed into the pipe that monitored the flow!

"Obviously Vavara, Szwart, and Malinari had been trying to get someone's attention, and they'd succeeded. And Trennier had provided them with a way out.

"Well, the rest is sheer conjecture. I'm trying to remember

all of this from a dream after all, and it's a dream I've tried so hard to forget! And even at the time it was fragmentary, as dreams usually are; and Zek, my Zek . . . she wasn't at her best. But who would be in her . . . in her situation?"

Once again Trask fell silent, choking on his own emotions. In a little while, when Liz quietly inquired if she should make coffee, he simply nodded. Then for a time no one said anything, not even Jake. . . .

14
Zek's Passing

IT WAS SEVERAL MINUTES BEFORE TRASK could continue, but eventually: "Let me try to tell it the way I saw or received it," he said. "It was night at the Refuge, two hours ahead of our time in London. Zek had been awakened by her pager, a call from one of the two-man night nursing staff. Bruce Trennier was already down in the sump; whatever the trouble was, he'd said it couldn't wait. The forecast said heavy rain, and the resurgence was prone to flash-flooding. If there was a blockage, the pressure could create all kinds of fresh problems down there.

"Which was why he had gone down at night, with a tool box, a powerful torch, and an ancient, battery-powered landline telephone that was probably on the blink, because contact was weak and intermittent. But even before Zek got to the duty room, she sensed that something was wrong. Not with Trennier, you understand—for she didn't even know about him—but just generally wrong. Zek was a very strong telepath, as I've said, and there was . . . what? A presence? A probing in the psychic ether? Some kind of interference? Whatever, something wasn't right with the 'static'—the term used by telepaths to define the background hiss and babble of thoughts emitted by the people around them—and it was something she'd never experienced before.

"Now, in E-Branch we have rules: we don't use our talents on each other, ever. Myself, I have an excuse: my thing's automatic, as was Darcy Clarke's before me. Darcy wasn't in charge of what he did—in fact he didn't *do* anything— his thing simply took care of him. He was a deflector, the opposite of accident prone, as if some kind of guardian angel was constantly on duty looking after him. Darcy could have crossed a minefield in snowshoes without getting hurt, except his talent wouldn't have let him. But don't think it made him careless. On the contrary, he used to switch off the power before he'd even change a light bulb. Or maybe that was just another form of his talent in action.

"My thing is the same: if someone lies to me I can't help but know it. It's not that I want to, not every time, it's just something that happens. But a telepath has a choice: to tune in on the thoughts of others or simply ignore them. And most telepaths can turn the static down or even switch it off. Which is just as well, or they'd never get any sleep.

"So in E-Branch we don't mess with each other. Let's face it, it has to be the easiest way to lose friends. If your partner is in a bad mood, you really don't want to know that you're pissing him off just by being in the same room.

"But Zek . . . she was the same with everyone. At work— in the foreign embassies, or working criminal cases—she was the best. Outside of work, she switched off; she wasn't interested in the many perverse little thoughts that are flying around out there. And it was the same at the Refuge. She had enough on her plate just working with those poor sick kids, let alone probing the minds of her colleagues. And incidentally, she was the only esper out there. It's quite some time since E-Branch maintained any real presence in Radujevac.

"I mention these things so you'll see why she didn't immediately switch on to the truth of what was going on. Zek didn't use her talent as a matter of course, only where it was needed. And as for Trennier being down in the sump: she didn't find out about that until she'd reached the duty room. And even then she wasn't much bothered. Not at first.

"For that wasn't the reason she'd been woken up; no, that was because, being E-Branch, she was the senior officer in situ at that time. And any problem with the kids, the senior officer had to be informed. That's what it was, the kids. And as far as Zek was concerned—half-awake and all—that's all it was. But they were really going to town. Or rather, they weren't. That's what was wrong with the static: not that its flow had been interrupted, but that it just wasn't there. It was as if . . . as if the kids had all come awake at the same time and were *listening* to something. But listening *intently,* to the exclusion of everything else. And whatever it was they could hear . . . they didn't much like it.

"That was why they were using their pagers, every last one of them; also why the duty room's switchboard was lit up like a Christmas tree, and why Zek had been woken up and called in for her opinion.

"But she didn't get to voice that opinion, for as she entered the duty room and saw the switchboard, two things happened simultaneously. One: she reached out with her mind—to one of the kids, a case she'd been working with and knew intimately—and two, the old-fashioned landline telephone jangled and went on jangling. Of course it was Trennier, but a damned insistent Trennier.

"First the kid, a Romanian orphan of maybe eighteen years. Zek broke into his mind . . .

". . . And someone was there! Not just the kid, but someone, some*thing* else. Something incredibly intelligent, that crawled and observed and was thirsty for knowledge, something that felt like cold slime, and left a cold, cold void behind it. And when Zek's talent touched it, she 'felt' a recoil, and then a question—'*Who?*'—as whatever it was tried to fasten on her, too.

"Then she was out of there, snatching her thoughts back as if they'd contacted a live wire, closing them down and erecting her mental barriers as things began to make sense.

"By which time one of the duty nurses was answering

Trennier's call. This was a male nurse, one whom Zek knew to be solid as a rock; but as he listened to Trennier's hysterical babbling over that tinny old telephone wire, so his eyes widened and his mouth fell open.

"Zek took the phone from him, told him to go and see what was wrong with the kids. The other nurse had already left, and now she was on her own—well, except for the terrified voice of Bruce Trennier, reaching up to her from the sump.

"He told her about the body in the monitor pipe, said that it had been shoved, or *crushed,* all the way in, almost its full length. But despite the awesome force that must have been exerted to cram it in there headfirst—because the pipe was only eighteen inches in diameter, and the male figure was . . . *big*—there was still some kind of horrible life in it; the feet kept twitching! And that wasn't the worst of it. Who or whatever had done this awful thing was still down there. Trennier had heard something, and he'd seen movement in the inky darkness between him and the open duct!

"And now Zek knew beyond a doubt what was happening here. She didn't want to believe it, but she knew anyway. In the eye of her mind, suddenly she could see the whole story: something had happened to stop the water flowing from Perchorsk, and the Starside Gate was open again. It was the only possible explanation. The children were feeling the influence of whatever Trennier was experiencing, and the 'darkness' between him and his only escape route had to be, could only be—

"—Wamphyri! How didn't matter, but they were back. Back in our world this time, and Bruce Trennier was down there with them. And the kids . . . their vulnerable minds had been discovered and explored by more powerful minds, or one more powerful mind at least. Sensing it as mice sense a cat, the orphans had reacted—not without justification. Knowing the Wamphyri, Zek knew that their thoughts were terrible things—knew also that the cat was already bunching its muscles, preparing to spring.

"Her mind must have flown every which way. Her re-

187

sponsibilities to the Refuge, the children, E-Branch . . . even to me, God damn it! The fact that out of the Refuge's double handful of staff she was the only one who knew anything about the Wamphyri. And the sure knowledge that if they broke into the Refuge, into Romania, the world, then that the nightmare would be on us all over again. All of these things galvanizing Zek into activity. But the right or wrong activity— who could say? She only knew she must do something.

"And how to tell Trennier, still hysterical on the phone, that he was already as good as dead or changed forever, so perhaps he'd care to volunteer his own life for the sake of everyone else's? For Zek knew something about the Refuge that no one else, not even the New Zealander, the engineer, knew: that some years ago E-Branch had installed the last of several failsafes, and down there in the sump there was a way to close this end of the loop for good.

"Powerful explosive charges in the ceiling of the cavern: a blast sufficient to bring down the roof of the place and permanently seal it. And we would have done it long since but the Gates were closed and the Wamphyri gone, and we needed the turbine to power the Refuge.

"There were two switches that had to be thrown, one inside the sump to arm the charges, and the other outside the reinforced concrete barrier that sealed the resurgence and channelled its waters; the exterior switch triggered the thing, obviously. But also, as a sensible safety precaution, there was a fifteen minute delay after both switches had been thrown. And last but not least by way of safety, both hatches had to be locked from the outside—in fact they could *only* be locked from the outside—before the electrical circuit could complete itself.

"Zek calmed Trennier down as best she could, gave him directions to the switchbox, told him to throw the switch and get out of there (*if* he was able), but she kept that last reservation to herself. For there was no time, no way she could begin to explain her fears about the Wamphyri. Not that the New Zealander would have understood; he was in too much of a funk. And who wouldn't be, trapped in the dark with the Utterly Unknown? At least Zek had given him something to go on, instructions of a sort.

"Then she hit the alarms, woke the staff, told them to take the kids and move out—all of this taking very little time and none of it making too much sense to anyone except Zek, who didn't have time to explain.

"And in that chaos of blaring alarms, puzzled, sleepy staff colliding with each other, and scared kids awake and crying in their rooms, the rest of it was up to Zek. Now she had to make her way to the basement, set the trigger, and wait at the open hatch for the engineer to come through—and hope that it was *only* the engineer who came through—before she closed the hatch and locked it, completing the connection that would blow the sump and whatever else it contained to hell.

"But if it wasn't the New Zealander who came through, what then? My God! What a *nightmare!*

"And now maybe you'll forgive me that I've tried to forget all this, all the panic and sweaty horror of it as Zek, my Zek, rushed to the basement levels, climbed down into the now silent engine room, and made her way down a spiralling steel staircase into the belly of the Refuge, to the reinforced concrete floor whose underside was the man-made ceiling in the natural cavern of the resurgence. In normal circumstances that floor would be trembling to the throb of pressured water, but the water was a trickle now and the place no longer vibrated.

"There in that cellar-like room, which now seemed vaguely threatening, a pair of cyclindrical turrets stood up knee-high from the floor. The carbon steel hatch of one of them had been laid back on massive hinges, revealing a dark throat that was more threatening yet. But looking around and seeing a niche in the wall, and a shelf bearing an extension telephone handset, Zek believed she knew how to approach this thing.

"First and foremost there was the hatch: it must be closed, and immediately. If Trennier was on his way out . . . he would go through hell when he found the hatch locked. But there was nothing else for it, and it was only a temporary measure. And trying not to think of the New Zealander's terrible situation, Zek wasted no time but closed the hatch, locked its wheel, then ran to the open end of the cavern, where concrete steps took her down to the ancient bed of the resurgence.

"From there she climbed rusting iron rungs to a place high in the wall of the cavern, where a deep crevice housed the trigger's waterproof switch. It was stiff—probably a little rusty—but she managed to throw it anyway, then rapidly retraced her route back to the empty, echoing basement.

"By now Zek was feeling shaky; the combination of fear and frantic physical activity had almost exhausted her, but at last the stage was set. By now, too, Trennier should be battering on the closed hatch . . . but wasn't. And if by now he'd thrown that switch, he only had eight to ten minutes to get out of there.

"Zek had an automatic pistol. Ever since being attacked on Zante, she'd been in the habit of carrying a gun; I don't think I need mention what kind of ammunition she used. Now, preparing her weapon, she stuck it in her waistband and took up the dusty telephone from its shelf in the wall niche. Neglected, its battery was dead, but its generator handle twirled readily enough. In a moment she had Trennier on the other end of the line.

"The New Zealander was still in a state—even worse than before—and he hadn't done what Zek required of him. Oh, he'd found the switch in its secret place, but he hadn't thrown it. Trennier wasn't a stupid man. An engineer, he'd taken one look at that switch and known that the sump was rigged for destruction. Knowing Zek, however, he was pretty sure that wasn't going to happen while he was in there, but still he wasn't taking any chances. And in a panting whisper, he demanded to know what was going on, what it was all about, and what it was that was keeping him silent but observant company down there? Something was watching him, he felt sure.

"She couldn't tell him, could only tell him once again to

throw the switch and get back to one of the ducts—either one, it made no difference—and climb out of there. As long as they stayed in contact, she would know it was him and no other; she wouldn't shoot him as he emerged.

"But telling him that was a mistake. *No other?* What other or others was Zek going on about? What did she know that Trennier didn't? Others that needed shooting? Others that were capable of stuffing a big man into an eighteen-inch pipe? What in hell *were* the murdering things down there in the dark with him, in the sump? But no, she needn't bother to tell him. And *fuck* the switch! He'd be going back to the duct right now—and up through the hatch—and God help anyone or thing that got in his way!

"Zek yelled into the phone then, screamed into it to get his attention, and finally she got it; but she knew she had to be hard on him. It was the only way. And so she told him about the hatches, how they were closed and she wasn't going to open one until she was sure he had thrown that switch! Oh, Zek knew she would let him out anyway, however it went, but she daren't let him see that.

"And so he did it, threw the switch; and Zek knew he had, because she'd reached out to him with her telepathy and 'seen' him do it! And now there was just fifteen minutes to go. . . .

"But in reaching out to Trennier, she had opened her mind—and it wasn't only his thoughts that came through the breach. Then, however briefly, she found herself listening to something else, the *Thing* that had terrified the children. It was a fleeting experience, momentary, but all the same it chilled her mind like a blast out of some frozen hell:

" '*Ahhh, see! Now he makes a move. Now he flees this place, and in so doing shows us the way out . . .*' That much and no more, before Zek closed her mind again. But more than enough, surely? Panicked, Bruce Trennier was on his way . . . and how many of the Wamphyri were following on behind him?

"But it also showed a degree of uncertainty on their part— showed that they weren't entirely sure of what they were up against in this world—for they hadn't simply taken Trennier and *made* him show them the way out. What would that cold Thing have learned, for example, from the damaged minds of the Refuge's children? Nothing, except perhaps something of the caring warmth and attention of the Refuge's staff. But that in itself might have been seen as a weakness, for on Starside such children wouldn't have been spared. Mentally, and frequently physically unfit, their only use would be as fodder for the beasts. Even on Sunside the Szgany would have thought twice before accepting such burdens, especially under threat from the Wamphyri. What could such children be, except an enormous hindrance? Yet here they were cared for? It spoke volumes for the inhabitants of Earth, but mainly that they were soft, riddled with unnecessary guilt, self-doubt, and pity for their society's underdogs. In Starside underdogs were eaten.

"What Zek didn't know, of course, was that Vavara and the others had already seen something of Earth's awesome firepower. At the Starside Gate, they'd clashed with General Mikhail Suvorov's men: an unequal battle, yes, but at the time they'd been an army. Now there were just the three of them, plus a handful of lieutenants. Not only that, but Malinari also knew that at least one of this world's inhabitants was a powerful telepath. While she wasn't of his order (but then again, who was?) still she was proof that the Hell-lands weren't entirely defenseless.

"The minutes ticked by, and Zek was on tenterhooks. Five minutes, six, seven. Even if she returned to the dry bed of the resurgence and climbed up to the crevice with the switch, still she couldn't reverse the process now. The clock was ticking and nothing could stop it, and the only way to delay it would be to open one of the hatches, a temporary measure and definitely the most dangerous of all.

"The basement was lit by half-a-dozen naked light bulbs in the ceiling. Since these were powered by a small emergency generator, their light was less than reliable. Through all of what she had been doing, Zek had worked in the flicker of these weak light sources, all the while conscious of the

Refuge's foghorn alarms, their muted blare carrying down to her through concrete floors and steel stairwells. Yet in a way the sound had comforted her, and even the flickering lights had reminded her of the world above, its relative sanity.

"Now it seemed someone was intent on denying her even these small comforts. For suddenly the alarms ceased, and at the same time the lights burned low, held for a moment, and went out. It could only be that up there in the chaos of the Refuge, someone had turned the alarms off. Whoever it was, he had inadvertently hit the basement light switch, too.

"And now there were only a few minutes left before the sump erupted in death and destruction. Zek couldn't even be sure that she herself was safe there in the basement, let alone Bruce Trennier in the sump. And she was tempted to reach out to him yet again and see what progress he'd made. She would have done so—but that was when the telephone jangled.

"Mercifully she'd thought to take a small torch down there with her. Three paces took her to the niche with the telephone, and in another moment she was asking: 'Bruce . . . are you alright? Where on earth are you?'

" 'At the foot of the duct,' he answered, and his voice was one long shudder. 'I've been dodging . . . God, *things!* I catch them in my torch beam, and they just sort of melt aside! But I can feel them there in the darkness. One of them . . . it doesn't seem to have a shape! It collapses in my torch beam, flows, reforms. And Zek—God, Zek—*they make my flesh creep!'*

" 'Bruce, come up,' she told him. 'But as quick as you can, and I'll let you out.'

"And then another slow minute until she heard him banging on the hatch that she'd closed. A moment to spin the wheel, her heart hammering and breath coming in panting gasps; the silence absolute, the darkness, too, except where her torch beam sliced into it. She hauled on the hatch, and he pushed from below, and in that last moment she thought to reach out to him, touch him with her mind. And she did—

"—But *his* mind was a blinding white agony, and his single thought was a scream that shrank even as it pierced her, gradually disappearing into the distance of mental oblivion. And as it ran and ran, with nowhere to hide, still it echoed her name: '*Zek!—Ah, Zek!—Zekkk!—Zekkkk!—Ah, Zek-k-k-k-k!*' Until it was gone. Then:

"Zek's strength was as furious as her fear as she tried to slam the heavy lid on Trennier. For in fact it *was* the New Zealander—his head and shoulders—emerging from the hatch. But it wasn't his mind that drove him; it wasn't his muscles propelling him up out of the darkness, for pain had robbed him of consciousness and all its attendant skills. Try to picture it. His body rising up, loose arms flopping up over the rim, blind eyes staring, back ramrod straight. The engineer was like some grotesque puppet . . . he *was* a grotesque puppet!

"For someone had an arm up inside him, at full stretch, and that someone's hand was gripping his spine from inside, holding him upright! A glove-puppet, yes, as he folded in the middle to topple out of the turret, and another's head and shoulders came into view. But such an Other!

"Zek's legs were rubber, her hand, too, where she forced it to reach for the gun in her waistband. She was stumbling backwards, away from this scene of uttermost horror, yet every move she made was in some kind of dreadful slow-motion. And the figure in the hatch wrenching its crimson arm from Trennier's body . . . blood flying, splashing Zek's face in a red slap . . . yellow eyes burning on her, seeming to burn *into* her, their cores blazing scarlet in a moment. They were like the holes in a Halloween mask, those eyes, but they were alive!

"He—*it*—came out of the hatch in one flowing movement, while another figure rose up behind him; all of this happening in a surreal slow-motion that was simply a trick of Zek's mind. For in fact it was very fast, and in her extreme of numb, gnawing terror, almost too fast to follow.

"She snapped out of it, put her hands together, aimed with the torch and the gun both. But even as she pulled the trigger, that bloodied arm swept the gun aside, sent it flying, and the torch, too. And a cold wet hand caught at her wrists, trapping both of them in its icy grip. . . ."

Trask had paused. His eyes were staring, unblinking. Gaunt and grey, he seemed to have collapsed down into himself a little.

When a crackle of static sounded from the radio, the duty officer gave a start. But then a tinny voice was heard, reporting the jet-copter's progress. "Bird One to base . . . ETA twenty to twenty-five minutes, over."

"Roger, out," said the D.O. into his handset. That served to bring Trask out of it, and:

"I suppose I'd better finish it," he said. And in a little while, lacklustre and robotic, but inured now, he carried on.

"Understand, this wasn't my dream—not all of it—though I'm sure that parts of it were. What I've told you so far is my . . . my *reconstruction* of the so-called 'Radujevac incident,' as I've pictured it time and time over in my mind's eye, and in my current nightmares. It's built out of details that Nathan Keogh gave us, out of . . . God, *evidence* . . . that we found at the Refuge, and lastly out of Zek's telepathic contact with me, while I lay tossing and turning during her final moments.

"Her final moments, yes . . .

"For that was when she knew it was over, when that bastard thing Malinari trapped her wrists, gripped them in his freezing cold hand, and smiled his dreadful smile at her. Smiled at Zek, inclined his head, and began reading her like a book. But every page as he absorbed it was torn out, discarded, went fluttering into oblivion. And knowing it was over, that was when she contacted me. Once before she'd done it, when she'd thought she was dying. But this time she was dying.

"In my nightmare I saw his face. Handsome, yes, but a vacant sort of beauty, superficial, cosmetic. Lord Malinari looked as he willed himself to look, young but not too young, dark but not too dark, thirsty and . . . and no way to hide it. Greedy for knowledge, and the power it would bring. Zek's knowledge, which she wasn't going to give him without a fight.

"At first she didn't look at him, could only stare at poor Trennier, sprawled on the floor in his own blood, his face alternating between glaring white and shadow, white and shadow, as her torch rocked to a standstill close by. At his bulging eyes, his gaping mouth. Poor Trennier, raped and dead. But—

" 'Ah, no,' said Malinari the Mind, in a voice like bubbles bursting on a pool of oil. 'Not dead but undead, or soon to be. He knows things—of metals, machines, and engines—and I would know them, too. But you . . . the things that *you* know are of far greater interest. Moreover, I see that I am not the first of my kind that you have known.'

"Zek could feel her knowledge slipping from her—slithering out of her and into him, like a greasy rope in a tug-o'-war—and she fed her thoughts to me that much faster. But Malinari would not be denied; he read her telepathic messages, too, interpreting them as best he might. As for her knowledge:

"It was as if Zek's past, her memories, her *understanding* of the world . . . as if it were all iron-filings, and Malinari's mind a vast magnet drawing them out of her. But she fought—oh how she fought—so that what came to me was of the moment, not of the past, as she allowed me to see how it was, and explained in a kaleidoscope of telepathic scenes how it had been for her, and how it would be for the world if I didn't receive her warning.

"But she knew that it couldn't go on—couldn't be allowed to go on—for he was taking too much, and if she let him he'd get it all. About me, E-Branch, our espers, their talents; Malinari would get it all, if she let him.

"By now the others were up out of the sump: Vavara, incredibly beautiful in Zek's mind, lit by her own radiance, alluring so as to further weaken Zek by her presence. And I saw her, but I'll spare you any description because I know that *any* description would be false. For the beauty of a vampire Lady is *literally* skin deep. Let me just say this: most women—young women, especially those of great beauty—would hate her; they would be irresistibly attracted to her, but they'd hate her. And even the most blasé man, a man drained by his excesses, sated to his full measure, would lust after Vavara.

"And finally Lord Szwart. A darkness . . . a flowing, oozing something . . . a shape without a shape . . . the ultimate in metamorphism . . . scorning any fixed form for the constant, ongoing, unceasing mutation of protoplasm which was his existence. A fly-the-light, but more so than any other Great Vampire: the closest comparison we could make would be Nathan Keogh's description of Eygor Killglance of Madmanse in Turgosheim, in a vampire world. But where Eygor was made of flesh and bone—albeit the flesh and bones of others—Szwart was of a far more elemental material. And most of it was darkness.

"Vavara, seeing Zek drawn up against Nephran Malinari, and jealous of any naturally attractive woman, said, 'Take what you will and finish it.' Her voice was beautiful as her lying form, as ugly as her words. And Szwart's was a hiss of air driven out through temporary lungs specifically created, as on the spur of the moment, to enable speech:

" 'Aye, get done with it. There are young ones up above . . . sweet meat for the taaaking . . . and a world entire to conquer.' But:

" 'No, ah no,' said Malinari, and moved his slender hand to lift Zek's chin. 'She fights me with a will of iron, and I desire what's in there.' And to Zek—and through her to me—'Do you know, the eyes are the windows of the soul? It's true, Zekintha. But to these fingers of mine, they are also the doorways to the mind. And I weary of this and would have it quickly.' He held up two fingers before her, aiming them at her, only inches from her eyes.

"Zek knew what he would do; but seeing his fingers vibrating, pulsing with purple veins, elongating and reaching towards her, she also knew what *she* must do. She volunteered a picture, thrust it at him, showed him the doom she'd planned for him and the others and seared it into his probing mind. Oh, she lied—described a devastation far greater than the truth, that would come ripping through the floor in rivers of fire and tortured concrete, threatening him even here— and perhaps Lord Malinari suspected it was a lie. But the way Zek's eyes were locked on that open hatch, out of which the last of three lieutenants was even now appearing, he couldn't take the chance.

" 'What?' he said, furious where he drew back a pace. 'And was this for me, for us?' Then he gathered her up, carried her to the hatch, and without pause . . . without pause . . .

"Headfirst she fell, down and down, and as Nephran Malinari slammed and locked the hatch, the time was up.

"That was when I woke up, drenched and shivering, hot yet cold, with Zek's last words still ringing in my mind.

" 'Goodbye, Ben,' she said. 'I love you.'

"And then a blinding white light, which I prayed was only the dazzle of my bedside lamp as my trembling fingers switched it on. That's what I prayed it was—

"—But it wasn't."

15
Charnel House

IT WAS PLAIN THAT TRASK COULDN'T GO ON, SO while he sat there shaking his head in a kind of numb disbelief, still seeking a reason for, or perhaps a solution to, his irreparable trauma, the precog Ian Goodly took over. In contrast to Trask's harsh, grating rasp, his voice was almost melodious:

"It was a period of unrest among the old USSR's satellite countries," he began, "one of many since the death of European communism. The former Yugoslavia, Bulgaria, Romania, they were all in a state of political turmoil, and

Radujevac stood at the crossroads, as it were, of all three nations. The Refuge was a kind of Sovereign Base Area—a British enclave, if you like—on foreign soil. But despite that, and as a result of its work, it was greatly respected and had achieved an almost diplomatic status. Of course, the British government had safe houses, embassies and the like, in all the former satellites. But because of the unrest access was always difficult, even to the Refuge.

"Well, Nathan Keogh arrived at our London HQ that night, and he was in the process of explaining what was happening in Sunside/Starside when Ben got there. At first Ben was overjoyed, even relieved to see him. Maybe this was what had sparked his dream; perhaps in some way he had anticipated this renewed contact with a friend from the once-hostile environment of the vampire world. But as Nathan's story unfolded, Ben's awareness—his sense of dread, of foreboding—returned in short order. It was one of those times that come to all esp-endowed persons, when out of the blue they're made aware of the other side, the downside of their talents. And now more than ever Ben's talent was telling him that Zek's telepathic message had been no mere nightmare. . . ."

As the precog paused, Trask levered himself off the desk, stood up straight, and closed his eyes. He breathed in until his lungs couldn't take any more, then made for the door. And no one said anything until he had made an unsteady exit.

Covering for his superior—though in fact Trask needed no such excuse—Goodly said, "Did you hear the chopper?" (No one had.) "Ben will want to see it safely down, and maybe . . . maybe talk to the pilot?" He offered a shrug which was followed by an awkward silence, until Jake said:

"Ian?" It was the first time he'd used Goodly's first name. "Will you finish it?"

Goodly looked mildly surprised as he answered, "Of course. All of this is for you, after all. But in any case there's not much more to tell.

"We had radio and telephone links to the Refuge," the precog went on. "Well, we *should* have had, but not that night. We tried but couldn't get through. And because of what Nathan had told us, we feared the worst. But Ben—denying, or even defying his own talent—he had to know for sure, of course. Several means were to hand.

"We called in our espers, everyone who was available, and put them to work. But long before the first of them arrived at the HQ, Nathan was volunteering his services. He'd been to the Refuge before and its coordinates were locked in his mind. But if Ben was right and the Wamphyri had come through the subterranean Gate—and if they were still there—what then?

"For Ben, the next hour was an endless anxiety attack; he sweated and agonized over danger-fraught decisions and equally painful but inescapable truths. Having faith in his talent, he knew it was already too late—but it was *Zek* who was there at the Refuge! And Nathan: he would have gone at the snap of Ben's fingers—indeed, he was the only one who could go, along that special route of his. And in fact we had to restrain him, order him not to. And Ben weighing all of this in his tormented mind, all the time knowing in his heart that it was too late, that it had *been* too late from the moment he'd started awake in a cold sweat at his home in Kensington.

"Then Millicent Cleary arrived; Milly is—*now* she is—the very best of our telepaths. And right on her heels our locator of long standing, David Chung. I'll never forget the scene in the ops room that night: Chung standing before the illuminated wall-map with the tip of his index finger touching the location of Radujevac, and his left hand holding Milly's. We frequently work in tandem that way. And after only a second or so, their reactions:

"How David snatched himself back, away from the wall. And how Milly snatched back her hand from his! For the locator had sensed something—something at Radujevac, at the Refuge—and she had picked it right out of his mind: the clammy feel of it, its evil taint. Mindsmog!

"Milly had hoped to contact Zek; firm friends and colleagues, they knew each other's minds. But now, there was simply no trace of Zek's telepathic aura, no indication of life. Hers was a 'flatline' on the monitor of telepathic awareness. And as for the overwhelming presence of mindsmog: it couldn't be denied or mistaken, and Ben's worst fears were corroborated.

"Of course, the Necroscope had his own way of looking into matters of that sort, but . . . no need to go into that here.

"Well, just like last night, I blamed myself. Why hadn't I seen it coming? What good is a talent that only reveals itself when it wants to? Why is the future so *bloody* devious? I blamed myself that I hadn't foreseen it, while Ben was in hell for *having* seen it! And the rest of the team, they were depressed that they'd had to confirm it. While at the Refuge, the mindsmog was rapidly dispersing. . . .

"After that, there was no holding Nathan. His father, Harry Keogh, had owed Zek favours. And Nathan himself was in her debt . . . not only was she a friend, one who had fought alongside him in Starside, but she'd even been involved with his discovery of the Möbius Continuum. No less than Ben, Nathan knew he wouldn't rest until he—until they—were sure. Not sure that Zek was dead, for all of us knew that by then, but sure that she would never be undead.

"And so we armed ourselves, and Nathan took us to the Refuge. But a refuge no longer, for now it was a charnel house. . . .

"Ben, myself, Chung, and Lardis—*huh!* Try keeping the Old Lidesci out of it; he'd loved Zek dearly—Nathan took us along the Möbius Route to Radujevac. It was some two hours, maybe two and a half, since Ben came awake from his nightmare. More than enough time for the . . . the *slaughter* of the staff and children. From what we saw, twenty minutes had been enough!

"Those poor kids, and the people who had looked after them; their torn, sometimes shrivelled bodies were already cold. They had been dead before Ben had driven his car even halfway in to the HQ. And I believe that seeing that for himself—that knowing there was nothing he could have done—was the only thing that kept him sane.

"There were no survivors. Thirty-six kids and eight staff, dead or . . . or disappeared. Gone from us, anyway. For you see, we knew only too well that the ones who weren't there . . . that they weren't survivors, either. And certainly they'd have been better off dead. For they were now undead, or if not now, then soon. There was no other explanation for their absence; unless they had simply been taken as food, for later. But if that was the case, why only adults, when the children had been murdered out of hand and left behind? Anyway:

"The missing staff, three of them—or rather two of them, since last night—were Denise Karalambos, a pediatrician from Athens, Andre Corner, a psychiatric specialist from London, and . . . and someone who isn't any longer a problem: Bruce Trennier, the engineer. As for why they were singled out, there are theories but we can't be sure. Trennier, as we've seen, found favour as a lieutenant. Perhaps the others are similarly situated. But anyone who feels sorry for them can forget it. They'd be better off dead—they're *going to be* better off dead. At least, that has to be our point of view. Not to mention our intention.

"But about Zek—and excuse me if I seem offhanded; it's simply that I find it best to be cold about certain things, for I'm sure my emotions would be just as fragile as anyone else's if I were to forget myself and let them hold sway— Zek hadn't suffered. When that blast hit the sump, she hadn't felt a thing. Down in the basement, everything was askew. The reinforced concrete floor had buckled upwards; the turrets had been blown off their bases like popping a pair of corks; the cave of the resurgence . . . simply wasn't there any more. The walls and roof were completely caved in, and it's a wonder that the rear end of the Refuge hadn't followed suit.

"The Wamphyri and their lieutenants must have felt it, too: that awesome blast. Indeed, any creature in that basement— any creature of normal flesh and blood—would have been stunned by the concussion or even killed by the shock of it.

But then, the Wamphyri aren't human, and in all probability it only served to enrage them further. Certainly they raged through the Refuge.

"The only good thing to come of it all, as far as I could tell, was that one of those bloody awful Gates was now well and truly closed. Oh, the Gate itself was still there, miles up the underground river, under the Carpathian foothills, but its single exit was finally blocked by two thousand tons of fractured concrete slabs and God only knows how much solid rock.

"So much for that, but what about the three creatures who had come through and were already in our world? What about them and their lieutenants, and now a trio of new thralls to aid and advise them in their Earthly ventures? And three very intelligent thralls, at that, who knew the ways of Earth?

"That, we believe, is the main reason why those three were spared . . . or cursed, depending on how you see it: because they could add to Malinari's intelligence of this new and potentially dangerous world. And we also see something of his cunning—and of his ruthlessness, too—in the murder of the innocents. It was simply a matter of leaving no one behind to speak about what they had witnessed.

"For you see, only six of the victims appeared to have . . . to have been *used*. And where they had been fairly well drained, the rest of them were just dead. But horribly dead. For most of them it had been instantaneous: stiffened fingers with nails as hard and as sharp as chisels had chopped through their backs or into their chests, to break their spines or crush their hearts. The terrible strength of the Wamphyri! But others . . . we don't think some of the others had it so, well, so 'easy.'

"I said that certain corpses were shrivelled. But 'shrivelled' doesn't say it all by any means. Lardis, when he saw those bodies, said it was Szwart's work. It wasn't simply a reduction of bodily fluids but of . . . I don't know, of the substance, the essence—the soul?—of the victims. The destruction of whatever it is that makes a person human, giving him shape, character, humanity, for Christ's sake! These pitiful things, they no longer had any of that. Picture the last apple on the tree, all wrinkled and dried out by the sun, all fallen in, with the last of its juices fermented and sick inside it. When it falls or if you touch it, its skin splits, and deep in its core the pulp is rotten and black. That's what they were like. . . .

"And there were others whose eyes were open, staring, quite empty, and for all that they were dead I couldn't help but feel that they hadn't known very much about it. Their bodies weren't shrivelled like those of Szwart's victims, no, but it seemed to me that their minds had been. And Lardis told us Malinari would have been responsible for that.

"As for the female victims: their pale dead faces were full of awe, amazement . . . rapture? Some kind of exquisite, delicious agony? It's true that I don't have the words for it, but I might have a name: Vavara.

"Well, enough. There are *no* words that can say how we felt. Appalled doesn't nearly cover it. And nothing we could do about it, not then, not immediately. What, we should alert the authorities, shout it to the world, initiate total panic and put the fear of God and all the devils of hell into every mortal human being on the entire planet . . . *if* we were believed? We couldn't do any of those things, and for obvious reasons. Can't you just picture the witchhunts? God, but we'd be back in the Dark Ages! Witch-pricking and human bonfires, and licences to torture and kill handed out willy-nilly, free to anyone with a grudge.

"Medical research would stop, stop dead—or undead! The laboratories would search for cures, of course they would, and spread the thing faster than a plague. Blood donors? You think we're short of blood now? Blood would become the most precious of commodities, and keeping it the first priority. People locked in their homes, making them impregnable fortresses, defending them with guns, silver, stakes, crossbows and whatever. And the filthy rich with their private armies, making the odd, eccentric hermit of, say, Howard Hughes's meager stature seem like a high-profile socialite by comparison.

"Borders. In the last fifteen to twenty years we've seen them open up. Britain has been cagey about controls, passports and such, thank God—but Europe? Can't you just imagine the panic, see the chaos as all the old rules and statutes were reinstated, the checkpoints rushed back into being, with armed guards at ports and airports, and not forgetting the reservoirs, farms, fisheries, and . . . and *anywhere* where food is processed? And how long before countries started blaming each other?

"When the shit—excuse me, the accusations—started flying, Russia and Romania would probably take the brunt of it, if only because the Gates are on their territory. But what about the U.K., Great Britain? We've known about the Gates for thirty-odd years! Or am I just talking about 'we,' the team, the organization—E-Branch itself, for God's sake—and our involvement? As for our Minister Responsible, the 'Invisible Man' at the top: *huh!* But haven't we all heard about this—er, how does it go?—this 'culpable deniability,' or some such gobbledygook? 'Damage limitation,' and the like? Does anyone care to guess what those things really mean? They're just ways of carrying on lying to cover up unpalatable truths that weren't told the first time around, that's all. And folks, what *that* boils down to is, *we* would get crucified! The end of E-Branch . . . and who would look after the shop then?

"And that's not the end of it. Hell, I've barely started! Sooner or later the world would find out that the Russians had actually *made* the Gate at Perchorsk, an experiment that didn't work out. And the same world would demand that they destroy it. Too damned late, of course, but destroy it anyway. Oh, really? What, with Mikhail Suvorov's henchmen in Moscow still waiting for it to pay off? They should shut down a potential goldmine just because the gold-greedy West couldn't stand the competition? And can't you just see the old Iron Curtain slamming shut again, and that old red flag flying as before?

"Oh, they might get the message eventually—when nights turned to nightmares—and then they'd destroy it quick enough. But how? As they were ready to do it the last time around, with nukes? For just like the rest of us the Soviets have made 'progress' in the last quarter-century, and I really don't care to speculate about what they might do now . . . but I will, if only to make the point and get this over and done with:

"Nuclear, biological, and chemical weapons; missiles with multiple warheads, launched through the Gate at Perchorsk. The total devastation of a world—Nathan's world—and Nathan and all his people, all the Szgany, with it. Neutron bombs, yes, so that all life would die but the gold would still be there, with no one and nothing to deny its plundering, its massive, planetwide *tomb*-looting! Which is fine, or not, except we don't even know if neutron radiation will kill the Wamphyri. Only that it will kill everything else.

"And meanwhile the vampires would be raging on this world. Because if we killed a couple of thralls, the Lords would make more. Survival, people: the damned survival of the damned! And how long before total embargoes—in effect sieges—were laid on entire islands, nations, continents, as the terror overtook them one by one? And how long then before the missiles and the neutron bombs were flying again, this time on our world? We've had 'final solutions' before, but there are holocausts and holocausts.

"I mentioned the Dark Ages, but I think we could probably be sent back, oh, a couple of centuries earlier than that. . . .

". . . So you see, we couldn't tell anyone. It was our baby, and we'd just have to handle it ourselves. But . . . if we handled it our way—E-Branch's way, the right way—then we might have a chance. And in fact, there were several clues that indeed we had a chance.

"It was a question of thinking it all through, then using our combined talents to check on our conclusions. Very well, so why had Vavara, Szwart, and Malinari left Starside to come venturing in our world? Where were the benefits for them? What was wrong with Sunside that they'd left it to their lieutenants and burgeoning vampire army in favour of Earth?

"But they were known on Sunside, indeed they were figures from legend there, and the Szgany knew how to fight them; fight them with alien weapons and the incredible skills of the Necroscope, Nathan Keogh. Also, *these* vampires were ambitious beyond the bloodiest dreams of almost any other Lords or Ladies of the Wamphyri before them. Perhaps the world of Sunside/Starside was too limiting in its scope. But Earth . . .

"They'd learned of Earth from Mikhail Suvorov and his ill-fated team of explorer-prospectors. They *knew* us: that without our weapons we were softer far than the Szgany of Sunside. And there were millions, indeed billions of us, spread out in many different nations across a world that was as wide as its horizons. Not merely a single strip of habitable woodlands between barrier mountains and burning deserts, but a huge and thriving termite's nest of sprawling humanity! A land of milk and honey—and blood, of course—stretching out forever.

"Better far, we didn't believe in vampires! In our world a vampire was a fiction, a creature in a book, a myth out of our superstitious past. Even in Romania, Hungary, or the Greek Islands, you'd have trouble finding more than a handful who *truly* believe in vampires today. In E-Branch, however, we have known for a long time that they never were a myth, that indeed there were vampires in our world once before and maybe more than once.

"And Zek, she knew it, too, and knew it better than most. She had actually lived in the Lady Karen's aerie on Starside! So perhaps the mentalist Lord Malinari took something from her after all, the fact that earlier invaders had learned an important lesson: in *this* world longevity is synonymous with anonymity. But having faced—or having sent their thralls to face—Mikhail Suvorov's firepower on Starside, maybe they'd known that before they set out.

"There's evidence of that last, too. Suvorov's party went through from Perchorsk, emerging into Starside through the surface Gate. But the Wamphyri chose the other route, the original or natural Gate into our world, probably because they knew that Perchorsk was once again a semi-military base and defended, and all of its weapons concentrated in one spot, the Perchorsk Gate itself. Hardly a good place to commence a covert infiltration!

"But the best evidence that Malinari and the others intended to keep their presence secret, at least for the time being, lay with those poor dead kids and murdered staff. For they had *not* been vampirized! No vampire essence—nothing of that sort—had been allowed to get into them. So plainly it wasn't the intention of the Wamphyri to start a plague. Not yet, anyway.

"But people *had* been killed, murdered by vampires, and the Old Lidesci wouldn't be satisfied until the bodies were burned. While he had found no trace of infection in them—not even in the six who'd been used, drained—still he was insistent. And since no one in this world has Lardis's experience in such matters, the experience of so many years, no one argued the point.

"What was more, the . . . the *cremation* that Lardis insisted upon fitted perfectly with a plan we were shaping, however gradually. For not only were we unable to bring the presence of the Wamphyri into the open, but we must actually disguise it, cover it up, *assist* them in their efforts to remain secret! Secret to the world in general, at least, but not to us, not to E-Branch. No, for we *knew* our enemy of old.

"There was fuel oil, plenty of it, at the Refuge. Ben saw to it that the entire contents of a fifty gallon drum went down the wrecked inspection ducts, then we punctured the rest of the drums and let the fuel leak through all the ground floor rooms. And finally we stood off while Nathan struck a match. That one match was all it took.

"It could only be the act of a maniac or group of maniacs, some kind of crazed sect. Or perhaps sabotage, the work of some anti-British terrorist organization. Or maybe a band of utterly ruthless criminals, determined to cover up their crime. At any rate, that was how it would look. . . .

"Well, Romanian rescue services are notoriously slow, and where the Refuge stood across the Danube from Radujevac . . . it wasn't the most populated or accessible region. The Danube itself was the most frequented route through the countryside. Fortunately for us there were no landing stages, wharves, or docks on the Romanian side, and the nearest fire engine was all of a hundred miles away!

"So we watched the Refuge burn, and eventually Nathan took us home again. But back in London we took our time before calling the authorities in Belgrade, Sofia, Bucharest, to tell them we'd had an SOS, a Mayday, from the Refuge, that a gang of raiders was sacking the place. It took them a couple of days to get back to us with their condolences; their security forces would do all they could to bring the unknown marauders to justice, of course, but since the Refuge had been gutted there was precious little to go on. . . .

"And meanwhile, we were busy. *I* was busy, bending all my efforts to scan the future as never before. But . . . the simple fact is I can't force what I do, can't control it. I see what I see when I see it, and that's it. And our locators were busy, none more so than David Chung. But where to look? There was no more mindsmog, and there were no borders in continental Europe. The three invaders, their lieutenants out of Starside and their 'raw' recruits, they could be anywhere. They could have crossed the river west into Yugoslavia, gone east into Bulgaria, headed north into the Carpathians, or caught a boat upriver for Hungary. In daylight hours they'd go to earth, or to any dark, safe place. But at night . . . no one travels as fast as the Wamphyri.

"Nathan suggested returning to Sunside for Anna Marie English, but to what purpose? The invaders were leaving no 'blight' behind them. As yet, they weren't vampirising anyone. Murders? But there are always murders, and there are always missing persons. No, we couldn't hope to track them that way. In any case, Anna Marie wouldn't have come back; she had dedicated her life to the orphans of the bloodwars, and to her man in Sunside.

"The mindsmog thing puzzled us a while: the lack of it.

For where there are vampires, and especially Lords of the Wamphyri, there is usually mindsmog: a tainted, impenetrable cloud on the psychic aether . . . unless that was something else that Malinari had stolen from Zek's mind? But of course it was! He had also been about to learn something of E-Branch from her—until she had deliberately shortened his interrogation by showing him his intended doom, which had precipitated and mercifully shortened her own.

"But just how *much* did he know? How much had he sapped from Zek's mind, her memory, her knowledge in general and especially of the Branch? We had no way of knowing. But it must have been sufficient that he and the others felt the need to lie low and control their alien mental emissions. Or perhaps we were wrong and they were simply being cautious, biding their time.

"Nathan stayed with us for five days, just long enough to look up a few old . . . well, acquaintances. But he was needed in Sunside and daren't delay any longer. And remember, his problem was as great if not greater than ours: a small army of aspiring Lords, lieutenants, thralls, and warrior creatures, left behind by our trio of Wamphyri invaders; an army which now inhabited the toppled ruins of Starside's ancient aeries, from which they raided on the Szgany as before. No, we had no claim on Nathan; indeed, our long-term debt to him could never be repaid. And so we had to let him go, with our best wishes—and as many weapons as he could take with him—back along the Möbius Route to rejoin the battle for his vampire world.

"And through all of that time, that terrible, frantic week, the only one of us who wasn't busy was Ben Trask. He had simply withdrawn from a world that would never be the same again, and I admit that I thought E-Branch had seen the last of him. Fortunately I was wrong, and when he returned he was stronger than ever—well, in some ways—but in his resolve, for sure.

"And now I'll tell you something that even he doesn't know. I was duty officer that night at E-Branch HQ—that night when Nathan brought Lardis through from Sunside, and Ben nightmared about Zek—and the moment that Ben came in and I saw the state he was in, I . . . I knew about Zek. I mean, I *knew*.

"Oh, I couldn't tell him, but where he was uncertain and dared not allow himself to be sure, I knew and hated myself for knowing. Just seeing him like that, Ben's future was immediately apparent to me. In one way it was the clearest picture of anyone's future that I'd ever seen, yet in another it was the vaguest—which was *how* I knew.

"For all I saw was how cold and lonely that future would be. . . ."

Goodly's delivery, the way he had told the story of the events of that night at E-Branch HQ from his own personal viewpoint—the obvious passion and compassion in this apparently reserved, indeed phlegmatic man—had brought him into far greater definition in Jake's perception; or rather, it had brought him into focus as a three-dimensional character in his own right. Previously a shadow or a soft-voiced cipher, he had somehow filled out. And Jake understood now that the precog had been a major part of this scene for a very long time.

Now, too, and also for the first time, Goodly's physical person had impressed itself upon the Branch's most recent however hesitant recruit. Ian Goodly: all of six-feet-four-inches tall, skeletally thin and gangly, grey-haired and mainly gaunt-featured. His expression was usually grave; he rarely smiled; only his eyes—warm, brown, and totally disarming—belied what invariably constituted an unfortunate first-impression appearance, that of a cadaverous mortician. Except, and as Jake was suddenly aware, you can't always tell a book from its cover. He would have done better to take more notice of Goodly's eyes than his outline.

Outside the ops truck, he cornered the precog and drew him away from the others into the shade of a tree.

"What is it?" Goodly asked, though he believed he already knew well enough. For just like Trask and Lardis Lidesci before him, he'd left several blank pages in his telling of the story. Jake was still fishing for the bits that would bring the whole thing into focus.

"Just you and me," Jake answered. "Just the two of us, and no one else to confuse the issue. Would you mind if I ask you a few questions? I mean, right from square one I've had this feeling that you're on my side, that you think I should be told the whole thing. The others are holding stuff back, but you're reluctant to do so. Am I right?"

Goodly smiled a wry smile, sighed, and said, "I'll tell you what I can. But even though you're right about my being on your side—or rather, about my talent being on your side— still I won't be able to answer all of your questions. The Branch comes first, and Ben Trask *is* the Branch. What Ben says goes."

"Some of my questions, then," Jake pressed. And he quickly went on: "So you're a precog, right? And this talent of yours, this precognition, it lets you see into the future?"

"That's the general idea," Goodly sighed again. "But only a very rough idea, for it's not nearly as simple as that. Haven't I made that plain?" And now he was frowning.

"Okay, fine," Jake placated him. "But you did tell me you'd seen *some* of my future, right? You did say that I'd be with you, with E-Branch, for quite some time to come."

"That's true, yes," Goodly answered.

"In what capacity?"

"I don't know."

"Okay, then is it going to be that way simply because Trask won't let me go off and do my own thing, or . . . ?"

"*Possibly* because he won't let you go," the precog answered. "He has to see how you work out, which could take a while. That could be—it obviously is—part of the reason why I've foreseen your continuing presence, yes. But what is this, Jake? Are you still uncertain? I thought you'd decided to stay?"

". . . Or, is it mainly because he thinks I'm going to be useful to you?" Jake ignored Goodly's last.

"Well that, too, we hope. But Jake, you're talking in circles. And I don't see—"

"I'm *getting* to it!" Jake growled, his attitude intense now. And after a moment's thought: "So tell me, is it me, Jake Cutter, who'll be useful to you, or is it this Harry?"

"Er, that was my meaning, yes," said the precog, "that the Necroscope would definitely be useful to us. But if you want me to pick and choose, I can't do it. I would have to answer, both of you—you'll both be extremely useful to us. I thought that he had been made plain, too."

"He's . . . what, contacting me, this Harry? Getting into my head to guide me, is that it?" Jake was pushing it now. "Or is he simply using me?"

"Using you? Personally, I would say he's keeping you safe. Wouldn't you?"

"But in my head, like telepathy? A kind of telepathic control?" Jake scowled.

"Telepathy?" Goodly seemed uncertain. "Something *like* telepathy, yes. But Harry had a different name for it."

"Had? Why is it that when we talk about this Harry everything has to be past tense?" Then Jake gave a snort. "*Huh!* Dumb question—because he's dead, of course!—which I can't see at all. For if he's dead, how can he do whatever it is he's doing to me? See, I don't believe in ghosts. They're a concept I just can't seem to wrap my head around. And as for Harry Keogh: he's something I don't *want* to wrap my head around, even though it's apparent he's already seen to that! But since he's obviously a disembodied voice out of the past, then it must be equally obvious that his talent was similar to yours. I mean, Harry didn't so much read the future as reach into it . . . is how it seems to me. But okay, fine, let's keep it going: So if what he's doing to me *isn't* telepathy, then what did he call it?"

"It wouldn't help you to know, not at this stage." Goodly shook his head. "In fact it could easily become an obstruction, a deterrent to your acceptance of . . . of everything."

Jake's frustration was mounting again. "A deterrent to my acceptance?" he snapped. "Don't you think there are enough deterrents already? It's nuts, all of it! I mean, what am I, some kind of psychic medium? If there was a reason, just one logical reason, why I should suddenly become this dead bloke's target, his focus, his genius loci, then I might be willing to believe at least some of this . . . this whatever. See, I know that what I've actually seen and experienced so far is real, but I don't know that a lot of what I've been *told* is real. I trust my own five senses, or used to, but I don't understand how or why I'm involved. I'd even *like* to believe what I've heard, if only as an alternative to considering myself some kind of psycho, some kind of schizoid nutcase. But . . . but . . . *but Harry is fucking dead!*"

"Well, in a *way* he's dead," said the precog, just as serious as ever, as if their conversation was utterly mundane. "But you see, Harry didn't view existence, life and death, as we do. There was a time when *he* really was two people. It was after he suffered . . . well, an *accident*, that his mind temporarily manifested itself in the identity of his own infant son. And later, he underwent another singular change. Best to think of it as a kind of metempsychosis, or—"

"Metempsychosis?" Jake cut him short. For despite being sure he'd never heard the word before, still he understood it; likewise another word that meant much the same thing. "You mean transmigration? Of souls? Like he was . . . what, some kind of body-snatcher?" And now suspicion was written plain on the younger man's face.

"It wasn't like that at all!" the precog protested.

"What?" Jake's voice was brittle now, cracking like glass splintering under the heel of a boot. "I don't give a twopenny toss what it was like! Shit, look at it from my point of view! This bloke's dead but he's trying to control my mind? And then what, my body? And if he ever got it, do you really think he'd want to give it back? And what about me, Mr. Ian bloody Goodly, precog? What the *fuck* about me? Is that why you can't tell me my future? Because the real me doesn't have one?"

"Calm down, for goodness' sake!" Goodly looked alarmed. "My word, but you've a very short memory, Jake Cutter!"

"Eh?" That had served to slow Jake down a little. "A short memory? How so?"

"Didn't Harry get you out of jail? Hasn't he saved your life twice already, and Liz's, too?"

Jake considered it, relaxed a very little, said: "But what does he hope to do with me, this . . . this ghost?"

"Well, perhaps that's one I can answer," Goodly told him. "You see, the Necroscope's principal tenet was that whatever a man does in life he will continue to do after death. He proved it, too: used it to discover the Möbius Continuum. You'll just have to take my word for that, for the time being anyway. But Harry's greatest claim to fame, or one of them, lay in finding and destroying vampires. Oh yes, the Earth was infested before this latest invasion. And believe me, Jake, without the Necroscope on our side, our world would have become an unimaginable hell-hole of a place a long time ago. So . . ."

". . . So, you think he intends to keep on doing what he did before," Jake nodded his understanding, all the while fighting hard to suppress his disbelief. "This Harry . . . he's trying to come back because he somehow knows *they* have come back, and he wants to go on killing vampires. He's the avenging ghost and I . . . I'm his gadget?"

The precog shrugged and answered, "And there you have it."

Jake shook his head, looked bewildered, said: "Come again? Didn't you get something backwards just then? Surely you meant there it has me!"

But Goodly was weary of this now. "As you will," he answered. And pursing his thin lips, he turned away.

Jake saw his mistake, didn't want to alienate someone who obviously gave a damn, and quickly said, "Listen, I appreciate everything you've told me. I'm not trying to mess you about—none of you—but looking for a little firm ground, somewhere I can safely plant my feet. The way I'm feeling, every step is like quicksand. And what you just said doesn't help any. What, I'm supposed to be happy with the notion of this Harry working his will through me, if not actually *on* me? Well, that's probably fine by you E-Branch people, all nice and safe in your own talented little skulls, but—"

"But there's no safe place in E-Branch, Jake," the precog cut him short, glancing back over his shoulder. "However, I did say you would be around for quite some time. Which, with the Necroscope—or something of him—on your side, seems a very fair forecast to me."

"But a ghost?"

"There are ghosts and ghosts," the other answered, walking away.

"But he's *dead*, for Christ's sake!" Made meaningless now, through repetition, still Jake's exclamation exploded from his dry lips. "And not just a ghost—not just any old spook—but one who has access to my mind!"

"In E-Branch," Goodly told him, without looking back, "we do believe in ghosts, especially in Harry Keogh. We have every good reason to. But that's something you don't have to take my word for, Jake. You see, I'm sure that before very long you'll believe in them, too. I, Mr. Ian bloody Goodly, precog, am very sure of it, yes. . . ."

16
A Meeting of Minds

JAKE WAS IN CHOPPER ONE WITH TRASK, LIZ, Goodly, Lardis, and a pair of technicians, Jimmy Harvey and Paul Arenson. Their next stop was Alice Springs (a "mere" eight hundred miles east) for refuelling. Chopper Two needed an hour's maintenance and would follow on behind. As for the vehicular contingent:

"They're heading south for Kalgoorlie," Paul Arenson, a gangling, blue-eyed blond of maybe thirty-three years was telling his younger colleague. "From there they'll go piggyback on a freight train to Broken Hill, then back on the road again to Brisbane. All except the big artic. It has to be the Great Aussie Bight coast road for the big feller. I calculate something like two thousand, three hundred miles all told. We'll be home and dry in less than five hours; that's taking it easy, including a stop to stretch our legs at Alice. But as for the lads in the big truck . . . just be glad you're not one of them. Five hours for us, and three or four *days* for them!"

The conversation buzzed in Jake's head, singing with the vibration of the jet-copter. The airplane was safe and stable, but with its paramilitary design it hadn't been built for comfort. Jake sat on the floor in the narrow stowage area towards the tail, where there were no seats. Half-reclining, his large, angular frame was cushioned by holdalls, sausage-bags, and various packs of personal belongings, some hard and some soft; it wasn't his idea of luxury. But tired, and even hoping to get a little sleep, he repositioned himself as best he could and let the aircraft's singing soak into him.

The "tune" was much too regular for a lullaby, and snatches of muted conversation kept drifting back to him, monotone lyrics that didn't fit the music but clung like cobwebs to his thoroughly weary mind. Cocooned in this odd mix of white noise and blurred babble, gradually Jake felt himself nodding off.

Liz Merrick was loosely belted into the rearmost of the seats, a gunner's swivelling bucket seat between wide sliding doors on both sides. Her long legs were up, flopping over the gunner's arm rests; the gun itself slumped nose-down, strapped in position. Glinting a dull blue-grey, and despite its proximity to Liz's lovely body, the weapon looked sullenly impotent. But the picture Jake kept in his mind as he drifted into sleep was that of a naked Liz with the gun between her legs. . . .

. . . But then he was *asleep, and* he *was the gun between her legs! And—damn it to hell!—he wasn't fucking Liz but was facing* away *from her out of the door. And she wasn't trying to ride him but was* firing *him* . . . *her arms round his waist, with one hand massaging his balls while the other, working his rampant dick, shot burst after burst of silvery, smoking semen at nightmarish vampire shapes that flapped in the chopper's slipstream, snarling their bloodlust as they fought to get inside the plane, to get at Liz, Trask, Goodly and the others!*

Barely asleep, Jake jerked awake. Liz was staring at him, her cheeks flaming, mouth half-open, eyes wide. And Jake didn't need a degree in psychiatry—or in parapsychology— to understand what had happened here. Whether as a deliberate voyeur or an innocent observer, Liz had been in his mind. She'd seen that last scene. And as for what it meant: that was his fear surfacing, his ongoing suspicion that Ben Trask was simply using him, now complicated by the notion that Trask was also using *her* as some kind of bait—like a carrot for a donkey?—to keep him happy as he plodded on. He could be right at that, or he could be wrong. But if Liz were the carrot, then what did Trask have in mind for the stick? Everything remained to be seen.

"I . . . I . . ." Liz mouthed words at him—mouthed them, but nothing came out—as she quickly, self-consciously, ashamedly slid her jean-clad legs from the gunner's arm rests and sat up straighter in the bucket seat.

Serves you fucking right! Jake snapped back, but silently, in his head. And he knew he'd reached her from the way her head jerked. *And now keep the fuck out!*

Following which, as his anger cooled, it took some time to get back to sleep. . . .

Snatches of conversation drifting back to him. But in his ears or in his head? Perhaps he was still on Liz's mind, and unsuspected even by the girl herself where she sat in her bucket seat midway between Jake in stowage and the others in their seats up front, she had become some kind of mental relay station. For in the few days she had known him Liz had established something of a rapport with Jake; it was possible that the sending technique she had used to taunt Bruce Trennier had "fixed" itself and was now developing more rapidly in her special mind. Maybe this was simply her way of making amends: by letting Jake in on the conversation. The conversation about him. Or was it something, or some one *else entirely?*

Trask's hushed voice, asking: "But why him?"

Lardis Lidesci: "Does the why of it really matter? If Jake has been chosen, he's been chosen."

And Ian Goodly: "There are certain similarities. Maybe we shouldn't overlook them. I'm sure mental characteristics—how Jake thinks—are more important than the purely physical way he looks. When we look at him we don't see Harry, that's true, but the Necroscope was a hard act to follow. Perhaps we should give more thought as to how Harry sees him. And there *are* similarities."

Trask: "Go on."

Goodly: "For one thing, they both lost loved ones. Both of them drowned, murdered, too."

Trask: "Granted, but that's where it ends. And as for losing a loved one, murdered, you could say the same about me. But where is Harry's humility? Where's his compassion, his warmth? This Jake . . . he's abrasive, a roughneck, spoiled and wild."

Goodly: "A roughneck? But in the right circumstances that would be—and it already has been—a positive bonus. A rough *diamond,* maybe. Surely the Necroscope would know better than to choose a weakling for a job like this?"

Trask: "But a hard-man? A killer, even if he does have his reasons?"

Lardis: "Me, I say they were good reasons. I like him! And I say it again, if he's Harry Hell-lander's choice, that's good enough for me."

Trask: "And me . . . well, within limits. So don't misunderstand me—I'm not arguing the Necroscope's choice—it's just that I don't understand it. I have this feeling that Jake's not only fighting us but fighting Harry, too."

Goodly: "Oh, he is, be sure of it! But aside from his manners and tendency to aggression, there *are* similarities."

Trask, dubiously: "More similarities?"

Goodly: "Indeed. For Harry believed in revenge, too.

Don't you remember? An eye for an eye? He was just a boy when he went after Boris Dragosani. If like attracts like— mentally speaking, that is—then I can well see how Harry would be drawn to this one. And that's something else you might give some thought to: if you want Jake firmly on the team, and his mind exclusively on the job in hand, you could do a lot worse than find this man, this Luigi Castellano."

Trask: "And then what? Let Jake go after him?"

Goodly: "This Castellano is rubbish and should be disposed of—we're all agreed on that. I think Jake will chase him down no matter what, which makes Castellano a distraction. But if he were to be taken out . . . no more distraction. And we would have Jake's gratitude."

Trask, mildly surprised: "Well, now! And just listen to the cold-blooded one! But you're right, and we're checking into it. Interpol and other friends abroad. If we could just bring Castellano to justice, that might suffice." ·

Goodly: "No, it wouldn't." (A sensed shake of the precog's head). "When he is dead, *that* will suffice. You know as well as I do how Jake dealt with the other members of that gang. Do you really think he'll be satisfied to see their boss nice and comfortable, all warm and well-fed behind bars?"

Lardis: "Anyway, in case I haven't already said it loud or often enough, I like Jake Cutter. And so does Liz."

Liz, heatedly: "I do not! Well, not especially."

Lardis, chuckling throatily: "See?"

Then silence for a while, the darkness deepening, and Jake finally adrift in dreams. And a strange cold current taking him in tow, steering him to an unknown yet oddly familiar destination. . . .

A riverbank, and below its grassy, root-tangled rim, the water swirling in the eddies of a small bight. A boy, sitting on the edge and leaning forward at what seemed an unsafe angle, dangling his feet close to the slowly swirling surface. His elbows were on on his knees, his hands propping his chin, and he appeared to be talking to someone. Perhaps to himself.

Jake's shadow fell on him, and the boy turned his head to look up at him. He didn't seem at all surprised by Jake's presence (but then, neither did Jake). On the contrary, he smiled a pale, painful, yet appreciative greeting. "Hello, there! So you came. Why don't you sit down a while and talk to me?"

"I, er, didn't like to cut in on you." Jake answered, not knowing what else to say. And then, because he wasn't sure what else to do, either—and wondering if he knew the other—he finally followed his suggestion, sat down, and asked him: "Er, do you think it's possible we've met somewhere before?" Beginning to feel the strangeness of it all, he looked the boy over more closely, perhaps even warily.

Apart from the obvious fact that the other had recently been fighting, there didn't seem to be anything especially odd about him. He could be any scruffy boy, though for some reason Jake found himself doubting that. Maybe eleven or twelve years old, sandy-haired, freckled; he wasn't skinny yet barely filled out his ill-fitting, threadbare, second-hand school jacket. The top button was absent from a once-white shirt that hung halfway out of his grey flannel trousers, and a frayed, tightly knotted tie with a faded school motto hung askew from his crumpled collar. His lumpish nose supported plain prescription spectacles, small, circular windows through which dreaming blue eyes gazed out in a strange mixture of wonder and weird expectation.

Then, suddenly aware of Jake's inspection, the boy looked down at himself, wrinkled his nose in disgust, said: "This will be the school bully, big Stanley Green's work. He's got it coming, has our Stanley. In about a year from now, or maybe two." And his lips were thinner, tighter, more determined.

There was dried blood on those lips, a gash in the corner of his mouth, but little or nothing of fear in his dreamy eyes, which were now other than dreamy and contained a certain glint. Indeed they looked older than the rest of him, those eyes, and Jake thought there was probably a pretty mature mind in there, somewhere behind that half-haunted face. But he could never in a million years have guessed how mature— or how wise in otherworldly ways.

And because the boy hadn't as yet answered his first question (as to whether or not they knew each other), Jake now felt the urge to remind and prompt him. "Er, son?"

But he needn't have concerned himself. Obviously the other had considered Jake's earlier question, and now took his prompt into account, too.

"Son?" he finally repeated Jake, and cocked his young-old head on one side. "And you're wondering if we know each other? Well, I've got to answer no to both questions. Uh-uh, Jake. You and I don't know each other, not yet. And I'm not too comfortable with you calling me 'son.' It's a case of—I don't know—what came first, the chicken or the egg?" There was no animosity in his reply.

"Eh?" Jake frowned. "Someone else just bursting with riddles? I don't need that right now."

"But it's a hell of an adventure," said the boy, sounding not at all like a child, despite his child's voice. "Er, working them out, that is. I've done my share of that, Jake." Then, sitting back and gazing directly into Jake's eyes, studying his face and perhaps more than his face: "So you're he. And you've been having a hard time of it, right?"

"Well, since you seem to understand what's going on here," Jake answered, perhaps peevishly, "why don't you tell me?" His dream might be working something out for him, resolving a problem.

And the other nodded. "Very well, I'm telling you: you're having a hard time of it. But that's just as much your fault as mine; you have a very defensive mind. And me, I don't have much of a mind at all! Or I do, but not all in one place, not all at one time. Oh, I *know*—I mean, I've known—a lot of things. But what I remember and what I've forgotten are completely random. Like a kind of amnesia or a bad case of absentmindedness. Except it's not. For you see, I'm really not all here. Or putting it more sympathetically, all of *me* isn't here. Which means that while I won't get things 100 percent wrong, I may not get them entirely right either. That's why I need a focus. But now, since you seem determined to reject me, it looks like it may be hard for us to get along, and harder still for me to get it together. So, how long do you plan to keep slamming the door in my face, Jake?"

"Who are you?" Jake asked him then, feeling a weird tingle in his scalp, an unheard of sensation of *negative* déjà vu: that it wasn't him but the boy who had been here—or somewhere—before. And Jake felt he knew where he'd been.

But the other frowned and now seemed as uncertain as Jake. "I . . . I'm all sorts of people and things," he said. "I'm Alec, Nestor, Nathan, take your pick. There's something of Faethor in me, or has been, or will be. And something of me in a whole lot of people. It all depends on the time, the date, the place. And time is relative: what will be has been, ask any precog. That's why we have to be sure it works out right, don't you see?"

"You . . . you're Harry Keogh!" said Jake, shivering without knowing why—until he remembered what Harry Keogh was. "You're the ghost they've been telling me about!"

"And you're the gadget," said Harry.

"But I don't want to be!" Jake felt himself riveted to the riverbank; he wanted to leap away but couldn't move. It was the dream, the nightmare—one of *those* nightmares—where try as you might you can't escape from the thing that's chasing you.

"I'm not chasing you," the young Harry protested. "You are chasing me. Chasing me away! And in fact he was wavering, physically (or metaphysically) wavering, his figure a mere outline, his face and form thinning towards transparency.

"But you're after my mind, my body!" Jake cried.

The boy, the dream-Harry, the ghost (who by now was beginning to *look* ghostly, insubstantial as smoke), gave a desperate shake of his almost immaterial head. "That's not me, Jake. It's the Wamphyri who want your mind, body, and soul. *I* am the one—or rather *we* are the ones, and maybe the only ones—who might be able to stop them. So don't send me away, Jake. Don't fight me off!"

And suddenly Jake realized that he could, that he *was* actually doing it: fighting the other off, sending him away.

"I . . . I can, can't I?" he said, his fear retreating.

"You very nearly did!" said Harry, sighing as he firmed up again. "Okay, so perhaps this is too strange for you, the wrong time and place, the wrong me. I didn't think you'd see any harm in a small boy, that's all."

"What, in a child who talks like a man?" Jake felt himself shivering again, but less violently. "A boy whose eyes are innocent as a baby's yet old as the ages? A boy capable of metempsychosis—who's *in* my mind right now—while I'm the helpless, intended vessel?"

"You're by no means as helpless as you think," said Harry, perhaps admiringly. "That mind of yours: stubborn as hell, with good shields you've never had reason to use, nor even suspected you had! Anyway, mind transference isn't something that I . . . that I have in mind? I've had my time, Jake, my lives—and I'm still having them—but I do get your point. So very well, let's try something else. . . ."

A moment ago it had been warm in evening sunlight that came in flickering beams, fanning through the trees on the far bank and setting the water sparkling out towards the middle of the river where the current ran fastest. Now, in a single instant, it was cold and dark; frost lay thick on the ground, and the river was a ribbon of ice, frozen and motionless. A full moon hung low in a windswept sky, and a trio of gardens fronted rich houses that reared to the right of Jake and the boy where they walked along the river path. Except Jake's companion was no longer a boy but a youth.

Jake started away from the stranger—stumbled, might have fallen into frosted brambles on the overgrown river-bank—but Harry was quick to take his arm, hold him steady. "It's okay," he said, to still Jake's cry of alarm. "It's a different time, that's all, an older me. But the same place, more or less. The same river. We were back there," he thumbed the air, indicated the path behind them, "a few hundred yards down river, sitting on the bank. It was summer and I was talking to my mother when you came by. Now it's . . . oh, quite a few winters later. I'm a little closer to your own age now, so perhaps we'll be able to get along that much better."

Closer to my own age? Jake thought. *But you're a good deal firmer, too. That's a hell of a strong grip you have on my arm, and how much stronger on my mind?*

But Harry the youth only shook his head in disappointment. "Hiding your thoughts won't help. I'm *in* here, remember? Well, at present I am, anyway, while you accept me."

"Jesus!" Jake gasped. "It's like something out of *A Christmas Carol!* When I wake up, I won't believe it."

"That's what I'm afraid of," said Harry. "Worse still, you may not even remember it. That's why we have to get things done while we can, and hope they get fixed in your mind."

"Things?"

"Until you trust me," the other answered, "until you allow me a little permanency, we'll have to move in stops and starts. We'll get nowhere until I know the whole story, and I won't be able to help you until you believe."

"Believe in a ghost?"

"But I'm not, not really. And Jake, you wouldn't—I mean you really *wouldn't*—believe how often I've been through this before! Oh, I've had trouble convincing others before you."

While Harry talked, Jake looked him over. It was the same "boy" for sure, but he'd be nineteen or maybe twenty years old now. Wiry, he would weigh some nine and a half stone and stand seventy inches tall. His hair was an untidy sandy mop that reminded Jake of Clint Eastwood's in those old Western movies of more than thirty years ago. But his face wasn't nearly so hard and his freckles were still there, lending him a naive and definitely misleading boyish innocence.

More than any other feature, Harry Keogh's eyes were especially interesting. Looking at Jake, they seemed to see right through him (the sure sign of an esper, as Jake was now aware), as if he were the revenant, and not the reverse. But they were oh so blue, those eyes, that startling, colourless blue which always looks so unnatural, so that one thinks the owner has to be wearing lenses. More than that, there was something in them which said they'd seen a lot more than any twenty-year-old has any right seeing.

But still Jake felt a little easier with all of this now. After all, it was only a dream. And since this ghost, or whatever it was, was conversational, why not talk to it? Or humour it, as the case might be.

"So, if convincing people is as hard as you make out, why do you put yourself to the trouble?" he asked his strange companion.

They had come to a halt before the gate in the garden wall of the central house. Lights in the downstairs room adjacent to the garden sent angular black shadows marching over the brittle shrubbery and garden path . . . the shadows of men, glimpsed only briefly before the patio doors were slammed and curtains jerked hurriedly across the wide windows.

For a long moment Harry made no answer to Jake's question; he stood as if transfixed, looking in through the gate's horizontal bars. But the house was mainly dark, where mere chinks of light escaped at odd angles from the corners and joins of poorly-fitted curtains.

Then the youth started, blinked his eyes in the pale moonlight, and breathlessly answered, "Why do I keep putting myself out? That's easy, Jake. It's because I was the beginning, and I have to be the end." Then he gave another start, and said:

"We can't stay here. That house there is where I was born. My stepfather has visitors—Boris Dragosani and Max Batu—and later, I'll be visiting him, too. Tonight is the night I killed him. But there are things you mustn't see, not yet."

"You . . . you killed him?" And now the cold that Jake felt wasn't entirely physical, if it ever had been.

"I will," said the other. "But I don't want to see it, and I don't want you to see it. So now we have to go. Another place and time. Are you up to it?"

"Do I have a choice?"

"You can always wake up, but I wouldn't advise it. It was hard enough getting into you this time. And if you're as badly frightened as—"

"Frightened?" Jake cut him off, his pride surfacing. "Maybe I am, but I'm also interested—very. I want to know where this is going, want to find out what it's all about. And since *they* won't tell me—"

"They?" (Harry's turn to cut in.)

"Ben Trask and his people," Jake answered.

"*Ah!*" said Harry, nodding his head and smiling knowingly. "I might have guessed. In fact I suppose I knew. You mentioned 'them' before, and obviously E-Branch HQ was where I aimed you that first time, when I first became aware of you. But that was then and this is now, and we have to move on. Since this was my home for so many years, we'll probably be back. But . . . my timing was years off, and I can't think why. It must be my memory, which is incomplete. You see, *I'm* incomplete! I'm not entirely here. Actually, I'm not entirely anywhere! It seems to be only the strongest of times and places to which I'm drawn."

"Maybe it's a variation on the old theme," said Jake. "The killer returning to the scene—*and time*—of the crime!"

"Very clever," said Harry. "And you could even be right—in a way. The lure of powerful times and places. Yes, I can see that. But a killer?" He shrugged. "I can't deny it, and I won't try to explain it, not now. It's like I said: this isn't a good time for me. So I'll ask you once again—"

And: "Yes." Jake nodded. "I'm up to it. I think."

"Very well." The other nodded. "But this time I'll try for a place of innocence."

"Er, before we go," Jake quickly put in, "can you answer a question or two? I mean, while I'm still steady on my feet?"

"I'm surprised you haven't asked them sooner," Harry answered, his eyes still anxious where they peered through the bars of the gate at the house.

"Why me?" Jake said. "Why not one of these people you seem to know so well, the E-Branch crowd? Surely they would have accepted you that much more readily. From some of the things I've heard them say about you, they hold you in some kind of awe."

"But you're young," said the other. "You're strong enough to face whatever it is that's coming. Ben Trask and the others, they're old now. And they don't need . . ."

"Yes?"

"—Redemption? No, that's not it. Let's just say they're not troubled. They're straight in what they have to do. But you *are* troubled. There's a lot of anger in you, Jake, an explosive strength. And that's what is needed. It's what we have to find a use for, but the right use."

"So I was chosen out of nothing?" Jake frowned. "Because I need saving? What if I don't want saving? You see, I still have a job to do, and one way or the other I'll do it. What I'm saying is, you're taking a chance with me. I might not work out the way you want me to."

"There was a certain element of chance in it, yes," Harry answered. "But there were also things I couldn't ignore. In the Möbius Continuum, down future time-streams, I've seen your blue life-thread crossed with the red of vampires where you're going to meet up with them. But where some of them blink out, expire, your blue thread goes on. Déjà vu, Jake! I just couldn't ignore it. I want to make sure that blue thread goes on and on, that's all."

Bewildered, Jake shook his head. "None of which makes any sense at all to me."

"But it will, when you understand the Continuum. When you command it. And when you're able to do . . . *other* things."

"Command it? This . . . this going-places thing? You're saying there's some kind of order to it? I can control it? And as for doing *other* things: frankly, that worries me. You're beginning to sound a lot like these E-Branch people."

"How's your math?" the other turned his back on the house, looked out over the star-shot river of ice.

"My math?" Jake's bewilderment grew apace.

"Your numbers, your reckoning."

"I don't get short-changed, if that's what you mean."

"We should talk to Möbius," said Harry. "Except we can't, for he's long gone. That's a problem. So I suppose you'll have to learn it parrot-fashion. From me. And that could be a problem in its own right, because what I do now is pretty much instinctive, intuitive."

"And not very accurate," said Jake. "And probably dangerous, too. What good's all this jumping about if it doesn't get you where you want to go?"

"But it does."

"But not this time!" Jake waved a hand at the house. "You said so yourself."

"Uh-uh," Harry shook his head. "You're all confused. You keep forgetting that this is only a dream—and your dream at that! I can guide these subconscious thoughts of yours, I can aim them, but I'm not flying you. I'm just the co-pilot. Deep inside you *want* to know about me, my times, places, and history. That's what's driving all of this, your need to know. So give me a little help to move on, won't you? I can't concentrate to best effect in this location. I'm not at all comfortable here."

"You didn't need help the first time," Jake reminded him, "when you moved us from daylight to night, from the riverbank to this place, and—"

"—And when you didn't expect it," the other pointed out. "But it's this mind of yours. It resists me—resists psychic or metaphysical interference—and its resistance grows stronger all the time. Maybe that's another reason why I was drawn to you: because you were a rare one with a talent of your own, if not *all* your own, just waiting to be developed. In fact a great many people have one sort of ESP-ability or another; in most of them it's usually stillborn, incapable of further development. But I suspect that as esper begets esper the powers of the mind will come more and more into their own. Evolution, Jake: that was how it happened to me, and also how it happened in Sunside. Szgany shields are powerful, too. They have to be, or the Szgany would be extinct. In you it was dormant, waiting for an opportunity to break out. But now that it has been awakened—perhaps by contact with me, my dart—or then again by E-Branch . . ."

"Your dart? That really *was* you, then?" Jake was managing to absorb some of this, at least.

"Part of me, something of me. Awareness, Jake, awareness! Do you know the easiest way to magnetize a piece of iron? You throw it in with a lot of big magnets, that's how. And as for you—"

"I was thrown in at the deep end," said Jake.

The other nodded. "Apparently. So now if you'll only relax a little, we'll move on."

And Jake relaxed. . . .

To anyone else these time and location shifts might be unnerving: from a summer day on the river, to a moonlit winter night, to a night-light in a tiny garret room. Unnerving even if they worked as intended, but this time it seemed something had gone wrong. For in the little room where the dreamer now found himself he was on his own and there was no sign of his host, (his ghost?) But Jake—one of those rare types who can often distinguish between dreams and reality—wasn't too concerned. If anything he was pleased. Or rather he was glad on the one hand (for the dream had been getting *out* of hand) and a little disappointed on the other. Just when he'd thought he was getting somewhere, learning something . . .

But you still are, said Harry.

Startled, Jake looked all about. But he looked too quickly and saw nothing. And at the same time it dawned on him that he hadn't so much heard Harry's voice as felt it. "Telepathy?" he said. "Does that mean you didn't make it? In which case, where the hell are you?"

I'm over here, said Harry. *Sucked into the most innocent of places. Innocent for the time being, anyway.*

The "over here" was a direction-finder as clear and clearer than any voice. And now that Jake looked again he saw what he'd missed the first time: a cot, standing on rockers in the corner of the small room, where the eaves came down low. And lowering his head a little, he stepped towards it.

Within the cot, an infant; the baby had kicked himself free of a soft woollen blanket, lay naked and chubby, exposed except for diapers. His face was angelic, and his eyes—

"You!" said Jake.

Different times, different Harry Keoghs, said the other.

"But a baby, you?"

Well I was once upon a time! But what you're looking at . . . no, it isn't me. On the other hand, I am in here. For this is a time when I was incorporeal, Jake, and my son's mind was like a black hole. It sucked me in, saved me until I could become someone else.

"He . . . he has your eyes," said Jake, because there was no other way to answer what he'd just heard. And yet it did ring a bell, for Ian Goodly had tried to tell him something similar.

He has my mind, too! Harry told him, gurgling happily— or unhappily?—in his cot. *His and mine both. And unless I'm mistaken we've arrived at a very bad time.*

"What, again?"

I was looking for innocence and found it. But if I'm right, that's just about to end. You see, this is the time, almost to the moment, when Harry Jr. moves on, becomes The Dweller. Which in turn means—

A woman's voice cried out from an adjacent room in the garret flat. A cry of uttermost terror! But:

Don't panic, said Harry, despite that his own mental voice was filled with urgency now. *That's his mother, but things are well under control. And we're almost out of here. Before that, though . . . Jake, I need the names of these invaders, the creatures I've seen crossing your life-thread in Möbius time. If you know who they are, I can probably trace their histories to discover their weaknesses, maybe work out some way for you to deal with them.*

(Sounds of crashing furniture came from the other room, and a single shrill cry: *"No!"* Followed by a dull thud, a low moan, and silence . . . for a moment. Then a padding, and a hoarse, low panting. Sounds such as an animal might make. A large animal.)

Their names! cried Harry in Jake's mind.

"Names?" Jake answered, his eyes on the door where it stood slightly ajar. "Lords Malinari and Szwart, and the Lady Vavara: Wamphyri out of Starside." He might just as easily have uttered an invocation.

Almost wrenched from its hinges, the door crashed inwards, and in a moment Jake's dream became a shrieking, hellish nightmare! "What . . . ?!" he gasped. And:

Yulian Bodescu! the Necroscope's revenant sighed in Jake's mind.

The thing framed in the doorway was or had been a man; it wore a man's clothing and stood upright, however forward-leaning. Its arms were . . . long! And the hands at the ends of those arms were huge and clawlike, with projecting nails. The thing's face was something unbelievable. It could have been the face of a wolf, but it was almost hairless and there were certain anomalies that suggested a batlike origin. The monster's ears grew flat to the sides of its misshapen head; they too were batlike and projected higher than the rearward-sloping, elongated skull. Its nose—or rather its *snout*—was mobile, wrinkled, convoluted, with black and gaping nostrils. The thing's skin was ridged, looked scaly; its yellow, crimson-pupilled eyes were deepsunken in black sockets. And as for its *jaws,* its *teeth!*

The creature—Yulian Bodescu?—ignored Jake, loped to the cot, and crouched over it. And the light in his or its eyes had the glow of molten sulphur, the fires of hell fuelled by eager anticipation! Taloned hands were already reaching for the helpless infant as Jake tried to snatch at a gun that was no longer there. Uttering a strangled curse, he leaped to the attack . . . or would have, except his limbs seemed locked in place.

A nice gesture, but useless, Harry told him. *And anyway, in the waking world it would only serve to get you killed! This is a scene from my past, Jake. Obviously we survived it, myself and my son both, but I fancy your dream won't. So one last word before we part: next time, try to be easier to reach. . . .*

The scene warped, began to melt away even as Jake strove to move his body—a single muscle, a fingertip—and failed miserably. He stood poised, inert, desperate to go to the infant's aid despite what the Necroscope had told him. He tried to shout a warning, managed a hoarse croak, a clotted gurgle, and all in vain. For everything was dissolving away. Terror, utter horror, can bring a man awake even when he knows he's only dreaming.

The last thing Jake saw before he surfaced was the beast: on its knees beside the cot, mad with frustrated rage, tearing the bedclothes to shreds. But of the baby Harry himself, nothing at all. . . .

And Jake gave a small glad cry and woke up. For somehow in the moment before waking he knew—he'd been *given* to know—where the infant had gone.

Along the Möbius route to E-Branch, of course.

Where else?

Part Three
The Start of It

17
Second Thoughts, and Others Less Mundane

NOTICING JAKE'S DISTRESS, LIZ HAD SCRAMbled from her gunner's seat into the narrow cargo area, crouched down beside him, and was now hauling on the lapels of his jacket, roughing him up a little. "Jake! Jake, wake up!" Then—as his eyes snapped open, startling her, and lightning reflexes and hands worked in combination to slap her wrists aside, then grab them—"You were shouting," she explained. "And now you're hurting!"

He let go of her, dragged himself into an upright, seated position among the jumble of packs, and mumbled, "What? Shouting?" Of course he had been shouting, because he'd been nightmaring. But what about? Already the waking world, in the shape of Liz, was obliterating his dreams, consigning them to innermost recesses of subconscious mind. But realizing something of their importance, Jake was reluctant to let them go. "What was I shouting about?" he demanded harshly, but too late. For even as his head cleared the nightmare was retreating, shrinking to nothing.

Then he looked about—at the piled packs, the chopper's interior, the faces of the men up front looking back at him— and remembered where he was. And as the fear went out of Jake's eyes it was replaced by a worried frown. His face was damp with sweat, despite that it wasn't any too warm in . . . the aircraft? In the jet-copter, yes. His orientation was still a little off, making everything feel and sound unreal. Then it dawned on him that the hiss of the horizontal jets was absent, and the crisp *chop! chop! chop!* of rotors had taken over. They must be descending, into Alice Springs.

"I don't know what you were shouting about," Liz answered him. "Most of what you said was pure babble, until just before you woke up." She went back to her seat and buckled herself in. "Then you mentioned Szwart, Malinari, and Vavara. But you were doing a lot of twitching, too. It was a nightmare, Jake. A killer of a nightmare, I'd say!"

A killer. Yes, she was right:

A grotesque thing—Wamphyri!—its taloned hands reaching to snuff the life from an innocent baby boy. And:

"Yulian Bodescu!" Jake gasped aloud, starting as if he'd been slapped in the face. "Does anyone know who . . . who Yulian Bodescu was?" But that final scene, too, was fading away, following the rest of the nightmare into limbo.

In their seats up front, however, Ben Trask and Ian Goodly exchanged secretive but mainly wondering glances and said nothing . . . not until they were on the ground and they'd stretched their legs, and made their way to the lounge and the airport's watering hole. . . .

Jake and Lardis sat at the almost empty bar, chewing nuts and nursing large beers; Liz, Trask, and Goodly had a small table, smaller drinks, and ate from a plate of sandwiches. Huge overhead fans did their best to stir the sluggish air and keep the atmosphere bearable. But even the local Aussies were sweating. It was that kind of summer. El Niño, drying everything to kindling.

Lardis smacked his lips in appreciation, sighed, and told Jake: "This has to be one of the few true benefits of your entire world." And then, noticing how the bartender was giving him curious looks, he added, "Er, of Australia, I mean. One of the true benefits of Australia. They certainly know how to brew a good beer, these Australians."

The bartender looked Lardis up and down, and said, "I saw that movie, too, me old mate, way back when I was a little kid. But it didn't influence me mode o' dress!"

"Eh?" said Lardis.

"Crocodile bleedin' Dundee!" The other shook his head and moved off along the bar. "Jesus, what is it with you tourists? Do yer think we *all* live in the bleedin' outback?"

Lardis looked down at his clothes, lizard-skin belt, machete, shad-hide sandals, and scowled. "Have I been insulted?" he wondered out loud.

But Jake's thoughts were elsewhere. "Lardis, tell me about Harry Keogh," he said. "I mean, I've heard Trask talk about his compassion, warmth, and humility, which you have to admit makes him sound like a pacifist. But if he was so humble, how come he ended up as a—a what? A vampire-killer? And I gather it wasn't only vampires he killed."

"As for Harry Dwellersire's history in this world," the Old Lidesci answered, having first made sure that the bartender was well out of earshot, "I don't know the entire story. That's why I was only able to talk about Sunside/Starside. But from what I saw of him . . . well, I wouldn't be too sure about Harry's 'humility,' or his compassion either. After all, Nathan Kiklu was a humble one, too, upon a time. Anyway, I only met the Necroscope towards the end, which wasn't a pretty end. . . ."

Then, abruptly, Lardis's tone changed, and peering at Jake suspiciously he snapped, "Now do me a favour and stop trying to wheedle things out of me, okay? What am I anyway but 'a bleedin' tourist,' eh?"

While at the table, also out of earshot, Goodly, Liz, and Trask were considering something else. "Yulian Bodescu?" Trask looked at Liz. "You're sure he said Yulian Bodescu? We thought so, too, but we were too far away to be sure. Now tell me, how in hell did he come up with that name? If he's read it or perhaps remembered it from something someone has said, why has it chosen to surface now, in a dream?"

Liz could only shrug and ask, "Is it really that strange? I mean, it's hardly the most common of names, now is it? To be honest, it's just exactly the kind of name that would stick in my mind."

But Trask was out of sorts with himself, and it showed. "I put you in that gunner's bucket seat, close to him, so that you could listen in on him," he said. "In E-Branch we know how important dreams can be. But you say you got nothing?"

"To *start* with," Liz's voice hardened as she began to flare up, "I don't—"

But the precog quickly cautioned her: *"Shh! Keep it down."*

"Well, I don't understand why we can't tell Jake about the entire Bodescu affair!" she continued in a lowered but emphatic tone. "And what's more," (looking at Trask) "I didn't much like what you asked me to do. To *start* with, it's not E-Branch policy to spy on our colleagues, and—"

"Don't go lecturing me about Branch policy—Miss!" Trask glared. "As for Jake Cutter: he won't be a colleague until I'm one hundred percent sure he's on our side. The man vacilliates, sits on the fence. I'm not even sure he won't make a break for it the first chance he gets!"

"—*And*," Liz continued, determined to be heard, "the last time I tried it he . . . he knew."

"He what?" Goodly stared at her.

"Jake knew I was listening in on him," Liz said, deflated now. "He was dreaming—something sexy, erotic, yes, and frightening, too—and when I broke in on him it woke him up. So how can I ask him to trust me when he thinks I'm constantly in his mind?"

"So you didn't try?" Trask said.

"That's not so," she shook her head. "I did try, but I was blocked. I couldn't get in. Or I could, but it was like walking through a fog, all dismal and distorted. I didn't get one single clear picture."

"Precisely what I didn't want to hear," Trask grunted. "So now I'll tell you why I'm not ready to tell him the entire Yulian Bodescu story. You know that a vampire isn't safe even when he's dead and buried? If there was anything we learned from the Necroscope, it was that. Even as we burned the very earth where Thibor Ferenczy had been buried, still the bastard was instructing Yulian Bodescu, telling him about E-Branch. After that, the damage Yulian caused us, the deaths, the pain . . ." He paused and shook his head.

And Goodly said, "So even at this stage you're not entirely certain that this is the Necroscope's work? You think that

Jake might be under the influence of someone or something else? Just as Thibor got at Yulian, so someone might be getting at Jake?"

"We have to remember what Harry was, and what he *became* at the end," Trask answered. "And not only him but his lover Penny Sanderson, and what both The Dweller and Harry's other son Nestor became."

"Vampires," Liz said, with a small shudder.

"Wamphyri!" said Trask. "All of them. The Necroscope died on Starside. And now something—three somethings—have come out of Starside to infest our world. And Jake is being influenced by a remnant, or revenant, of the Necroscope himself. Let's not forget that just as Harry sired Nathan Kiklu, he also fathered Nestor. Two sides of the same coin, do you see? And do you wonder that I'm cautious? Why, of course I'm cautious! I should let something like *that* infiltrate E-Branch, get in amongst us, learn our secrets, use them against us? No, I don't think so."

"And if you're wrong?" said Liz.

"I *hope* I'm wrong!" Trask answered. "I *believe* I'm wrong, and I *want* to be wrong. But if I'm right I'll be alive, and so will you, Liz. Look, you've read about Harry but you never knew him, you haven't seen what he could do. Not the *other* things he could do. I have, and I don't want to see powers such as those fall into the wrong hands. That could mean the end of us all."

He sat back in his chair, let his brooding eyes rest speculatively on Jake and Lardis at the bar, but only for a moment. Then he finished by saying, "So that's that. For now let it go. Let's all of us let it go. But Liz, try to remember what I've said. And the next time I ask you to do something, don't be so damn quick off the mark to question my motives. . . ."

Meanwhile, at the bar, Jake had asked the bartender for a sedative, something to help him sleep during the next stage of the journey. And after the man had gone off to fetch him something:

"Haven't you had enough of sleep?" Lardis asked him.

Jake looked at him. "Sleep is a funny thing," he said. "Do you know what my doctor told me, when I was laid up in hospital in Marseille that time, after I'd got myself trampled on?"

"But how could I possibly know?" Lardis answered, as yet a long way from mastering the vagaries of the English tongue. "It isn't as if I was there with you, now is it?"

"Anyway," said Jake, "I had things to do and wanted to be out of there, but they wouldn't let me go. And this doctor told me I needed to rest, get some sleep. He said there were different kinds of sleep: a kind that comes from physical exhaustion, and another from mental. And that even when you've done no physical or mental work, there's the kind that tells you your body and brain have been mobile for too long without a decent break. Sleep is a medicine—the best you can get—following injury or mental trauma, yet too much of it can be debilitating rather than curative. You can walk and talk in your sleep, and in some cases solve intricate problems. Sleep can be induced, resisted, prolonged, or interrupted, but no one can do without it for too long. . . ."

As he fell silent, Lardis said, "*Phew!* Ask a simple question!"

Jake nodded his agreement, said, "I'm not usually so long-winded, but it's been on my mind—not so much what that doctor said about sleep, but the things he left out. At the time those things didn't apply to my case. Now they do."

"I'm learning a lot about sleep!" Lardis grunted. "Tell me more."

"It produces dreams," said Jake. "Often they're enigmatic, unsolvable, and they're usually unremembered because they don't mean anything. Are you with me?"

"And I'm learning a lot of new words, too!" Lardis sighed. "But go on, go on."

"But from time to time," Jake went on, "from time to time, they *do* mean something. They're like—I don't know—clearing houses for all the jumble of our waking hours. And when the rubble has been cleared away, sometimes there's a silver nugget or two left over."

"And you've been pros—er, prospec—er . . ."

"Prospecting?"

"Right! Right?"

"Aboard the jet-copter," Jake answered, "I'm sure my dream—my nightmare—meant something. And I want to get back into it." He offered a weary shrug. "I must be crazy, right? To look forward to returning to a bad dream? But anyway, what the hell? I may have been sleeping, but I didn't get much rest. I'm still dead on my feet."

"It's the heat," said Lardis. "It drains a man's strength. I'm tired, too . . . we all are. On Sunside I'd probably be under some tree right now, asleep in a deep cool forest. But I've had trouble with my dreams, too, Jake. The fact is, I'd probably be nightmaring about the hell that's brewing in Starside! And that kind of sleep . . . well, you're right: it can't cure anything."

"Me, I'll risk it anyway," Jake muttered. "Just as soon as I'm back on that chopper."

When the pilot declared the jet-copter refuelled, the two technicians were the first out across the asphalt. Jake and Lardis were next, and tailing them Trask, Goodly, and Liz. They had at least one hundred and fifty yards to walk to the helipad.

"Funny thing," Goodly reported as they left the embarcation building and set out into the sizzling sunlight, "but what Liz said suddenly makes sense. There's Jake in plain view, not forty yards ahead, and I can't read a thing of his future. Not any longer."

"But isn't that normal?" Trask was immediately concerned. "Aren't you always telling us that this talent of yours isn't controllable, that you can't just switch it on and off?"

Goodly nodded and said, "Right. But I should at least be aware of something. My original prediction, that Jake would be with us for some time to come, hasn't changed. The future doesn't chop and change like that; what has been foreseen is inevitable . . . or it should be. It's *how* it will be, its circumstances, that can change. But now, with Jake, I can't sense a damn thing! It's as if there were nothing there."

"Like he's shielded?" Now Trask was even more concerned.

"I suppose so, yes," said the precog.

"Huh!" Trask grunted. "It's the same for me. I thought I was imagining it. I still know the truth of him, the reality? But I'm no longer sure whose truth it is."

"Harry's dart?" Goodly wondered. "The Necroscope had powerful shields. Has he perhaps passed them on to Jake?"

"Yes, Harry was shielded," Trask answered. "Him, and the traitor Wellesley, too. But Nathan also has shields, and likewise—and especially—the Wamphyri! So Harry isn't the only one who could have passed this on, whatever it is. And I can't help thinking: maybe it hasn't been passed for the best possible reasons. I mean, why should he want to keep us out?"

And Liz put in: "Maybe it's not deliberately or aggressively active, but just . . . active?"

"Like something new, feeling its way?" Trask said. "Well, it's possible, I suppose."

"You could always check it out," the precog said. "David Chung can locate us—any one of us—just like snapping his fingers. He'd soon tell us if we have something of *that* nature travelling with us."

"Mindsmog?" said Trask.

By which time Liz was thoroughly alarmed. "Or it could be just his taint!" she now broke in. "Harry's taint, I mean. For he was after all—"

"—We know what he was," Trask quickly cut her short.

"And we knew *then* what he was," Goodly said, taking Liz's side. "And we accepted it. You especially, Ben. It was you who let him go, remember? When Harry's house—his last vestige on Earth—when we burned it to ashes, you could have killed him then."

"I could have tried," said the other.

"But you didn't."

"We all have our talents," Trask argued. "Maybe mine told me it wasn't possible."

"And maybe it told you to let him live," said Goodly. (As Trask's closest friend, he was the only member of E-Branch who had ever been able to talk to him as openly as this.)

"I was younger then," Trask answered gruffly, "and a sight more foolish. The Necroscope could have been lying when he said he was quitting Earth for Starside. Talent or no talent, I didn't have the right to take that chance. But I did. Foolish, as I've said."

"Younger I remember," the precog nodded. "But foolish? If Harry hadn't lived, what then? Who would have stopped Shaitan, and given his life for us in the vampire world? And what would have been our fate then? The chance that you took paid off."

But now the jet-copter loomed, with Jake leaning out and down, offering a helping hand to Liz. And: "We'll just have to let it go for now," Trask murmured, his voice almost inaudible even to his companions as the engine coughed into life and the rotor blades began slicing the air overhead. "But that doesn't mean we'll stop watching. And sooner or later, we'll see what we'll see."

What he didn't tell them, keeping it back for the moment, was that in fact he had already contacted David Chung by telephone from the airport. From now on they wouldn't be the only ones who were "watching."

And while Chung, the Branch's top locator, would still be far distant in the purely physical sense, psychically he would be very close indeed—and closer in both senses when he found a relief to take over his duties, allowing him to join up with his colleagues in Brisbane.

. . . so damn hard to get in?! The hinted question but definite exclamation rang like a shout in Jake's sleeping mind, startling him. But he immediately recognized the "voice" and said:

"You? I was hoping you'd come by."

You could have fooled me! said the ex-Necroscope. *But for that tiny piece of me that will be with you always, I wouldn't know where to find you. Even with it, it's hard to*

*get through your shields. Still, maybe that's a good thing.
I'm sure it's going to be, eventually.*

"But where are you?" Jake had been waiting for everything to straighten up but nothing had, so that now he wondered: *And for that matter, where am I?*

He was floating. Not surprising, really, for he had often dreamed he could fly, and as often been disappointed on waking up to discover that he couldn't. This must be a different version of the same thing. But floating in darkness?

You don't recognize the place? Harry Keogh's disembodied voice asked him.

"A place?" Jake answered. "But there's nothing here. Nothing at all." And as he lazily turned (or at least he *felt* like he was turning) on his own axis, he could see that what he had said was literally true. There was absolutely nothing here. As if this were the bottom of a bottomless pit, or the darkest of dark nights, or—

Or the kind of nowhere and no-when place that the universe must have been like before there was light? Yes, I know, said Harry. *Once experienced, however, there's no forgetting it. So when we were here last you must have had your eyes shut. I can understand that. It's always been the same, and for just about everyone who ever tried it—including me! So now let me welcome you to the Möbius Continuum. No gravity or light or matter at all. Not even a sound unless we make it, which* isn't *advisable. Not here.*

"And this is it? Your way of . . . of getting about?"

This is it. But it's still only a dream. Your *dream, Jake. And the only thing that's real about it is me.*

"So how did I get here?"

I influenced it, and you dreamed it. I just wanted you to see it through my eyes, and maybe get used to it. For you see, you've been lucky on three occasions now. Three times when you thought you were in danger—two of which you really were—I was close enough to help you out.

"My escape from jail?" Jake nodded his understanding. "And the next time from Bruce Trennier, right?"

Right. But as my dart—let's call it my metaphysical

intuition—becomes a more accepted part of you, there'll be less room for the actual me. Already you've reached the stage where you're almost able to shut me out. But before you can do that, you still have a lot to learn.

"About the Möbius Continuum?"

For one thing, yes.

(Jake was still turning; he didn't know which way was up, but he wasn't at all dizzy from it). "And that's why I'm here?"

You tell me. You dreamed it! But it's as good a starting place as any.

"You did influence it, though?"

Yes, but you must have wanted it. Wanted to visit, wanted to know.

"To know how to use it, you mean?"

Exactly. And how not to misuse it.

"Eh?"

Well, if this were really it, the Continuum, you'd probably be stone deaf by now. You see, you don't talk in the Möbius Continuum, Jake—not in a place where even thoughts have weight.

"Thoughts have weight here?"

They do in the physical world, too. Ask any telepath, or any scientist for that matter. Those tiny sparks that jump the gaps in your brain, Jake? If they didn't make the connections, you couldn't think. Have you never wondered why geniuses have "weighty thoughts?"

"But that's just an expression, surely?"

But in the Möbius Continuum it's reality. Well, of sorts. A parallel reality, at least.

"So . . . I've no need to talk?"

Not at all. Thinking will suffice. But here in your dream it makes no difference—because you aren't talking anyway. Or at best you're only muttering to yourself.

"You're making me feel like a cretin!" Jake burst out. "I don't know where I am or how I got here—or how to get *out* of here—and you're telling me I have a lot to learn about it? A lot to learn about nothing, about nowhere, about emptiness?"

Oh, it isn't nothing, Jake. It isn't nowhere, but a route to every-where and-when! Let me ask you to do something for me . . . actually, for you. Just keep quiet for a moment or two, and float. And feel it! Feel the Möbius Continuum!

Jake did, and felt it. "It's . . . big," he said then, feeling very small. "It's . . . huge! It knows I'm here, and it doesn't especially want me here. But *where* here?"

Everywhere! said Harry. *Or anywhere. Anywhere you want to be, want to go, as long as you know the coordinates. Come with me. Just* come, *and you'll see.*

"You mean follow you?" And suddenly Jake was afraid. "But I can't even see you!"

I'm in your head, Jake. Just let go.

"Of you?"

Of everything.

And Jake did it, let go. He sensed motion in himself, and also felt himself come to halt. At a door.

A time door, said Harry. *A door on past time.* And:

"But this is even more like a . . . a . . . *ahhhh!*" said Jake. Because now he was standing on the threshold, looking back into the past. And while it wasn't deliberate he was echoing what he seemed to be hearing:

A concerted *"Ahhhhhh!"* like some unending one-note chorus, the vocal product of a vast choir of angels echoing in a sounding church or cathedral. And yet Jake only *seemed* to be hearing it; it was in his mind as a result of what he was seeing, which must surely be accompanied by just such a *sound*—the sound of life, of evolution, from its prehistoric source to this present moment, this very NOW.

More like A Christmas Carol? Harry finished it for him. *I suppose it is, in a way. But this isn't a ghost of the past, it* is *the past—as viewed in Möbius-time.*

Looking out, looking back, through the door, Jake saw what appeared to be the core of some vastly distant nova, an incredible neon-blue bomb-burst, whose streamers were lines of light. A myriad endlessly twisting, twining, frequently-touching lines or neon tubes of blue light, all reaching out from that central explosion, expanding towards him, rushing upon him like a luminous meteorite shower. Except the tracks didn't dim but remained printed on space—indeed, printed on time! And all Jake could say was, "W-what?"

The blue life-threads of humanity, of all Mankind from its very beginning, Harry told him, quietly. *And that central nova: that is the beginning, the source, the birthlight a quarter of a billion years ago, when our ancestors crept out of the soupy oceans to evolve primitive lungs on volcanic-lava beaches.*

"Life-threads?" Jake whispered. He had scarcely heard the other, was merely repeating him like a man in a dream— which of course he was.

The tracks we've left in time, Harry answered, *like metaphysical fossils. A photograph of Man's snail-trail, his evolution from his humblest beginnings. The proof of it is there, Jake, right before your eyes. For see, one of those blue life-threads connects with you. Follow it back far enough and you'd see it blaze into being, a pure blue glow to light you on your way through life. The moment you were born, yes . . . And:*

"You don't appear to have a thread," said Jake. But since the explanation was obvious, he quickly went on: "If I were to trip and fall through this door, I might fall all the way back to the Big Bang!"

No, Harry told him. *But if you willed it you might travel back through all your ancestors to the beginning of life. Awesome, isn't it?* And before Jake could answer:

Back there some little way I saw your blue thread crossed by scarlet. But the vampire threads stopped right there, while yours sped on. It was Bruce Trennier and his brood, when they died the true death.

"At which time," Jake frowned, "—what, just yesterday?— I had already received your dart. Some kind of paradox?"

He sensed Harry's shrug, his irritation. *But that was one of the reasons you received it! Time is relative; what will be has been. You think of time as having been, or as being now, or as still to come. But the way I see it times are just different places, all within reach. It's the fourth dimension, Jake. And the Möbius Continuum lies parallel to all four. As for paradoxes: they'd be rife if we could actually change the past or see the future. That's why precogs like Ian Goodly have such a hard time of it. It's why they are allowed to know something of what will be, but never how it will be.*

Jake looked again through the door and made a futile effort to follow the track of the neon-blue thread that flowed out of him where it twisted and twined its way to his origins. Perhaps he would see what Harry had seen: scarlet threads crossing it in Möbius-time and coming to an end there. But among all the myriad lives that had been, his was soon lost to sight.

"All the world's past," he said.

This time I helped you find it, said Harry. *The next time—if you should ever need it—you could well be on your own, so try to remember these coordinates. As for future-time doors: that's easy. They point the other way, that's all! You'll work it out* (a barely suppressed chuckle,) *in time.*

"I . . . I shouldn't be here," said Jake, suddenly dizzy. "I mean, no one should be here."

That's a normal reaction. (Jake sensed Harry's nod.) *Anyway, we have to be moving on. Those names you gave me: I found a connection, someone who knew their owners.*

"N-not in this world, you didn't," said Jake, as the time door closed. "They were Wamphyri and came out of Starside."

True, said the other, *but they didn't come alone. I . . . I have been advised to look up someone who came with them. And I think you should meet him, too.*

More motion—an acceleration—that Jake sensed rather than felt. "W-where are we going?"

To the Refuge.

"But it isn't there any more."

Its ruins are.

"But why there?"

To talk to someone who died there.

"Someone who died? Past tense? But we can't be going into the past. The past-time door has closed."

That's right. And anyway it's not physically possible, not for you. You couldn't materialize there. No, we're going to the Refuge in your present, your now, your dream.

"But if this someone is dead, how can we . . . ?"

Too many buts, said Harry. *And anyway, we're there.*

"There" was an awful place to be. Jake was up to his knees in cold water, in a darkness almost as deep as that of the Möbius Continuum itself. The water—river water from the resurgence, he supposed—slopped around his legs and roved on, while the unseen ceiling dripped cold moisture down his collar. The atmosphere was stale, still foul with a lingering stench of smoke, spent explosives, and . . . other tastes and taints.

As Jake's eyes grew accustomed to the darkness, he began to make out certain features of the cavern . . . and saw that it was more than just a cavern. It was the sump, what was left of it in the aftermath of Zek Föener's horrific, heroic death. Now he remembered Trask's story, also something of what Harry Keogh had said: that they were here to talk to someone (a dead someone?) who had come through from Starside with Malinari and the others. And:

Oh, he's here, the incorporeal Harry told him, causing Jake to start yet again. *Zek, too, but she has company. Good company, as do a majority of the dead. A Great Majority. When Zek is . . . when she's* accustomed *to all this, then I'll return and talk to her about old times, remind her that we'll be together again—all of us—eventually. But that might take some time yet, for Zek was very much alive. She was one of my very dearest friends right to the end. Which reminds me of our reason for being here . . . to talk to the other fellow.*

Harry's voice had dropped to a low growl; it seemed to Jake that an unaccustomed darkness had crept into it, and a very uncharacteristic threat. So threatening, in fact, that in another moment his mind went into overdrive as he identified the source of his main concern, which until now had mainly been lost among the minutia and maziness of dreaming: the fact that Harry Keogh was here to talk to someone who was dead.

"The other fellow?" Jake repeated his still unseen companion. "I thought Zek was alone down here? And anyway, how can—you—we—talk—to . . . ?" But by now everything was coming together that much faster, including things Jake really didn't want to think about, but which were there anyway.

Like the meaning of a certain word or name: Necroscope. And what the precog Ian Goodly had told him about Harry: that he didn't view life and death the way others do, and his means of communication was *similar* to telepathy, but he had a different name for it.

Like what? Like necromancy?

"You're a necromancer!" Jake gasped, before he could check himself.

No!!! The incorporeal other's denial lashed him, like a cry of rage in Jake's cringing mind. *Whatever else I am or may have been, I'm NOT a necromancer! Never call me that again!*

And now another voice out of nowhere, but sweet as a breath of fresh air to fan Jake's feverish mind. And despite that he'd never known her, still he knew her: Zek Föener!

Necromancer? Ah, no, (her voice was a sigh). *Just call him Harry, and know him for a true friend. And as for this— this blessing he gave us, letting us comfort each other through the long lonely night of death—do you take it for an evil thing? Then you're mistaken. It's our one light in this eternal darkness. And you may simply call it dead-speak. . . .*

18
Korath's Story

I KNEW THAT YOU'D BE BACK, HARRY, ZEK SAID. *from the moment I saw you ride away on that big American motorcycle, with Penny, on your way to Starside, I always knew you'd be back. I sensed you in Nathan; it wasn't really you but . . . but a like-father-like-son thing? This time it really is you. And you're as different from the dead now as you were from the living then.*

Zek, Harry answered, his deadspeak voice crestfallen now. *I didn't mean to disturb you. That's the last thing I wanted.*

But you of all people should have known, she scolded him, however gently, however fondly, *that what we do in life we continue to do in death.*

"And you were a class act," Jake cut in. "A telepath, and a good one."

She was the best, Harry told him. *And apparently she still is, except it's no longer telepathy but deadspeak.*

Your ma was your spokesperson in the long ago, Harry, Zek reminded him, *but it looks like I'll be taking over. The Great Majority haven't forgotten you, and I know they'll never forget your son, Nathan. But you'll appreciate that toward the end . . . well, there were problems.*

Problems Jake doesn't know about, Harry quickly put in. *He doesn't need to know. He's having a hard time accepting some of these things as it is, and I don't want to—you know—put any additional strain on his faith in me? Also, if you're to become a spokesperson, it will be on Jake's behalf, not mine. You see, I have very little of permanence here. Already this is taking a great effort of will. As Jake takes on my work there'll be even less need for me, and my presence that much harder to maintain. As for Nathan, (a touch of*

253

sadness now in that ethereal voice,) *I've never met him. He received his ultimate awareness through me, it's true, but he was, is, and will always be his own man.*

"And I won't be?" said Jake anxiously.

See? said Harry, a tinge of sarcasm showing. *He's one very suspicious man, this Jake Cutter.*

"If you're hiding things from me, how can I be otherwise?" Jake countered. "First Ben Trask and E-Branch, and now you. So what are these problems that I don't know about?"

All in good time, Harry answered. *It takes time to become a Necroscope, Jake. With me it was accidental—or perhaps it was in my genes, my birthright? I'm not sure—while with you it's just blind chance. But that blue thread of yours, in future time...?* (Jake sensed a deeply-etched frown, the shake of a puzzled head.) *Anyway you're it, or you will be, so get used to the idea.*

"I'm it? You mean a Necroscope?"

No, I mean the *Necroscope,* the other answered. *You don't know how rare this thing is! There will be just the one Necroscope, you. In this world, anyway.*

"And if I don't want to be 'the' Necroscope? If I have my own way to go, which to me is just as important?"

For long seconds there was silence, until Harry said: *Then it could very well be that you can kiss your world goodbye.* His deadspeak voice was very low again.

"You don't leave me much choice, do you?" Jake answered, a little bitterly. "Why don't you just—I don't know, scan the future, use a future-time door, or some such—and see how things turn out without me?"

You're going to have to start listening, said Harry. *Look, you can't trust the future. The past, yes, because it's fixed. But not the future. The one thing I* can *tell you is that you'll be meeting up with vampires—Wamphyri! The question is: do you desire to meet them on your terms, or on mine? With your meagre knowledge, or my experience and skills?... Assuming you can develop those skills, that is.*

Jake thought about that, but in fact there wasn't a lot to

think about. He believed Harry Keogh now—believed in his own five senses, too,—also in certain *extra* senses, which had now been so compellingly demonstrated—and he completely believed everything that Trask and the others had told him. In total, it left him with only one conclusion: that it was real, and he was up to his neck in it.

And up to his knees in this dark water, and still not entirely sure what he was doing here. But while listening to these dead voices in his head, his dream, Jake had also looked about, obtained a picture of where he was. It could only be that Harry was showing him this place telepathically, for it was in no way dreamlike. It was totally real.

The caved-in ceiling, sagging in places and in others bulging upwards from the furious force of powerful explosives; the collapsed stanchions, great tangles of shattered metal and concrete, cratered from the blast and blackened by fire. And back there along what was once the course of the subterranean river, the way completely blocked where the original cavern's ceiling had succumbed to man-made convulsions and its own great weight of fractured rock.

Dramatic, but not what we're here to see, said Harry, satisfied now that Jake had at least accepted his involvement, if not the all-important role he was to play in what was to come. *So now come this way, to where he died.*

Harry was in Jake's mind, guiding his feet; all Jake need do was follow where the other led:

To the solid, twelve-foot-thick, reinforced concrete wall of the dam which contained the dynamos and sensitive equipment that once supplied and monitored the Refuge's power.

The once-smooth face of the concrete wall was gouged and pitted, blackened in places, but it was still intact. Built to withstand the pressure of the water, it had also withstood the pressure of the blast.

That's close enough, Harry said, bringing Jake to a halt where the water was a little shallower. *There could well be . . . remains down there, under the water, that you wouldn't want to step on.*

"Remains?" Jake said. But no need, for the more he conversed with the other in this way, the more he was given to understand that *like* telepathy, deadspeak frequently conveyed more than was actually said. The remains that Harry referred to were those of the lieutenant or thrall that Malinari and the others had used to block one of the outlets, by which means attracting attention to the sump and making possible their escape.

As that fact dawned, Jake stiffened; the short hairs rose on the nape of his neck as he took a pace to the rear, wrinkled his nose in disgust, and swallowed to ease the sudden, involuntary constriction of his throat. The water seemed to gurgle more blackly, viscously, around his calves, as he saw the curved rim of a steel conduit projecting from the dam wall.

Perhaps mercifully, he could only see the uppermost curve of the pipe, while the bore itself—and what it contained—remained hidden in the swirl of black water.

Jesus Christ! Jake thought, and at once sensed Harry's reproval.

Try not to do that, Jake! For expressions have crept into common speech that never should have.

"But . . . they stuffed a man, one of their own, in there?" The concept was horrifying. But not nearly as awful as the new voice that now joined the conversation.

A man? (that deep bass voice rumbled and grunted). *Was I a mere man, then? Korath Mindsthrall, a mere man? Ah, but don't let my name mislead you, for then you might consider me a mere thrall, too! Aye, and so I was at first. But all that was thirty thousand sunups agone, when first Lord Malinari found me in Sunside. After he recruited me, then, I was his thrall, next a lieutenant, finally his chiefest lieutenant. I stood alongside Malinari during his years of power, of treachery, when his name was a curse even in the aeries of the Wamphyri! I was banished with him out of Starside into the Icelands, and we suffered the ice together in the company of frozen beasts. I was there with my Lord at the freezing, and at the melt . . . and this is my reward.*

Jake had backed off, found himself a dry ledge of concrete fallen from the ceiling and crept up onto it. He sat there hugging his knees, shivering, but not from the cold. That was only in his dream. The real cold was in his mind, in the awful voice from beyond the grave. Or rather, from beyond death, for Korath Mindsthrall had never known a real grave.

"And is this . . . is this your secret?" Jake was appalled, as much by the cold dread, the loathing in his own voice as by anything else. "Is this what it means to be a Necroscope, 'the' Necroscope: to suffer deadspeak and talk to things like Korath? His thoughts are . . . corruption! Not the things he says but the way they feel. I can't feel you, Harry; you're there in my head but unobtrusive, not so much an intruder as a guide. But Korath . . . I can *feel* his thoughts like slugs oozing in my head, polluting my mind!"

He sensed Harry's grim nod of agreement. *Exactly. Just as his rotting body polluted this water, before his flesh sloughed from his bones. But this is where he died, and this is where he is. Now maybe you can understand why Ben Trask was reluctant to tell you everything. It's not every man who could bear to speak to the dead, Jake.*

"It certainly isn't this one!" Jake gave his head a wild shake. "In fact all I want right now is to get the hell out of here!"

NO! NO, WAIT! Korath Mindsthrall begged. *Don't go! Don't leave me! Before you there was nothing, only darkness and loneliness, and the sure knowledge that I was shunned. I have listened to the teeming dead whispering in their endless night, and I know they whisper warnings of me: that I am a vampire, a* terrible *creature best left to its own devices. Well, and so I was a vampire. But now . . . I have no devices! I have nothing. Why, even my flesh has melted from my broken bones and is gone from me! Have you no pity, you warm ones? I may not harm you. I am nothing. DON'T LEAVE MEEEEEE!*

And just as suddenly the loathing was gone and Jake found himself pitying this Thing. Until Harry told him:

That, too, is a mistake. Vampires are the greatest cheats and liars imaginable, devious beyond measure. This one, Korath, is no exception. Later, we'll ask him why Malinari

257

chose him—"his chiefest lieutenant"—to block this pipe, when he had at least three others to choose from. On a whim? Hardly. You don't indenture or instruct someone for as long as Korath Mindsthrall claims he was in thrall, just to kill him out of hand. Malinari had a reason.

NO! Korath howled. *That is a lie! No, no—forgive me—not a lie but . . . but a misconception? Malinari had no reason; he was never required to reason! He was The Mind, and whatever he willed be done. Flesh was needed to block this pipe, and my flesh . . . it was pliable and available. That was enough. Say no more.*

So, said Harry, *your flesh was pliable—*

But not that pliable! The vampire cut in. *You cannot possibly imagine the agonies that I . . .*

—And you were compliant.

I was not! (Korath denied it.) *I did not know! Lord Malinari sent out his thoughts; they touched upon the man who tended this place and understood machines. But The Mind was clever and careful. In Sunside there are Szgany who know when the Wamphyri are near; they close their minds, think no thoughts and so hide themselves from the Great Vampires. Perhaps in this strange new world there would be men like that. Ever stealthy, Malinari ensured that his presence went unsuspected. And he took knowledge from this engineer, and learned the ways of the sump, which was my downfall! My master told me the pipe was a way out. He bade me crawl inside to make sure the way was clear. When my shoulders would not go, he and Vavara and Szwart summoned their furious Wamphyri strength to break the bones in my back and shoulders and drive me home like a stopper in a bottle. . . .*

Zek? Jake? said Harry, and there was something new in his low deadspeak voice. They knew what it was: that he spoke only to them, that he was shielding his thoughts from Korath Mindsthrall. *Let me handle this. Zek, it probably isn't going to be pleasant, so by all means leave it entirely to me. Korath will say things you don't want to hear. And so might I.*

I'll absent myself, she answered him at once. *I've had my fair share of dealings with vampires, as you know, and I don't need reminding. Jake, I look forward to working with you if or whenever you need me. Meanwhile there are others I should talk to, and let them know you're here. You won't be alone, Jake.*

Before the dreamer could answer there was an emptiness in his mind where Zek had been, or not so much an emptiness as an awareness of her leaving. And: "How about me?" he asked Harry. "Any chance that I could perhaps 'absent myself', too?"

None at all, Harry told him. *You don't have to join in if you don't want to, but you should at least listen. If I can, I'll get Korath to tell us his story; or more importantly, his master's story. And those of Vavara and Szwart, too. If you're going to defeat your enemies, Jake, you need to know them. Why don't you just take it easy this time out and listen in? Learn something about the Wamphyri and their ways, and learn it from the horse's—or the vampire's—mouth?* Without waiting for an answer, he spoke again to Korath:

I've a mind to leave you "to your own devices," yes. Just as the teeming dead advise. But that would make me as cruel as the master who crushed you and left you here to die. And so I'm tempted to stay with you awhile, and converse with you in your loneliness, which you must know will last forever and ever. But on the other hand—having had to do with vampires before—I see no point in talking to one who is bound by his very nature to tell me nothing but lies.

Korath's answering cry immediately went up: *Ah! Ah! Have mercy! Have mercy! Pity me, I pray. For a moment then I thought that you had gone, I thought you had left me! Then I felt your warmth—though yours is not so obvious as that of your friend, er, Jake?—and so knew you were still here. Now hear me: I am a gruff and violent vampire, that is true, but I was not always this way. I was made what I am, by Malinari! Made by him, and now unmade by him. So what more harm can he do me? Who or whatever you are, talk to me. Only allow me to bathe in your light, which burns like a candle in this intolerable darkness, and ask of me what you will. I shall not lie. As men are known to speak the truth on their deathbeds, so I shall speak it from beyond.*

I want to know about Malinari, said Harry. *And Vavara and Szwart. I want to know* all *about them, from the beginning.*

And Korath eagerly answered: *None knows their stories better than I. But . . . such tales will take time in the telling.*

I have time, said Harry. *Well, within certain limits. And so do you.* You *have an eternity of time.*

One question, said the other.

Ask it.

Why?

Because I would exterminate them and all that they stand for, Harry answered, truthfully and ruthlessly. *Their kind are not wanted in this world.*

Good! said Korath, his voice gurgling with phlegmy anticipation. *Why should they have life, having deprived me of mine? In Starside we acknowledge four states of being/unbeing. These are, one: the void before birth. Two: the time of warm-blooded life such as the Szgany of Sunside enjoy it. Three: a "higher" condition known as undeath, when a man's existence might possibly reach to eternity. And four: the true death, which is nothing less than a return to the primal void. But I, Korath, have found the last to be a lie. It is a darkness, aye, but never a void. The true death is an absence of motion, but not of mind. I think! I am! But immobile, forgotten, lost in the long, long night, I have no peace. So why should the ones who put me here have peace? Why should they have anything? No, I will not lie to you, Necroscope.*

Then get on with it, said Harry. *Begin with Nephran Malinari, since he would seem the most dangerous.*

Wrong! said Korath. *For each is as bad as the others. Why do you think they were banished out of Starside?*

Doubtless I'm about to find out, said Harry. *But I'll warn you now: while time is not of the essence, don't try to spin it out. I'm not long on patience and could be about better things. Is that understood?*

It is indeed, the vampire answered. Then:

Without pause Korath got on with it; and by virtue of the nature of deadspeak—also because the ex-lieutenant's tale was illustrated with vivid mind-pictures—Jake found himself listening in. Along with his mentor, he soon became absorbed in the narrative. . . .

"It was hundreds of years agone," (Korath began) "though to me, having spent so much time in the ice—frozen and stilled, and preserved even in my thoughts—it stands out in my memory like yesterday. Or perhaps yestereve.

"I was of the clan Vadastra; indeed, I was the son of the chief, Dinu Vadastra. Our place was in the forest many miles to the east of the great pass into Starside. We toiled in gathering and growing, in the breeding of domesticated livestock, and in hunting and fishing. Being settled—unlike the majority of the Szgany, who are nomads—there were no bounds for my father to beat. In any event we were not troubled by foreign settlers; indeed our land was shunned by all the neighbouring tribes. For you see, my people were supplicants who gave of their goods (a portion, or 'tithe' as you would say) to Lord Nephran Malinari, called Malinari the Mind, out of Malstack in Starside.

"Now, do not ask me if I enjoyed our situation. I was born to it and knew no other way. Likewise the Vadastras as a tribe; only the old men of my people had been travellers, who in their time had known the ways of the true nomad. The life of the supplicant suited *them* to perfection; the Wamphyri had no use for ancient, withered flesh or desiccated blood. And so the elders were safe so long as they could work, gathering the wild honey and fruits of the woods. My father was also safe, for while he had not as yet grown long in the tooth, still he was the chief of his people, whom Malinari had appointed keeper of the tithe . . . for which reason he was greatly feared and in most matters obeyed without question. In most matters, aye.

"And my father, Dinu Vadastra, was a hard man: tall, broad, and a bully. When lesser men complained of the 'theft' of their wives, sons, or daughters taken in the tithe, he would deal very harshly with them. Why, they might even find *themselves* listed as troublemakers and, regardless of the draw, destined for Malinari's great aerie when next his tithesmen did their rounds.

"There was a girl I loved . . . at least I *think* I loved her, but all such things are a mystery to me now. Love? That is for the warm ones. Now there is—or there was—only lust. When my master and his lieutenants hunted among the so-called 'free' tribes of Sunside, oh, *then* there was lust! *Ahhhhhhh!*

"But please forgive me my meandering mind. For I see that you do not wish to know that. . . .

"As for this young girl whom I may or may not have loved, more anon. Let it suffice for now to say that she was my downfall. The first of them, anyway. . . .

"Now understand, Malinari was not greedy—at least, not when the Wamphyri were at peace with one another and no bloodwar was raging—but he was ever choosey. His tithesmen, lieutenants all, knew that he wanted only the best out of Sunside. No curdled honey, bitter plums or scrawny beasts for Malinari, and no snaggle-tooth boys or bow-legged girls, either. And my father was always hard put to fix a 'fair' tithe. He might on rare occasion slip in a barrel of less-than-best plum brandy, a crippled shad or a brace or two of game left hanging just a day or so too long, but never anything outrageously offensive. And he was the same in his dealings with human flesh.

"Loners, if they saw our campfires in the night and came down from the barrier mountains to warm themselves, were ever welcomed. They would be given food and drink—aye, and a lot of the latter—before being tapped on the head and laid aside for the tithe. And if the cart or caravan of some lone traveller's family group should happen onto Vadastra territory, well that were reckoned a bonus. For then fewer of our own would be needed for the list.

"We were some three hundred and eighty. The number rarely rose by more than a dozen or so, and when it did was as readily reduced. In any given year, perhaps fifty babies would be born; with any luck half would grow to adults while the rest would be borne away into Starside. My Lord Nephran Malinari . . . was reputed to have a sweet tooth for basted infants.

"But I must not jump ahead of myself, for at that time he was not my Lord as such. Or rather, I was not as yet in thrall to him.

"Where was I? Ah, yes: the tithe:

"Married men who sired no children for a year or two were wont to find themselves shortlisted. And as for women who were barren: their future, or lack of such, was guaranteed. Likewise any troublemakers, of course. Thus the tribe maintained itself, barely, and the tithe saw to it that we were never too large or small. Once in a three-month Malinari's tithesmen would come on their flyers over the mountains from Starside, and now and then the master himself would accompany them on their visits.

"And now to this girl, whom I may even have loved.

"My father kept her back from the tithe, for me. Alas that he had crossed so many of his own people, who suspected that he was biased in certain of his duties—in the quarterly drawing of the tithe-markers, for instance—and there were plenty who would pay him back, who would like to see *his* loved ones on the list. Or rather his loved *one*, this selfsame Korath, whose poor mother had died giving birth to him.

"But the girl Nadia . . . she and her mother were gatherers, as were most of our women, and both of them were among the comeliest of Vadastra females. Nadia's father had been a talented hunter, until nine months agone when his marker came up in the draw. That had been that, if not quite as *easy* as that.

"For he was young and strong as a bull shad; he had to be knocked down, bound in all his limbs, and even gagged before he would be still! And because of accusations he'd made concerning my father—the way Dinu had looked at his wife—there might be some who suspected that their chief had 'fixed' certain matters in his own favour. Make of that what you will, but I won't deny that from then on Nadia's mother was Dinu's . . . or should I simply say that she submitted to Dinu, and leave it at that? But his? His property? His obedient woman? Ah, wait and see. . . .

"The fact was that Melana Zetra had loved her husband, and when she was over the horror of his being taken in the tithe—and when she was close to my father, *and* after she had covertly investigated the way he worked the list—then she made up her mind to act. I cannot state Melana's reasons for doing what she next did; perhaps it was madness brought on by grief, but if so she had hidden her condition extremely well. Or then again, she may have been crazy like a fox and simply biding her time.

"My best theory is that she would be with her husband, Banos, again, regardless of the conditions, and had determined to sacrifice herself to that end. Banos had been taken by Malinari of the Wamphyri; now Melana would be taken also. But along the way she would settle a few old scores. The Szgany can be devious in their own right, and I cannot help but wonder if that is where the Wamphyri get it: is it perhaps in the blood? For the blood is the life, after all.

"But if this secretly incensed or maddened Melana would be with her husband in Starside, why not make it a family affair? What of her daughter, Nadia? Would she be safe on her own with the Szgany Vadastra, or better off in Starside with her mother and father? Being comely, it was unlikely she'd be fodder; why, given time she might even become a Lady! Could it be any worse to be undead *with* the Wamphyri than to live under the constant threat of being stolen away or eaten *by* the Wamphyri? And what of an informer? Might not he, or she—as a supplicant in the fullest, truest meaning of the word—gain favour in the red-litten lamps of their eyes? I suspect it was a mixture of all of these imponderables that motivated the maddened or scheming Melana to do what she did next.

"The time of the tithe was at hand, and Dinu Vadastra had

calculated correctly that Malinari would come with his lieutenant tithesmen out of Starside. It had been some time since
The Mind himself had deigned to venture forth from Malstack across the barrier mountains into the velvet of Sunside's night.

"The skies were clear and the moon tumbling on high; all
the familiar constellations were twinkling in the smoke of
our signal fires, while low over the barrier mountains the star
of ill-omen—the Northstar, which lights the aeries of the
Wamphyri—bathed the peaks with its silvery-blue ice-chip
gleaming. A fine night, aye, for some. . . .

". . . As it might have been for me if not for my now
barely-remembered love of Nadia Zetra. Still, I cannot blame
her, for I am sure that Nadia knew nothing of her mother's
plan. If she had . . . it's more than likely we would have fled
from our fate, becoming loners; or we might have journeyed
west and joined up with some band of true Travellers in their
constant evasion of the Wamphyri; or perhaps we would
have been happy simply to be free a while, together she and
I, and let the future take care of itself. Oh, a great many
possibilities, if Nadia had known.

"As for my father: if *he* had so much as suspected . . . then
Melana's life were forfeit long before the first of Malinari's
flyers touched down on Vadastra soil. But of course none of
us knew, except Melana herself.

"And so to the preparations.

"All was in order. As the dusk settled in, Dinu had called
for the tributes (in fact the ransom, for the life of the clan
Vadastra) to be displayed on trestle tables to one side of the
clearing, where he had tallied them as was his wont. Six
barrels of oil, six of white wine and six of red; six of good
plum brandy (and all of it *good* plum brandy, mind, because
Malinari was coming), and six more of wild honey. A pair
of young bull shads, freshly butchered, fifteen brace of pi-
geon, and five of wild boar; and a very special prize indeed:
a live, caged wolf of the wild, a bitch at that, and pregnant
to boot! The Wamphyri are especially fond of wolf cubs
basted in their mother's milk, and of heart-of-wolf and wolf

meat generally, which they swear by as an aphrodisiac and positive aid to their longevity. As if they needed such!

"And meanwhile Dinu's specially chosen squad of bully boys was out and about, to ensure that certain *other* tributes—of the human variety—were not fled. For while the tithe-markers were already drawn, the unfortunate parties had not been named for fear that they would make off into the night. Thus, as the time drew nigh, the wailing of mothers and daughters, the curses of men and the sobbing of their sons could be heard in and around the camp, as one by one the various listed 'names' were informed of their misfortune by Dinu's tithe-takers.

"Some were already known, of course: the troublemakers in their cages, and outsiders who had wandered inadvertently onto Vadastra territory. But the three males, three females, and six infants of the clan itself, their naming was left to last, for the reasons stated. Then they were gathered in by Dinu's bully boys, chained and gagged before they could voice any great complaint or cause commotion, and tethered to await the coming of the tithesmen and their vampire master, Lord Nephran Malinari. As for the babies: they were wrapped in bundles on the trestle tables, along with the other wines, victuals, and sweetmeats.

"Myself: I was with Nadia, 'safe' in my father's caravan. From peepholes in the withe walls, silently and scarce breathing, we watched and waited as instructed. For my father liked to keep his prized ones (I still find the idea of 'loved ones' hard to envisage) well out of sight of the Wamphyri, so as not to arouse their interest. Likewise Nadia's mother, Melana Zetra; Dinu had advised her to remain out of sight, hidden in her caravan, lest being comely she attract unwanted attention.

"And in the fifth hour after sundown they came.

"The skies had been clear, as told, and only a warm breeze, like the breath of the dreaming forest, to tease the flames of the campfires and stir the branches of the trees about the central clearing. But the Wamphyri have their own weird ways with nature; they work their will on air, earth, and water as acid works on metals, etching them to their design.

"We had seen it all before: the mist gathering on the high peaks and rolling down like some vaporous avalanche, all milky-white in the moonlight. The sudden flurry of cold air down from the barrier mountains, beating on the flames of our fires as if to smother them, and lashing the gentler winds of the forest to frenzied flight. And suddenly, from behind the peaks, the first stain of dark clouds writhing blindly out of the north, feeling their way like snaky fingers and obscuring the glittering Northstar as they came.

"And in those clouds, riding on high, swooping and fluttering like withered leaves caught in a flurry—yet unlike leaves *directed* and with purpose—the scaly flyer mounts of the Wamphyri!

"And oh, the moaning and gibbering of those plague winds, as the creatures that rode them—and the Ones who rode *them*—came on, gliding, descending, trapping the air in the scoops of their webby membrane wings, and settling to the foothills over Vadastra territory . . . except, as by now you have surely reasoned, these lands were Vadastra in name only.

"For in fact they belonged to Lord Nephran Malinari of the Wamphyri. And Malinari had come to collect his tithe. . . ."

19
Malinari

IN THE GLOOM OF THE WRECKED SUMP, IN THE dark of Jake's dream—which was in fact much more than a dream, indeed a metaphysical connection through Harry Keogh to an ex-lieutenant of the Wamphyri—Korath Mindsthrall continued his story:

"There were vampires and vampires. In Starside's great aeries of the Wamphyri as were, I saw some who were hideous beyond description, too monstrous to look upon even through a thrall's eyes.

"In general they would keep to their manlike outlines, but would shape their various parts to their own design. Their ears were often carved and fretted into fanciful sculptures; convolute nostrils might be pierced and hung with rings of gold; arms lengthened to extend their reach in battle, and teeth permanently enlarged until speech itself was difficult. Lords frequently kept battle-scars as trophies; a flayed cheek might be made to heal so that the white of the bone showed through; a gouged eye could be grown elsewhere than the face.

"In those days there was a young Lord called Lesk the Glut because of his appetites. Stolen as a child out of Sunside, he grew to a youth, became a lieutenant, eventually slew his master for his leech. But Lesk was a madman, and the stolen leech only enhanced his madness. When his murdered master's familiar warrior hesitated to answer to Lesk's command, he actually did battle with the thing . . . *and* killed it! He won the fight but lost an eye, which he grew again upon his shoulder.

"Organs such as these were rudimentary. Some Lords deliberately affected an extra eye at the nape of the neck . . . sufficient to give warning of an attack from the rear. And these eyes would be lidless, so that they could never close in sleep.

"I mention these things so as to illustrate the hideousness of which I have spoken. But in fact those Lords—and occasionally Ladies—who affected such alterations or mutilations were usually the weakest of their kind; they only made themselves to look ugly so as to present more fearsome facades in battle, and so perhaps to avoid battle entirely.

"Take for example Volse Pinescu, called Lord Wen, which was surely the greatest possible misnomer. What, just *one* wen, when in all likelihood Volse was the ugliest of all the Lords of the Wamphyri? For it was Lord Wen's habit to foster hairy blemishes, running sores, and festoons of boils all over his face and form in order that his aspect would be that much more terrifying. Do you see? No clean man or thing would strike him for fear of the drench which must surely ensue!

"Even amongst the highest ranking vampire Lords, there were several such as Lesk and Volse. But then again, there were also those who had no need for such deceptions and affectations. And Nephran Malinari was one of them.

"For he was vain and he was handsome ... ah, but this, too, was a facade in its way. For The Mind was a monster underneath, even as monstrous as his mind, if you'll forgive this puny play on words. But at least in his *appearance* Lord Malinari was less the beast and more the beautiful human being; more truly, well, 'lordly,' as it were. But for something so very terrible to be so beautiful, surely that were the ultimate deception?

"Back to that night:

"Seven great flyers had landed on the rim of a broad ledge, a false plateau in the foothills overlooking Vadastra territory. Malinari's mist (for you may be sure it was of his manufacture) rolled down to flank him and his, then spread out and descended to the forest. It was met by a lesser mist that sprang from the soil and woodlands themselves, so ringing in our rude homes and their central clearing. And all about us a sea of white-lapping mist; and in the clearing itself a ground mist—but unlike any natural mist, sentient and sick-feeling—writhing and twining about the cabins and long-immobilized caravans where the latter were all propped on their empty axles. Malinari's thoughts were in the mist; they felt things out, searching for treachery. But there was none. Or at least, not towards Malinari.

"The wind had fled south and the night was still again. As the mist slowly dispersed, the flyers launched from their foothills ledge and came gliding on stretchy membranous wings.

"Now, the flying mounts of the Wamphyri are monstrous creatures, though not so much for any kind of malevolent activity on their part as for their appearance and nature. For while at first glance they seem like giant, long-necked and long-tailed bats, on closer inspection . . . plainly they are made from men! Their wings have enormous span, with the alveolate, once-human skeletons of arms, legs, and grotesquely *extended* fingers and toes all visible through the sheathing, grey-gleaming membrane of their envelopes. The creatures have massive hearts, to fuel the muscles that power their great wings; other than that they are little more than airfoils of flexible cartilage and hollow bone in sheaths of light, lean meat. In short, they are mainly wings with very little mind. Built to fly and obey—with their tiny, walnut brains linked invisibly, mentally, to their riders—they do nothing but what their masters will. Oh, they have bits in their mouths and reins for guidance, but only for emphasis when mental commands go lacking a ready response.

"So, now you understand me when I speak of 'flyers, descending towards our clearing on their stretchy membrane wings.' As for their riders:

"These soon became visible. Three of the seven—those in the middle of the V-formation—were at ease, arrogant, haughty in their ornate leather saddles; the others were young lieutenants, eager, forward-leaning, and feral-eyed. It was probably the first time they had been allowed to venture forth with Malinari's tithesmen. But the figure to which every eye was drawn was that in the dead centre of the aerial tableau. To him, and to his mount.

"That central flyer was by far the largest, strongest, and most elaborately fashioned; a handful of good men—perhaps as many as six or seven—had gone into its construction in Malinari's vats of metamorphosis in Malstack, in Starside. Gliding down towards the clearing, the huge but human eyes in its half-human head at the end of that long, snaky neck, swung this way and that, seeking an acceptable landing place; while black and seemingly vacant saucer eyes in its belly lidded themselves in preparation, so as not to suffer damage in the landing.

"Ah, but when I speak of eyes, do not let me forget those of the rider where they glowed like small scarlet lamps in his face. Of course they did, for this was Lord Nephran Malinari—Malinari the Mind himself.

"His flyer's wings formed themselves into air-scoops; its tail—the elongated, knuckled spine of a man—swung this way and that, keeping balance; coiled tentacles like springs extended down from belly cavities, their sensitive tips tracing the contours of the ground. Then, with a sighing of air and a folding of wings, the thing set down light as a feather. And flanking it, six lesser beasts likewise touched down, their lieutenant riders out of their saddles and striding to their master's side all in a few liquid moments. While for those same moments Malinari sat there as if in contemplation, reins loosely clasped, one elbow on the pommel of his saddle, and chin in hand.

"Then, stirring himself up, he swung lithely down from his mount, sighed, and said, 'Well, and here we are.' Simply that, the merest murmur of a sound; yet powered by Malinari's mentalism, every man, woman, and child in the entire Vadastra settlement heard it! And to every mind he touched—despite that his voice was brandy deep and honey sweet—a certain fetor clinging. For with all his powers of deception, even Malinari could not hide the underlying stench of blood.

"His mentalism had its limits. Spread thin as this, it was good for seeking out enemies or Szgany in hiding, but very little else. So that having displayed it he now dispensed with it. And the swift withdrawal of his probes felt like water clearing from one's ears after surfacing from a dive in a deep pool. And now, too, he called for my father Dinu in a voice both rich and strong. But while the brandy depth was still there, the sweetness was all used up. For now it was time for the business.

"The Vadastras (all except the few favored ones, who were hidden away) were gathered as a clan on that side of the clearing farthest from the barrier mountains, so positioned that all eyes had been enabled to follow the arrival of Malinari and his tithesmen. My father, who stood central and to the fore of this gathering, came with all speed in answer to

Malinari's call and prostrated himself before his acknowledged master. And the vampire Lord stood there a little while, looking down on him, perhaps enjoying his grovelling.

"But, *ahhhh*—this Malinari was *handsome!* He was all of an hundred and sixty years old, but looked no more than forty. His hair was black and shone like a nighthawk's wing—as well it might, being greased with the fat of Vadastra women! Swept back from the broad dome of his head, behind pointed ears which were not as large or misshapen as the webby, conch-like ears of most Lords, and with its jet ringlets curled on his caped shoulders, while its gleaming black curtain fanned out down his back like the hair of a young girl, or the decorative head plumage of the black eagle . . . why, it loaned him the haughty looks of a great hunting bird—a *veritable* nighthawk, aye! And for once it was no deception; for as much as he was anything, Malinari was certainly the bird of prey.

"And his face, its deathly pallor . . . the deep-sunken eyes under arcing eyebrows . . . cheekbones jutting . . . the high brow rising . . . slightly flattened nose whose convolute flanges were almost imperceptible . . . the lean cheeks and perfect bow of his bloodred lips. The red of blood, aye, to match the fire of his eyes. In any other man or vampire the fiery lamps of Malinari's eyes would be less than ornamental, but they suited The Mind to perfection. Indeed, they loaned his cheeks a ruddy semblance of warmth, of life, while in fact he was the cold and cruel master of something *other* than life, but not yet death.

"And tall: he would be two long paces tall, and then some. And slim as a wand, yet strong as a dozen of our best, who were only men. I knew this last for a certainty, for there never was a weak Lord of the Wamphyri. But Malinari's strength wasn't of the flesh alone; not only brawn, but brain; not merely muscle, but mind. He *was* The Mind!

"And, 'Up,' he finally commanded my father. 'Up, and show me my tribute.'

"There was no kissing of sandalled feet, nor yet of hands,

as my father came erect; no touching of any sort. Such were The Mind's powers that even a touch could prove harmful, draining a man's knowledge or erasing part of his memory. And anyway Dinu was Malinari's trusted servant who would not dare hold anything back from him. This was how it had been between them for many a shameful year. Shameful, aye. For if I've not already said that I loathed this cringing, sub-servient existence, surely by now I have hinted as much?

"Anyway:

"My father was big, burly, bearded, and blustering. Rumor had it that he was a bastard, too, but I never heard it bruited in his presence. Puffed up with his own importance, yet somehow managing to bow and scrape, he led Malinari and his men to that side of the clearing where the trestle tables were bowed a little from the weight of the tribute. Here Dinu Vadastra had been as clever as he dared to be, so arranging the trestles that the centre spans were bound to bow a little under any extra weight! Whether or no his ploy fooled any-one, it certainly looked good. And indeed Malinari seemed impressed.

"Then he and my father conversed. And because Dinu's caravan stood very close to the trestle tables, and the night being so still now (and likewise all those who were not di-rectly involved, keeping *very* still), Nadia and I heard their every word.

" 'Dinu, chief of the clan Vadastra,' Malinari spoke to my father. 'It appears you had word of my coming. I would even say you *must* have had, since you've responded with this oh-so-excellent tribute! What's more, try as I might I cannot remember the time when my tithesmen brought home so handsome a bounty. What? Why, I could even be forgiven for thinking that perhaps they've been robbing me all this time. My own lieutenants, like ungrateful dogs, thieving from the house that shelters them. . . .'

"He stared at his men—glared at them with eyes of flame, lengthened his jaws and yawned at them a little—so that they all drew back a pace . . . until he grinned a wolf's grin at them, then threw back his great head and laughed until his hair shimmered all down his back.

" 'Ah, but see, I have made a joke,' he said. 'For all and all, my lieutenants, thralls, and familiar creatures know that to thieve from me is to bid farewell to all this. My rules are made simple, so that even a dullard may understand them. In my manse in Starside dwell many starveling warriors who have their needs no less than men; from time to time they enjoy the occasional tidbit, and to a monster they are especially fond of tidbits that kick and shriek and spurt red. . . .'

"And after a pause, turning to my father: 'Dry work, this joking,' he said. 'Are we perhaps thirsty, Dinu Vadastra?' And he beckoned to his side a junior lieutenant.

"By then, as might well be imagined, my father was *very* thirsty. He produced a tray of beaten gold, and three goblets of that same common metal which he filled with white wine from a barrel. This was ever the ritual: that Dinu play the part of one of Lord Malinari's food-tasters. For like all of the Wamphyri but more so than most, The Mind was susceptible to silver in however small a measure—indeed to *granules* of silver, to the very *dust* of silver—and likewise to garlic, whose mere reek was guaranteed to cause nausea and copious vomiting. Thus Dinu would take the first sip, which would provide him with an early opportunity to declare the wine fouled; next the tithesman, who being a vampire would not only taste any poison but react violently to it; and finally Malinari, first inhaling deeply of the wine's bouquet through his snout's fleshly funnels, before gulping it down. For however much he affected lordly airs, and, on occasion, a 'flowery' or 'delicate' mode of speech, still Lord Malinari's table manners were dreadful!

"So on through every barrel, a taste from each; the brandies, too, and even the honey. And while my father was sensible enough to drink but sparingly, still he was staggering a little towards the end. As for the foodstuffs—the wild grain, roots and fruits, animals and such, aye, and bairns, too—they were not tested, though for a fact Malinari lingered a while over a fat boy child whose black eyes smiled at him in all innocence, while the monster's own crimson orbs flared that much brighter in his face. . . .

"Then on to the wolf-bitch in her cage: 'A prize indeed!' Malinari approved. 'I may keep her and her whelps both,' and he made as if to stroke her through the bars. But growling low in her throat, she snapped at him, and Malinari withdrew his hand with no room to spare, saying, 'Or perhaps not. For wolves are plaguy, treacherous beasts at best. But fine strong meat, Dinu Vadastra, I'll grant you that. And on that same subject, where, pray, are the rest of my animals—the ones who walk upright?'

"With which the unfortunate ones, all sorted and chained in a row—a man, a girl, a youth, a woman, and so on—were trooped out for Malinari's inspection. They had been caused to void themselves (for the sake of "cleanliness,") then had been washed, groomed, and clad in good fur robes fastened with golden clasps. And there they paraded, most with bowed heads, but a few of the younger men muttering (however unwisely), and the adult women sobbing, and this or that young girl far too prideful, too aware of her lithe Szgany sensuality, head tilted and dark eyes fluttering, daring to gaze on Malinari and even hoping to impress him. Ah, but The Mind was not easily impressed.

"He walked the line—or rather flowed along it, with that deceptive grace of the Wamphyri—and his tithesmen with him, senior men to the fore and juniors well to the rear. And whenever Malinari paused to look closer at one of his male acquisitions, then his senior lieutenants would step forward and take hold of the man, forcing wide his jaws so that the Great Vampire could examine his teeth. Then they would unfasten his gold clasp, displaying his naked body, and sometimes Malinari might indicate his approval of a youth's long limbs and broad shoulders, murmuring, 'This one is for the making, I think. In Malstack, my vats stand empty.' Or, 'This one is a fighting man, tall and well-muscled, aye.' Or again, he might say nothing at all, but simply shake his head. For there was always the provisioning.

"In a while he came to one of those *too*-proud girls, who

dared to gaze upon him, and paused. Again his senior tithesmen moved forward, one of them reaching for the clasp at the girl's throat to open her robe. But she was a beauty, and the lieutenant too eager. Noticing this, Lord Malinari caught his hand and stayed it, then narrowed his eyes in a frown, saying:

" 'Ah, but see how your blood courses, Stefanu. Why, I can feel it pulsing through your veins like a raging river! And so you're a lustful one, are you? But you know—now that I think of it—I have often wondered why, when I send *you* out to collect my tithes, I get so few virgins?'

" 'Master, I—' said Stefanu, trying to back off. But Malinari held him, saying:

" 'Ah, *ah*, be still!' And he touched the index finger of his free hand to the man's brow. Stefanu groaned, jerked, began to lift his right hand where it was sheathed in a murderous gauntlet. This was wholly a reflex action, nothing more, but Malinari had seen it. His eyes blazed up at once, like coals under the bellows, and as his jaws elongated and his lips curled back from scythe-like teeth, so Stefanu fell to his knees and begged for mercy.

"Then for long moments Malinari's index finger trembled on his lieutenant's forehead, and his face writhed in a passion as he read the man's thoughts, at least the ones that were important to him. Until suddenly, straining as if from some enormous effort of will, he snatched back his hand and snarled:

" 'Oh, you miserable, lecherous man! Consider yourself fortunate, for while I have had your thoughts, I've left your mind intact. Not out of any love for you, Stefanu Mindsthrall—ravisher of my women before I've so much as seen them—but because I may soon have need of you. And treacherous? Did I not see you raise your hand, your wargloved hand, against me? Did you dare think to strike me? Perhaps you did! And so for now . . . *begone!* Remove! Take yourself from my sight. Get to your flyer and wait for me there, and consider your treacherous ways: what you have done this night, and to whom, and what it would be like to live out the rest of your life floundering and drooling, mindless in a pit of your own wastes—which might *yet* be your get from all this!'

"He released Stefanu, and when he had wriggled away, stumbled to his feet and fled, Malinari said to the girl, 'My dear, give me your hand.' She obeyed him at once. And using his mentalism he saw what only he could see, then asked her, 'Are you truly a virgin?'

" 'Oh yes, my Lord,' she answered. And Malinari nodded and smiled.

" 'Had you said no,' he told her, 'I might have made you a lieutenant's woman, for your honesty. But I abhor liars, however pretty—especially little whores who would attempt my seduction by trying to hide their thoughts from me. Wherefore . . . no high station for you, young lady, but there are common thralls in my manse who will enjoy instructing you. Or you them, whichever!' And wrinkling his nose, he shrugged and turned away from her.

"Malinari's inspection was over. And now he told Dinu Vadastra, 'I am not displeased. Not with you and yours. But you've seen how I deal with them who would deny me my due. So now tell me truly: was this the best you could do?'

" 'The Vadastras have never made finer wines or brandies,' my father answered. 'As for the foodstuffs, no better flesh may be bred or hunted, no purer honey or sweeter fruits foraged. On my word, my Lord, this is our best.'

" 'And what of the tithe in human flesh?' Malinari glanced at the robed ones in their chains. 'Are these also the best you have to offer, or do you hold something in reserve?'

" 'Again I've done my best,' Dinu told him. 'But certainly I must have a reserve—of good blood, good flesh for breeding—lest the Vadastras falter and become useless to you.'

"And Malinari nodded and said, 'This was always our understanding, aye. But Dinu, take heed, hard times are coming, and my needs are great. Do you see this dark cloud hanging over us, like a portent of ill-omen? What say you, chief of the Vadastras? It seems to me it bodes not well.'

"And when my father glanced at the heavens—indeed

there was a dark and hovering cloud, which until now had gone mainly unnoticed. It turned slowly in the night-dark skies over Vadastra territory, and within its writhing mass, riding the laden air, darker shapes seemed hidden.

"So that Dinu's voice was less certain, small and faltering, as he inquired, 'W-w-what does it mean, my Lord?'

"But The Mind's 'cultured' tones were grown very deep and menacing now, and his scarlet eyes more truly aflame as he answered, 'It means that despite our—what, our friendship?—and despite that you have been a true and honest man . . .'

"At which point there sounded a small commotion; a fluttering figure appeared at the rim of the tableau, and: 'What? A true and honest man, this Dinu Vadastra? This so-called chief? This great thief? I say wait, give me but a moment to show you that you are *wrong*, my Lord!' The voice was shrill and female.

"And Nadia, where she huddled close to me in my father's caravan, started and gasped, her hand flying to her mouth. For she had recognized the voice: that of her mother, Melana Zetra, who came hurrying now from her hiding place. And:

" 'But what is this?' Malinari arched his eyebrows, and his forehead creased in a frown. 'Someone dares to raise her voice, to interfere, and to command Nephran Malinari to wait?'

"For a moment Dinu Vadastra was stunned; likewise the rest of the clan, including Nadia and myself. But as Melana came in a rush, her hair awry and her face gaunt with fear— the terror of what she was about—it was observed that she wore a robe of offering. And indeed she was offering herself, of her own free will, to Malinari and his tithesmen! Ah, but she was offering a deal more than that.

" 'What?' said Malinari again, in utter amaze, as she threw herself down before him, clawing the earth at his feet. 'Is she a mad thing, that she interferes with the tithe?'

" 'Mad with grief!' Melana cried, tearing her hair, throwing off her robe and kneeling there naked. 'Mad with rage, and with outrage. For I have been cheated and used badly.

My people too, and even you, my Lord, cheated! All of us—by this man!' And she pointed a trembling finger at Dinu.

"It was the beginning of the end. And any observer could be forgiven for thinking that Dinu was himself Wamphyri—the way his eyes popped out like plums in his face, and the way he bared his teeth—as he threw himself upon Melana and bore her down. His knife rose over the tangle they made . . . until Malinari took it from him, tossed it away, then grabbed Dinu by the scruff of the neck and drew him upright.

" 'Speak up!' he commanded Nadia's mother. 'How have I been cheated? Oh, be sure I could learn it my way, but the process is harmful and your chief might easily lose all powers of reason. Moreover, I would like him to hear for himself what may yet harm him even more. So say on, woman: tell me how Dinu Vadastra has betrayed me.' He looked at my father dangling in his grasp, his sandalled feet barely touching the ground, then grunted and thrust him away, sending him sprawling to the earth. Dinu would have attacked Melana again, at once, but a pair of lesser lieutenants were at his side, their gauntlets ready. And so he kept still.

"Then Melana spoke up, and the complaints she listed were the selfsame grievances that every decent Vadastra man, woman, or child capable of reasoned and intelligent thought had carried in his or her heart for long and long, without ever daring to give them substance. She spoke of the chief's many prejudices, and of his favourites—such as herself—who remained hidden away, secret and undisclosed to the Great Lord of Vampires, when his tithesmen came out of Starside to collect his tribute; and of Dinu's treachery to his own tribesmen: how, if he were jealous of a man's prowess, or if he should be bested in some piddling campfire argument, then the better man might expect to find himself listed for the tithe. So that for long and long, no one had dared say Dinu no.

"Melana went on and on, as if she would never end. For as my father's odalisque, she had been privy to a great many wicked things in his caravan—all of his conspiracies with his cronies—in the time since her good husband, Banos, was taken in the tithe. And so she lashed Dinu with her unforgiving tongue, which all the while gathered fire and passion; for Melana knew that one way or the other it was all done with now, and so she might as well do her worst.

"Then, towards the end, she spoke of her man, Banos Zetra; but here she broke down, sobbing her heart out when telling how Banos—a hunter whose contributions to the tithe had been significant—had been carried off to Malstack in Starside simply because Dinu Vadastra had fancied his wife for himself, and for no other reason.

" 'And here I kneel before you,' she finished at last, 'the living proof of all that I have said. But my man is in Starside and there's no place here for me now, for which reasons I would venture over the barrier mountains with you and yours, into the dark. And what of the ones that Dinu has hidden from you, great Lord? My daughter, who he saves for his own worthless son. Aye, and that selfsame son, Korath, who skulks like a whipped dog in his father's caravan there?' At the last she threw herself flat on the earth, sobbing and clasping Malinari's feet.

"And Malinari was silent for a while, as he considered all that he had been told. But meanwhile his men were not idle. Two of them were at the withe door of my father's caravan; finding it barred from within, they tore it from its hinges. And one of them poked his head in and saw us, calling out: 'They are here, my Lord. A youth and a girl, huddled in the dark like mice. The woman spoke the truth.'

" 'So,' said Malinari, and his voice was doomful quiet now, even as quiet as the strange dark clouds circling overhead. 'If she spoke the truth, then someone has lied. Bring these mice to me.'

"But my father cried out, 'My Lord! Have mercy, I beg you! He is my son, and the girl is his woman, and—'

" '*And* . . . you kept them from me,' said Malinari, silencing him with a glance. 'I was not shown them, nor asked if I wanted them. You desired no mercy of me then, only now. Like the child who steals a plum, then asks if he may have

280

one. Or in this case two plums . . . or three, if we include this good brave woman.'

"He stooped and caught up Melana's robe, took her shoulder and drew her to her feet. 'Cover yourself,' he said. 'I believe there may be a position for a hard-working woman—as an overseer of women—in Malstack in Starside. Moreover, I know of a certain thrall called Banos, who has not taken any woman of the manse in all the time he has served me. And Banos has served me well . . . unlike several I could name.' He gloomed on Dinu Vadastra, then across the clearing to where a certain senior lieutenant sat all morose astride his flyer.

"And though Melana fastened her warm robe about her, still she shivered. She had felt the weird cold when Malinari touched her, the tendrils of sentient ice that flowed from his fingers. Yet still she was the brave one. 'What of my daughter, my Lord? My beloved child, still innocent despite this unworthy Korath's vile embraces?'

"Malinari looked at her and raised an eyebrow. 'You should be aware,' he said, 'of the thin line between bravery and utter folly. I'm not much known for listening to complaints, and even less for granting wishes.' But then he sighed, and said, 'First let me see this girl, this—'

" 'Nadia,' Melana told him.

" 'As you *will*,' Malinari nodded. 'This Nadia. And for that matter, this unworthy Korath, too.' And his lieutenants dragged Nadia and myself before him. Thus I came face to face with Lord Nephran Malinari, of the Wamphyri!

" 'Are you your father's son?' he questioned me.

" 'Eh? Er, pardon?' (For how to answer such a question?)

" 'Eh? Pardon?' He mimicked me. 'Are you a cheat and a liar like your father, Dinu Vadastra?'

"Well, I wasn't like my father to that extent. But big and brawny I was, and perhaps a little stupid, too. 'I'm no cheat,' I told him. 'And no man calls me a liar.'

"When he moved I did not even see it! But I felt his clout, the thud of his back-hander against the side of my head, making my ears ring and knocking me off my feet. Well, it seemed plain to me that I had offended him. Now it was time to die—but not without a fight. I sprang up—and was at once pinioned by the men who had brought us from the caravan. But struggle as best I might I couldn't shift them or throw them off. And Malinari, he laughed, saying:

" 'Hold still and listen. You are big and handsome, and you are strong as a bull shad . . . and you are mine! Unworthy? Well, maybe. We'll wait and see if blood runs true. But first there's work for you, a chance to prove yourself, in Starside.'

"He turned to Nadia. 'You're the image of your mother. But are you as brave? Will you come into Starside, of your own free will, to be a vampire with your father and your mother there?'

" 'I have no other life, Lord,' she answered.

" 'But you will have,' Malinari told her. 'For you shall be a stable-maid, tending my flyers in their pens, in Malstack.'

"Then in a trice, in a flowing motion too fast to follow, he leaned to her neck and bit her! It was the work of a moment, to put his life—or undeath—into her, then into her mother, so that swooning, they collapsed on the earth. And finally Malinari turned once more to me.

"Held fast by his men, and stiffened by my terror, I could do nothing but stand stock-still, like a shad in the slaughteryard, with my eyes half-shuttered.

"But no, he merely wrinkled his nose at me, and his lieutenants did the rest. . . ."

20
Dark Lords of Starside

KORATH MINDSTHRALL WAS IN JAKE CUTTER'S mind as surely as his own thoughts, so that rather then having the story related to him, it was as if Jake lived it.

And that's dangerous, said Harry Keogh, "awakening"

Jake to his true position in the wrecked sump of the deserted Romanian Refuge. Except that wasn't the true picture (or his true location) either, for in fact he was only there by courtesy of Harry's mind-link. Jake's living, sleeping, dreaming body was airborne in a jet-copter flying east, somewhere over the Australian Simpson Desert.

"Dangerous?" Jake said, hugging his knees where he sat on a slab of concrete fallen from the ceiling, watching the black waters of the sump gurgling by. "What is?"

To let a vampire—even a dead one—get that deep into your mind, Harry answered darkly. *That's what's dangerous. And I think our friend Korath is stretching things out a bit.* But:

I am telling it the way it was! (Korath's "voice" again, protesting.) *You have asked me to tell you about Malinari the Mind. How may I comply without describing his deeds, defining his wickedness?*

Very well, Harry told him. *That's accepted. But I'm sure you can do it a little faster. Our time is limited here.*

I shall do my best, Korath answered, grumblingly. *But in any case, the rest of that night is a blur, for I had been bitten, vampirized by Malinari's lieutenants. The scenes . . . they all flow into one in the eye of my memory. Perhaps I desire to forget them, for what remains of them is . . . not pleasant. And the Vadastras were my people, after all.*

Then he was silent for a moment or two, until in a little while he picked up the thread of his story. . . .

"The bite of the vampire brings about a weakness, a lethargy, a heaviness of limbs and thoughts alike. If Malinari himself had taken my blood—and in the process transfused something of his essence—then I would remember nothing at all until much later. But I was strong and his lieutenants were only thralls. Oh, they were powerful men, and each and every one an aspirant, but they were not yet Wamphyri!

"Nadia and her mother, I saw them carried off towards the flyers while I reeled between the two who had recruited me. And Malinari, seeing that I was conscious, nodded his approval—of me, my strength, I suppose. But my senses were swimming as from drinking too much brandy; if one of his lieutenants had let go of an arm, I'm sure I would have fallen.

"Then . . . I remember . . . or I seem to remember . . . Malinari's voice raised, calling to my people, the entire Vadastra clan where they huddled at the far side of the clearing. 'Come join me,' he called. 'Eat, drink, partake of my tribute. For I shall free you of tyranny this night. This hated chief—this Dinu, of whom I've heard complaint—he is no more. Nor shall I require any more of you from now on. For I perceive that you have given enough. I free you, to be as you will, to do as you will, and to go where you will. Malinari has spoken . . . so let it be.' And his eyes burned brighter yet as he used his mentalism to reinforce his message, sending out his vampire thoughts to touch upon their minds.

"And drugged though I was—or rather, tainted with the essence of vampirism which now flowed in my veins—even I saw the pictures that Malinari painted in the minds of the people. Indeed, I may even have seen them more clearly *because* of that essence; but by that selfsame token I knew that those pictures lied:

"The glad bright faces of the young ones where they wandered hand in hand through the woods. The campfires where musicians played their bazouras and tambours; and meat roasting on spits while the menfolk clapped and young girls whirled in the dance. And wheeled caravans, trundling through the woods as of yore, bearing a people as free as the air; or at least free of Nephran Malinari, if not the rest of the Wamphyri. True travellers again, aye, in the forests of Sunside—

"—And all a lie.

" 'Come, bring your cups,' Malinari cried. 'Come drink with me, to your freedom!' And his men went among my people, leading them to the tables laden with tribute.

"But supported between them who had converted me, with my poor sick head lolling this way and that, I saw how the strange dark cloud—that cloud of ill-omen—was settling towards the clearing, and how a ground mist was once more gathering in the earth.

"As for my father: it cannot be said that he had been a good man, but where he grovelled now under the sandalled foot of a brawny lieutenant . . . who can say what thoughts passed through his mind? One thing for sure: he knew Malinari for a great deceiver, and his mind-pictures for lies. Also, he knew that he was done for; or in Malinari's own words, that the 'hated chief' of the Vadastras was 'no more.' Wherefore, what had he to lose? At least he might make a quick end of it.

"Squirming free of the lieutenant's foot, Dinu sprang up, pointed at the hovering cloud, and cried, "He brings his warrior creatures! He calls them down upon your heads! He destroys the Vadastras entire! Flee for your lives! Flee!'

"Too late, for again Lord Malinari was employing his mentalism, and now his pictures told the truth:

"Warriors circling in the shrouding cloud, held aloft on their fully-inflated gas bladders, extended air-scoop mantles, and spiralling updrafts from Sunside's night forests. Now they channeled gas to their propulsors, trimmed their mantles, came sputtering and issuing their poisonous vapours, descending towards the woods about the central clearing. And flanking them, controlling their tight aerial formation, a host of manta flyers, their eager thrall riders gauntleted to a man, and their purpose all too obvious!

"The tithe? *Hah!* Don't talk to me of tithes. Never such a tithe in all the history of Sunside. The tribute? But Malinari had come to claim the greatest tribute of all: an entire clan!

"The people fled. Coughing, choking, sickened by the vile exhaust fumes of Malinari's warriors, they fled for the forest . . . but again, too late. For the night was now a greater nightmare than ever. Hideous beasts were descending on the caravans and rude dwellings about the central clearing, flattening them to the earth. Vampire thralls slid down ropes dangling from the flyers. The people were surrounded. There was no escape!

"And through all of this, that demon Lord's laughter ringing out. And my father on his knees now, wringing his hands and asking, 'But why, Lord, why? Tell me this is not of my doing.'

"Above the thunder of raging warriors, the cries of lusting lieutenants and thralls, and the screams of the doomed people, Lord Malinari heard him. He swept back his robe, took his gauntlet from his belt and thrust his hand into it, answering, 'Your doing? Yours, Dinu? Do you truly think that anything you could do would be of any moment in this world? Because you were devious, is that your meaning? No, you fool, nothing is of *your* doing! Why, there never was a supplicant chief in all Sunside—from here to the furnace desert—who was *not* an enormous liar and cheat! It is your nature, even as it's mine.'

" 'But Lord, if not to punish me, why do you do this thing? Towards what end . . . ?' Dinu's jaw had fallen open; his eyes were wide in a face that craved understanding.

" 'It is the provisioning,' Malinari told him. 'But a *great* provisioning! My manse is a fortress where in times of peace we do well enough. But soon the peace will be ended. I am building an army, Dinu, and my needs are great. For in Starside a bloodwar is in the offing, and bloodwars are built on blood. In this case, yours!'

"With which he flexed his hand inside his glove, until all its hooks and blades stood out. And he cried out to his men and monsters: 'Take the young and healthy alive as best you can. As for the children, the middling-old and the dodderers—they are fodder.' Then, to my father:

" 'And you, Dinu . . . alas, you're middling-old.'

"His gauntlet of bright metal made a downward-sweeping arc in the smoky firelight, then gleamed red—dripped red—where he held it up to the reeking night. Almost as red as his eyes.

"And after that I saw no more . . ."

". . . Until I awakened in Malstack, my Lord's manse in Starside.

"Now, an aerie is an aerie, and all of them much alike. Or

at least they were in the olden times. Since when it seems some terrible vengeance has visited itself upon Starside; for I have seen the cadavers of those same vast dwellings, like the skeletal spines of giants, lying sprawled and broken where they fell on the barren boulder plains. And only hollow stumps remaining, mute revenants of castles that once were mighty.

"However, and in the time of which I speak: The Mind's manse stood far out on the plains, at the rim of that great clump of carven stacks, spires, and towers whereof the vampire Lords were wont to fashion their homes. Guarding its lower levels—in the scree jumbles at its foot, and in its high-walled, gantletted approaches—Malstack had many flightless warriors faithful only to Lord Malinari, who was after all their father. Lean and hungry, they were ever watchful.

"Within: there were wells in the aerie's basement, flabby siphoneers in the stubby turret of its roof, and in between all manner of levels to house Malinari's men and monsters, his vats of metamorphism and other workshops, stables for his flyers and warriors alike, launching bays, barracks for the soldiers, kitchens, workplaces, and quarters for specialist thralls such as weavers, metal- and leather-workers, and even musicians. Music, aye! For The Mind had something of an ear for Szgany tunes. The stringed bazoura with its swift, sweetly liquid notes was like a balm to ease the pain of his troubled head. For his mentalism was all things to Malinari: a blessing and a bane. One thing to hear the mere *voices* of men—when you have the power to stop them with a command or simple gesture—but something else to hear their very thoughts, so clamorous loud in your mind that you must struggle *not* to hear them!

"That was the curse of Malinari's mentalism: that it was there whether he wanted it or not. That while giving it direction, controlling it, took a great effort of will, shutting out its generally useless babble—the tumult of an entire aerie's thoughts—were almost impossible! And when the sun was up and the barrier mountains rimmed in gold, many a sleepless day for my master if not for the musicians who laved his mind with the songs of Sunside.

"But I fear I have strayed. For I was speaking of Malstack and now have returned to Malinari. Or perhaps not, for this was what you wanted: to learn about The Mind and his ways. And anyway, and as I've said, an aerie is an aerie, and all much of a kind. Enough of Malstack.

"So, what else can I tell you of my master as was? Let me think a moment. . . .

"His origins? Oh, yes, I know of them also. For with time, after I had proved myself as a thrall, rising through the ranks to become a lieutenant—and when during the bloodwars I became the first of his lieutenants—we got to be close, Malinari and I. Well, as close as master and slave can get. And upon a time, during a brief lull when we took respite in Malstack, I remember he said to me:

" 'Do you know, but what is in the blood usually comes out in the flesh?'

"To which I replied, 'Master?'

" 'Your father,' he said. 'Do you know how he became chief of the Vadastras?'

" 'I was a child at the time,' I answered, 'But yes, I remember. You made him the chief, my Lord.'

" 'And do you know why?'

" 'I have no idea, Lord.'

" 'Several reasons. One: because he desired the job. Among Szgany supplicants it takes a strong man—a man with a strong stomach—to be a chief and give away his own people. Two: because he was big and insensitive and a bully born, which I suppose is much the same as one. And three: because Dinu was rare among men, one of a small number that I could bear to converse with. Or rather, with whom I conversed on a level, without concerning myself whether or no they lied, and so not caring.'

" 'I am trying to understand, master,' I told him, since it seemed he required an answer.

" 'I divine men's thoughts,' Malinari explained. 'When they think against me, then I am . . . angered. And when I am angered, then I lose good men. Wherefore it sometimes serves me well *not* to read them! And I tell you, I lied to your father when I told him that his devious ways were known to me. Suspected, perhaps, but never known for a fact, not until the night when that woman he'd used betrayed him. Not that it mattered greatly; the Vadastras were doomed anyway, fuel for my bloodwar. Let me make myself plain: your father's mind was closed to me. As is yours.'

" 'Mine, Lord?'

" 'Indeed, for what is in the blood comes out in the flesh. You are heir to Dinu's mental processes . . . your minds are much alike, so that *your* thoughts, too, are vague and shadowy things to me, which I read as through a writhing mist. Oh, I could get to them more directly; should we say, by *contact?* With the very brain that holds them? For as you are surely aware, these fingers of mine are especially gifted in their own right. Alas, but that would probably mean the loss of yet another good man. That is a luxury which I cannot afford.'

" 'No, Lord,' I said, and I admit I backed off a pace. 'No, indeed, Lord!'

"But Malinari merely tut-tutted and shook his head, then winced and twitched a little as was sometimes his wont, saying, 'No, no! Have no fear, Korath. For while the rest of this manse of mine is filled with men and creatures—creatures with minds *that make noise and babble and uproar in my head, even when all else is silent!*—you seem as empty as those great dark spaces out between the stars. Oh, yes, and I like you for it.'

"Then in the privacy of my master's chambers, we would sit and listen to his music together—and I would try my best not to think. . . ."

"He told me of his beginnings.

"His father was Wamphyri: Giorgas Malin, who sniffed out even the craftiest of the Szgany by tracking the aura of their fear. He wasn't a mentalist as such—he read no minds—but he was *sensitive* to sentience, and knew when intelligent, fear-filled minds were close by. He sensed the shuddering and trembling of the very brains of his prey, even when they themselves were still and silent. Wherefore Sunside's nomads feared Malin worse than any other Lord; for despite their skill at cloaking their thoughts, he was usually able to discover them. In short, his talent had been similar to that of his son. Indeed, it had been the source of Malinari's mentalism.

"Or it was one of them. For of course Malinari was right: what's in the blood will out in the flesh. But it takes two to make a bloodson, a vampire born of woman, and The Mind's mother was a Szgany healer, whose power was in her hands. Do you understand the principle? She could cure the sick and the fevered by holding them, stroking them, by balming them with her lullabies and her loving touch. Ah, but I see that there are such in your world, too . . . faith healers, yes. And I also see that some are fakers, here as in my world. But Illula was the real thing.

"So, hunting in Sunside one night Giorgas found Illula the Healer—who had no man, for she had given her life over to her calling—and saw that she was beautiful. He had heard of her; the Wamphyri had their spies in Sunside, and little escaped the notice of the Starside Lords. However, there was no requirement for a healer in Giorgas's manse or in any of the aeries, for common ailments were unheard of among the Wamphyri, whose systems are so imbued with evil that lesser evils can gain no foothold. I exclude, of course, the various mutations, autisms, metamorphisms, and madnesses, with which the Great Vampires were ever afflicted, if afflicted is the right word. For apart from lunacy—oh, yes, and leprosy, the so-called 'bane of vampires' these other conditions were rarely considered illnesses at all; they were simply facts of life and longevity. For where men in their old age are prone to aches and pains, vampires in theirs are prone to all manner of weirdness.

"At any rate, while Illula's skills were of little use to Giorgas, her beauty—not to mention her virginity, which was a rarity in females of an age, even in Sunside—was a sure fascination. And of course he had the latter from her, then had her to wife. Yes, for Giorgas wanted sons to manage his aerie, and where better to get them than from a handsome woman? According to Lord Malinari, his sire was not without good looks himself; which perhaps accounts for The Mind's darkly handsome appearance.

"Ah, but the rare combination of Malinari's parents' talents accounted for a lot more than his merely physical attributes. . . .

"So, Illula the Healer was vampirized, and of course suffered the sleep of change. When she awakened, she was Wamphyri! And Giorgas's manse now had both master and mistress. But if men should be careful in choosing their wives, how much more careful in the making of vampires? Especially Great Vampires.

"Anyway, Illula was Wamphyri, and a deal of Giorgas's essence circulating within her; even the first nodes and filaments and foetal foulness of a parasite leech, gathering to her spine to suck on its marrow. That is ever the way of it. But as if to compensate for such depredations, the burgeoning vampire invariably accentuates the senses of the initiate. Not only the five mundane senses, but also—when such enhancement is of benefit to the parasite—any additional senses. . . .

"Illula and Giorgas shared a bed, and, of course—being his wife now and a Great Vampire in her own right—she clung to him through long Starside days, when the spires of the tallest aeries glowed golden in the seething rays from Sunside. And when her Lord started or moaned in his sleep (for even the most terrible of the Wamphyri are prone to nightmares, and some even more so, which usually spring from memories of their own conversions or initiations), then she would employ her healer's hands to soothe his brow and her soft-crooned lullabies to drive away whichever terrors invaded his dreams. But in the twilight before the night—when despite her ministrations he would come awake showing little or no benefit from his rest—then Illula would be nonplussed; and Lord Malin, he would laze around Malstack as if suffering from a crippling malaise ... which he was. And she was it.

"The fault lay in her once-healing hands, her once-calming songs, her once-balming presence. For now, enhanced by Giorgas's vampire essence and her ascension, her healing powers were reversed. Before, where Illula had given life— or at least given it back—now she drew it off. She battened on it like ... why like a vampire, naturally! For even if she would have it otherwise, her vampire would not. And there never was a vampire who *gave* of life, nor would there ever be.

"Thus Giorgas's life-force was drawn from him, and while he grew weak she grew strong, and her vampire stronger still. Wamphyri, aye, and what a monster she would have made. Except that wasn't to be.

"For she was pregnant by Giorgas, and on the day he died gave birth to a boy child whom she called Nephran, because that is the Szgany word for a wrong that may not be righted. And she knew that bringing *this* child into the world was wrong, but her mothering instinct made her keep him. As for his surname: certain tribes (Illula's being one such) used 'ari' as an alternative to 'son'. Thus instead of Malinson, he became Nephran Malinari.

"And as he grew to a man so the strange mixture or mutation of the joint skills of both of his parents—that which had been in their blood—came out in his flesh and grew with him. But unlike his father's half-mentalism, Nephran's was whole and wholly monstrous, and unlike Illula's healing touch, his was an evil life-devouring Power right from the beginning. And in combination these altered talents matured into the form which made him what he was and what he still is: Malinari the Mind.

"His love of music, he got that from his mother. Likewise his blinding headaches: she also passed those down to him. For as a healer in Sunside, that had been her payment—or lack of payment—for the good works she did: something of the illnesses of her patients transferred to her, presumably so that they might be cured! But in Nephran these migraines were made worse, complicated by the tumultuous, pounding thoughts of others.

"Well, and there we have the man. As for his mother:

"As time passed Illula's mind slowly slipped from her . . . or at least, the problems started with her mind. But gradually she developed so many illnesses in her body, boils and bruises, cankers and gangrenes, aches and pains and general disabilities, that her vampire was hard put to keep up. Let her parasite cure one disorder, another would spring up in its place. In Illula's more lucid moments, she would try to explain these things away: they were all the ailments she had cured in Sunside, now coming out in her. For her capacity for good had been robbed from her, and with it whatever was in her that kept these evils at bay.

"She might have died a slow death, or Malinari might have seen fit to put her away, but it didn't come to that. Illula's time was up and she knew it. When her son was eighteen she gave him Malstack, took a flyer and flew back to Sunside in the twilight before the dawn. Over the barrier mountains the sun found her, and she and her flyer both paid their dues in smoke, steam and stench.

"Well, and so much for Nephran Malinari's beginnings."

With which, finally, Korath was finished. For a while, at least . . .

Korath, you've done well so far, said Harry. But his dead-speak voice was noticeably fainter now. And before the extinct vampire could begin preening, Jake queried:

"Are you all right, Harry?"

I am . . . called *to many places,* the other answered. *I can be me as a boy, and as a man, or I can stand off and watch myself as I was. But I'm not much for doing what's already been done. And there are places to be where I need to be a lot more completely than I am here. None of which will make much sense to you, I know. But physically, I can effect very little here, except I do it through you.*

And Korath added, hopefully: *And through me?*

But Harry shook his incorporeal head. *You are less than*

I am. You can affect nothing, unless someone were foolish enough to let you get too deep into his mind, into his bones— which isn't going to happen. Jake, be warned: this Korath was a four-hundred-year-old vampire. If you should ever need to speak to him again, don't open your mind to him, not all the way. Never let him in, or you could end up carrying him with you forever.

And Jake shivered, hugged himself, and said, "Don't let it worry you. I can't see me returning to this place without damn good reason." And the water gurgled darkly, and the sump stank of nitre and stale explosives, of horror and death and crumbling, shock-stressed concrete.

Then . . . you are finished here? Korath's doomful voice trembled. *And is this my fate, to be left alone down here forever? Why, you have not even thanked me, much less pardoned me for being what I was made to be!*

Thanked you? Harry said, his voice still far-distant and faintly echoing. *Pardoned you? How many women did you rape and vampirize when you and your master "hunted" the Szgany in Sunside? How many good men have you killed with your gauntlet and your bare hands?*

Agghhh! Korath cried. And: *Ah, no, don't . . . don't remind me!* he pleaded. *That wasn't me! Or it was, but I was driven to do these things. I was driven by . . . driven by my . . .* (But here he came to an abrupt, stumbling, tongue-biting halt).

. . . By your leech? Harry finished it for him. *Your leech, Korath?* And then to Jake: *Do you see what I mean? Nothing more devious than a vampire, even when he's dead. This one had developed a leech and was ready to ascend. And Malinari was right to recruit him, for he was obviously the right stuff.*

"But he *is* dead now," Jake answered. "And being dead, what more mischief can he possibly get up to?"

I sometimes wonder if you listen at all! Harry told him. *I can only hope you'll remember some of this when you're awake.*

"Lord, who would want to?" Jake replied, then shivered and hugged himself tighter yet. "And talking about being awake—or if not awake at least out of this place—aren't we just about finished here?".

Jake, (Harry sighed,) *try to get this fixed in your stubborn head. I'm not sure I'll be back. I may not be able to come back. So while I am here you had better be taking in everything you can. And whatever else you do, remember that in future time I've seen your blue life-thread crossed by the red of vampires. So like it or not, one way or the other, it's coming.*

And Harry's deadspeak voice—despite that it was fainter yet—was so sincere, so urgent and fraught, that finally Jake had to take note of what it was telling him. With which he resigned himself yet again, and said: "So . . . what's next?"

Korath isn't finished, Harry answered, with something of a sigh—but different this time because it was a sigh of relief, not one of frustration. *We still don't know how he—how they—ended up here. We've only heard half of the story, and we still don't know very much at all about Vavara and Szwart.*

Jake might have contradicted him, for he had learned something of Vavara and Szwart himself, from Lardis Lidesci. Before he could speak, however:

Nor are you going to know much about them! (Korath's surly voice.) *Not from me, anyway. For you are ungrateful, and I have spoken my last.*

Not your last and not nearly enough, Harry told him. *Bluster all you like, Korath, but I say you will speak.*

Oh, and are you then a necromancer after all? Korath queried, sarcastically. *If so, perhaps I should point out that I've neither living nor dead flesh for you to worry with your pincers and hot irons.*

That's very true, Harry replied. *But I think I could probably find a bone or two, washed clean in this pipe—if I were a necromancer. But I'm not, and anyway there's no need. For you know as well as I that as little as you are now, if we take our leave of you, then you'll be even less. Or is our company worth nothing? In which case we must assume that you prefer this endless darkness, this eternal silence, and*

Brian Lumley

leave it at that. And leave you *forever and ever.*

After a long moment it seemed that Korath sobbed, but very quietly. Until finally he answered: *But you're a cold and cruel one, Harry Keogh.*

And Harry told him, *Ah, but I had good teachers. And they were vampires, too. So say on while you still have the chance, Korath, and while we are still here to hear you out. . . .*

21
A Dark Lady . . . And A Darker Lord

"FUELLED BY BLOOD, NEPHRAN MALINARI'S bloodwars were a terrible scourge on humanity," Korath picked up the threads of his story. "For as long as he ravaged on Sunside to provision fortress Malstack, so must the rest of the Wamphyri forage, lest Malinari's army so outstrip theirs as to whelm them under. Thus the Szgany suffered as never before—at least not for sixty thousand sunups—" (twelve hundred years) "since the mythic and immemorial time of Shaitan the Unborn's great wars, before he was unseated and banished north to the Icelands.

"The Mind's foes were many, his friends few. Even the latter were not his 'friends' in the human sense of the word, that sort of comradeship being so rare among the Wamphyri as to be a myth in its own right! But at any rate, his dubious allies were Vavara—a Lady in all but name, for she would not accept that men call her 'Lady' for fear it might damage her status by making her seem less than a Lord—and Szwart, which was the only name that suited a Thing such as he. Szwart, which means darkness! For indeed he *was* darkness, literally the darkest of all the Lords of the Wamphyri; something which I shall endeavor to explain in a little while. But for now, so much for Malinari's allies. Oh, there were a handful more, but Nephran, Szwart, and Vavara (who insisted upon the status of a man despite her obvious, indeed devastating feminine charms and attributes), they were the generals, the triumvirate, the Big Three.

"Then there were The Mind's foes, the enemy proper; first and foremost, Dramal Doombody, the most powerful of the Wamphyri of that period. Some thirty years earlier, at the pinnacle of his power, Dramal had contracted leprosy from a comely Szgany woman in which the disease had seeded itself but was not yet manifest; since when he had accepted to be known as 'Lord Doombody.' For of course his body *was* doomed, no matter how long it might take the great 'Bane of Vampires' to run its course.

"As to Dramal's surname prior to his long-term but inevitably lethal error, I have no knowledge. But I do know that his aerie, Dramstack—one of the most massive of all the stacks—was avoided generally as a pesthole, even in my time. Nathless, before Dramal's leprosy began wearing on him—which is to say, for the duration of Malinari's war— he shared his stack with a lesser 'colleague,' Lord Zaddok Zangastari, who had the topmost ramparts and the aerie's penultimate level (called Zadscar, because it was his headquarters, and also because of its external figuration of slanting gouges) for his own. Not that Zaddok was in any way careless of his health, but this sharing was an expedience of war: since Dramstack (including Zadscar) stood close to Darkspire, Lord Szwart's manse near the centre of the clump, it were better that two armies occupy Dramal's vast aerie, thus presenting a powerful front across the dividing gulf and threatening Szwart's forces with a partial siege at least.

"But as for battle tactics . . . I cannot admit to any great authority. These things I mention were overheard and remembered from those occasions when Nephran's war-council of three—himself, Szwart, and Vavara—met in whichever of their aeries to consider and order the ongoing hostilities. So let me not stray but get on with naming names:

"After Dramal and Zaddok came Lord Belath, a young

Lord who had just the one name, with no sire's name and no cognomen. Perhaps there was some secret in his ancestry that he did not wish divulged. As for a descriptive name or device which might best characterize him—there were some who fancied him 'Belath the Beast,' though I'm certain that no one ever suggested it to his face. Need I say more?

"But if Belath were beastly, then what of Lord Lesk, known as Lesk the Glut? For Lesk was a young berserker, only recently ascended, who was given to abandon himself as totally in battle as in his gluttony. Easily offended, he had even been known to take umbrage at his own personal warriors! If they were idle in answering his call, Lesk would work himself into a frenzy, challenge them to combat and beat them soundly . . . before returning them to their basics in his vats of metamorphism. And when his fury was in abeyance and his mood improved, then he would find time to rebuild them all over again. Thus while The Glut could never be reckoned one of the great schemers, he was most certainly a mighty engine of destruction.

"Nor were the vampire Lords alone in their awful strength and monstrous habits; many of Starside's Ladies were certainly their peers in malign intent, and a deal more devious and treacherous in their scheming. Vavara, who took sides with Malinari (we shall get to her, aye), was only one such; there were plenty of others who came close equals in malevolence. For example: Lady Jemma Freydaskith, of Hagspire.

"But surely the name of her manse says it all! Jemma *was* a hag, and a lustier, more ancient, wicked and withered hag there never was! Similarly, and where the name of her aerie describes her nature, surely the Lady's surname describes its origin. For there was only ever one Freyda among the Wamphyri, and that was Freyda Ferenc in the days of Shaitan the Unborn. Jemma Freydaskith knew the myths associated with the Lady's name; she likewise associated them with her own peculiarities of habit—her idiosyncrasies?—and so claimed direct descent from that ancient line. Now normally this would be disputable; the Wamphyri were bad record-keepers; living so long (*some* of them), history was yesterday to them;

they saw no point in looking back beyond their own immediate forebears. But Jemma was reputed to be more than seven hundred years old! Since no one else had memories of that primeval time, who was there to dispute her claim?

"Anyway, while true histories, pedigrees, and lineages were scarcities among the Wamphyri, certain myths were such as would live forever. Just so, and the myths surrounding Freyda Ferenc—while the Lady herself was long gone into oblivion—were of that order. Obviously she had been a Ferenczy, which in itself loaned authenticity to Jemma's claim, insofar as the Ferenczys were present in every Starside myth and legend (or at least the few that existed), even the most ancient of them. And what with Jemma's—predilections?—it seemed certain that something of Freyda's blood had found its way down the ages to her.

"For Freyda Ferenc had been gross of face and form, a veritable troll, with the thick skin of a trog and the fangs of a warrior! Men, even the most powerful of Lords, shrank from her person (likewise from her smell: she never washed), who for her hideous pleasure was known to suffocate male and female thralls alike with her sex! Which of itself were surely quite enough to make her a legend in her own time and a mythical figure in mine . . . but there was more.

"Freyda was that merciful rarity: a Mother of Vampires who, when she was ripe and in her final confinement, produced an hundred eggs, being so depleted during the which that she withered to a wisp and expired. But her spawn, all save one egg, was diseased and likewise died. The lone survivor fused with Bela Manculi, a Szgany thrall, and Bela became heir to Freydastack.

"And so to the final proof of Jemma's lineage, if such were needed: her sire had been Lord Bela Belari, or 'Bela's son'—an ancient in his own right—which might well make Jemma the great-granddaughter of Freyda Ferenc! Anyway, and having eschewed her father's name, 'Freydaskith' was what Jemma had called herself for thirty-five thousand sunups, during which her lifestyle had more than adequately supported her claim to the noxious ancestral connection in which she revelled . . .

"I have digressed! Yet by your silence I'm encouraged that I have interested you—

"—But on the other hand I sense your impatience, too, so now let me get on with it—which I would, gladly, except there is one more Lord of that era who was or is worthy of mention . . .

"Shaitan the Unborn, before his banishment, had spread his spawn far and wide in Starside. And in those mythic times there were even Lords who were more trog than man . . . which in itself speaks of Shaitan's depravity. But there again, among the Wamphyri, miscegeny, incest, bestiality, and other perversions could scarcely be considered uncommon. And anyway, who am I to criticize? For Shaitan was after all the *first* of all, and no one to show him the way when he strayed or say him nay when he erred.

"Thus, despite that he was gone, his line lived on. Bloodsons and a few -daughters bore Shaitan's name and likeness down the march of years. And each and every one of them proud of the connection, even as he had been proud in his time, with a pride that knew no shame, for which ultimately he had paid the price. But his heirs cared nothing for that, cared only that they were spawn of the spawn of Shaitan the Unborn, the first Great Vampire, the one true Lord and sire of the Wamphyri.

"And just as the first of his vampire progeny had borrowed from their illustrious forebear's name in the earliest days of Starside mythology (Lords and Ladies such as Sheilar the Slut, Shaithar Shaitanson, Shailar the Hagridden, Shaithag the Harrower, Shang Shaitari, and Shaithos Longarm), so in my time his descendants—or perhaps I should say descendant, for by then there was only one of 'pure' or direct line of descent—continued this great vanity. And that one's name was Shaithis.

"Shaithis was a 'young' Lord then, little more than a hundred years of age. But of course he could be as young or as old as he willed it; simply a matter of rigidly controlled meta-

300

morphism. And Lord Shaithis—who took no other name or sigil, but deemed his titular connection a blazon and statement sufficient in its own right—willed himself forever young and handsome.

"So he was, indeed beautiful, despite that he was as evil as any of the Great Vampires, and probably more so than most of them; and clever, too, skilled in controlling the lesser Lords, who were a rabble, adrift, and of little strategic consequence under Dramal Doombody. And not only men—Shaithis was also good with monsters. His vats bred many a nightmarish warrior.

"These and other attributes of leadership were proven during the course of Malinari's bloodwar of a thousand sunups, so that Shaithis rose even to the rank of Dramal himself, becoming his right-hand man and equal. And while many Lords were lost in that holocaust of blood, Shaithis went from strength to strength, until everyone supposed he would be a Power one day . . .

"And he probably was, but alas I was not there to see it. For my master and his allies were the losers. Malinari, Vavara, and Szwart, they were whelmed under, their great aeries sacked, their possessions looted, and their thralls and creatures converted.

"Well, as was the way of it in those days, they were banished north to the Icelands forever. And I, Korath Mindsthrall, my master's chief lieutenant . . . I went with them, of course.

"As to how it happened:

"In the beginning, Nephran Malinari was short of friends. And this had always been the case, ever since his mother Illula flew off into the sun and left him Malstack for his own. It was his weird talent that cost him the 'companionship' of the other Lords and Ladies. They could not trust him; they even feared to be close to him, who could be into their minds so easily. Also, his stack was a mighty fortress filled with men and beasts, and it was suspected that his ambitions reached beyond his station. Which of course they did, like the ambitions of all of them who were Lords. For lust, greed, and territorialism were ever their way of life.

"But isn't it true that a man who cannot make friends will usually make enemies? And as easily as that, the rumours sprang up: that Malinari was searching out allies and making ready his aerie for a bloodwar to rival the mythic wars of yore. But when I say 'easily,' that is not to say quickly; I would remind you that time is of small concern to the Wamphyri, and in fact the enmity that developed between The Mind and the others took decades in its shaping.

"Thus, when Malinari ravaged among the supplicant Vadastra clan on the night that I was taken and my people destroyed, his terrible tithe-gathering venture wasn't alone of his initiation or invention; Lord Doombody was also provisioning, and likewise the rest of the vampire Lords.

"Aye, for the simple truth of it was that they each feared each other. And fear fuelled fear, do you see?

"So naturally when The Mind first observed how his mentalist talents had isolated him, indeed he commenced searching out others who might also be under threat, to enlist their aid. Nor were they hard to find:

"The Lady Vavara, for one, but I use the term 'Lady' where she would not because I have *seen* and *been close* to her; and to see her . . . There never was a more perfect definition of femininity, though whether or no she affected her outward appearance (as for instance Shaithis, by means of metamorphism), of that I have no knowledge. Yet if she *was* Nature's handiwork . . . then why was that work so perfected in a female of the Wamphyri? It is a paradox to which I have no answer. But I find it hard to ascribe so much beauty to Nature alone.

"So, I have seen and been near her—*too* near and once too often, for I believe it was Vavara bade Malinari ram me in this pipe!—yet I cannot recall her clearly to memory. Perhaps that in itself defines her beauty: that its power is such as to maze common men, and no less common women. But here another paradox: for despite that she was *that* beautiful—a beguiler, a gorgeous witch, a sensuous sorceress—still she was unsure of herself, uncertain of her beauty. I can offer no other explanation for her habits, that a goddess (albeit a demon goddess) such as she was so offended by the concept of beauty in others that she could not bear it, and so was wont to remove the breasts, lips, noses, and other parts of her female thralls to make them ugly!

"There, in a nutshell, we have Vavara. And just as my vampire world was separated in two parts that were opposites, Sunside and Starside, so was she separated: her luminous exterior from the dark and swirly deeps within.

"She was Malinari the Mind's first choice as an ally; not because he lusted after her but because he knew that certain of the other Lords did. And Vavara had determined she would not be any Lord's woman, nor would she ever take a man until she found one who was at least her equal in desirability. An unlikely occurrence, for she was the one who had described Shaithis—generally considered godlike—as a mere 'lump' of a man! Oh, she took men, be sure, but they were her thralls and easily disposable in the unlikely event of complications.

"And Vavara, too, had heard rumours of a bloodwar in the offing, and also how Lesk the Glut had been boasting of what he would do to her after he'd sacked Mazemanse, her spindly, fretted, many-spired aerie where it stood not far from Malstack and Lord Szwart's Darkspire. How he would put out her ruby-red eyes to kill their fascination, singe her eyebrows, her long lashes, and the hair of her head to make her a hag, then fuck her every opening into great holes fit only for shads in the rut. *Hah!* So much for Vavara's 'beauty', if Lesk the Glut had his way! Is it any wonder she sided with Malinari?

"And finally there was Lord Szwart. But if I have found it difficult to describe Vavara, how then Szwart who was and still is literally indescribable? For of course all three of them are extant still. . . .

". . . I see by your silence that you would have what I know, despite that I know so little. So be it; what knowledge is mine shall be yours, no more nor less.

"As to who or what Szwart is: the best that I can offer—he is Wamphyri! But he is the *essence* of Wamphyri, distilled or filtered by the foulness of his forebears, mutated beyond recognition not by Nature but necessity, more leech than Lord, and a fly-the-light in the fullest sense of the word.

"The flickering light of candles, torchlight, firelight—the light of man-made combustion—these are the only kinds of light his eyes can bear, and even then not with complete impunity. But if the light matches the fire of his eyes he is fairly safe. Brighter than that, he knows pain! And any who would give Szwart pain . . . let him first pierce himself with silver dipped in kneblasch, fasten boulders to his neck, slit his wrists, and leap from the topmost battlements of the tallest aerie! Then he might be safe from Szwart.

"And only let someone declare enmity towards Szwart—let him broadcast his aversions or discuss them with his peers, and then have his words find their way *back* to the night-black master of Darkspire—and no matter who this loudmouth might be, whether high or low in the Wamphyri pecking order, be sure that Szwart would do his damnedest to put a stop to such mutterings.

"Aye, and when Szwart did his damnedest . . .

"There was one Narkus Stakis, Lord of Narkslump, a collapsed pile on the western fringe of the clump, who from the onset of all the rumour-mongering and side-choosing had voiced abroad his detestation of Lord Szwart. Precisely why he held Szwart in such low esteem, who could say?—perhaps he'd had wind of Lord Doombody's provisioning and other preparations for war, and the accompanying rumour that Dramal intended to root out all 'deviants' (which is to say his enemies, real and imagined) from the ranks of the Wamphyri.

"If that were a fact, then the proximity of Szwart's Darkspire to Dramal's Dramstack in the core of the clump would seem certain to make Szwart just such an enemy. For if Lord Doombody wished to expand territorially (assuming that this was his real purpose) he must first annex Darkspire, Szwart's gloomy, shadow-shrouded manse across too small a gulf of air. And so, and also because Dramal controlled a large percentage of Starside power, the very inferior Narkus Stakis had determined to side with him—whether or no Dramal required him as an ally.

"Alas for him that he made known his decision, especially his disinclination towards Szwart. . . .

"Lord Szwart was black; his aerie was black, and shadowed for the most part by mighty Dramstack; his warriors and flyers were black, and the black of night was his medium. Lord Stakis's Narkslump, more a great cleft knoll than a stack proper, stood in the western fringe of the cluster and low to the earth, and its silhouette against the northern auroras was more a ragged hump than a fang. Gloom was its constant companion.

"On the night that Narkus died a great drift of cloud obscured the moon and stars, and Starside was never so dark. The clouds sweeping north out of Sunside were black and swollen in their bellies, pregnant with rain that lashed at the aeries of the Wamphyri. There had been fantastic lightnings over the barrier mountains, and the wide forests of Sunside would be awash in the aftermath of the storm. Not a good night for raiding on the Szgany, not with the air full of ozone, when careless flyers and riders might so easily attract hellfire from the sky to singe them and send them plummeting. For which reasons most of the Lords and Ladies stayed to house. Most of them.

"But throughout the night several watchkeepers in aeries near the western rim, where they looked down on Narkslump's split dome, had noted how Lord Stakis's nightlights—the braziers within his battlements, behind the merlons and embrasures, and the torches in his watchtower turrets—were going out one by one, as if extinguished by the torrential rains. Except they were still going out long after the rains were done.

"Came morning; the Wamphyri stayed abed while the accursed sun rose up and up, to its zenith, when the spires of the highest stacks were lit by its rays, and many-layered curtains were drawn against its lethal heat. The day passed as all days must; soon it was night again, and the Lords and Ladies up and about. Lights burned in all the aeries—except Narkslump.

"And slow but sure the truth became known. A small handful of thrall survivors came on flyers and on foot, over the barren boulder plains to neighbouring Scarstack and Lurelodge, begging refuge from the master and mistress respectively of those middling manses. A body of men flew out from Scarstack to Narkslump and down into its landing bays. And later, in the midnight hour, they reported back to Lord Oulios the Scar on Narkslump's condition as they had found it. Also on Narkus's condition, as they had found him, his three lieutenants, and the body (or bodies?) of his thralls.

"Word spread swiftly abroad, to all the stacks of the Wamphyri. And now certain things were remembered from the previous night:

"In Dramstack, when the rains were at their worst, how the aerie's *Desmodus* colony was startled from its roost. A thousand great bats, all chittering and panicked for no apparent reason, whirling, colliding, and scolding where they circled the fretted ceiling of their cavern lair. And Lord Dramal Doombody, nodding in his private chambers, startled awake by confused mental messages from these bat familiars: *A dark shadow—a stranger, doubtless an enemy—has passed close by. Though he was cloaked in darkness, we sensed him, his eyes burning on Dramstack. They seethed and were full of hatred!*

"But Dramal's watchmen, huddling miserably in their drafty turrets and cold stone niches, and his flightless guardian warriors, rumbling behind the earthworks and on the boulder-strewn approaches to towering Dramstack, had seen nothing but a fleeting shadow: that of a cloud, they said. And cold, wet, and dull, they failed to wonder why the shadow had sped west rather than north.

"And so Dramal had ordered his familiars: *Go back to sleep! You nightmared. The pounding rain and lightning shook you loose from your dusty perches. No stranger is come to harm me or mine in Dramstack.*

"Not him or his, no. . . .

"A similar disturbance had been recorded in Karl Szorkala's Karlspire. And further west, in the grounds of Lady Sasha Lureswain's Lurelodge, one of her earthbound warriors had reared up and buffeted ineffectually at a dark blur of a shape that fluttered to a landing just beyond the bounds of Sasha's demesne—in Lord Stakis's territory, aye.

"And so to the report of them that flew from Scarstack to Narkslump, when they returned to Oulios the Scar in his high place. Narkslump was intact, as were its flyers and warrior creatures, all dutifully in their places, however nervous, unattended, and unfed. Vampire thralls, however—male and female, eunuchs and fighting men alike, some twenty in all— lay dead in their beds or at their various places of duty: in the walls and corridors, on the causeways, and in Narkus's harem. Likewise Narkus himself and his three lieutenants, all dead in their quarters.

"Well, Narkslump was scarcely a fortress such as towering Dramstack. And Narkus lorded it—or he had used to—over a mere dribble of men and monsters compared to the greater Lords in their lofty aeries. Even a small invasion force, if its components were stealthy and well ordered, could have infiltrated Narkslump's defenses under cover of the storm. But that wasn't the way the survivors in Scarstack and Lurelodge told it.

"According to one of them, a sentry on the night in question: 'The night was dark and overcast; residual rain dripped from rooves, buttresses, causeways, overhangs. I was cold, wet, uncomfortable in my niche. And I admit that I stayed well back, to avoid getting wetter still. But it was also a night of shadows. When I came out one time to scan abroad, I looked down on the lower ramparts where a colleague was keeping watch. Failing to see him, I assumed that he too was avoiding the worst of the drench. But I did see a shadow— or I thought it was a shadow—that flowed swiftly along the walkway and disappeared into a niche, then returned and continued along the ramparts. A stain, a blot on the stone, a shadow, aye . . . but mobile?

" 'There again, the clouds were fleeting and there were so many shadows, and I have only a thrall's eyes. A lieutenant's eyes might have been keener, better suited, but lieutenants do not guard the walls. My Lord Stakis's eyes would certainly have noted any weirdness or peculiarity, but he was in his chambers.

" 'When next I looked out and down, my colleague's brazier was out; a hiss of steam rose up; I assumed that there had been more rain, or my friend had been negligent of his fire. And the night was even darker.

" 'My duty station was lit fitfully by twin torches ensconced under slate awnings that fended off the rain. I replenished them with fresh faggots before returning to my niche and snuggling deeper yet. Time passed; perhaps I heard a grunt or call—a gurgled cry?—from the north flank. But in any case I ventured out again, to the northernmost point of my picket, where I leaned from an embrasure to look down on the adjacent flank. In the misted gloom of a landing bay, there was no watchman to be seen, but the steam of his extinguished brazier rose up!

" 'It was time I made report. But only recently recruited, my vampire skills were weak; I was not yet linked to my master. If I cried out with my mind alone, Lord Stakis would not "hear" my alert, and deep within the rock he couldn't possibly hear my voice. Wherefore a dilemma: should I desert my position and go to the Lieutenant of the Watch, who I knew to be a very difficult man? And if I did, and nothing was found amiss, what then?

" 'I leaned out again and looked down . . . and at once drew back! For traversing the scarp directly below me—coming diagonally upwards across the treacherous, rain-slick face of the rock and scarcely pausing to negotiate the way—I had spied a lumpy shadow like a dark blot against the lesser darkness. But did I say dark? The shadow was *black!* And where it merged with other shadows it disappeared completely, only to emerge a moment later, always climbing towards my battlements station.

" 'Now I knew to run and make report—or at least to run,

if nothing else! But already the shadow was stretching itself, groping like the fingers of some phantom hand towards the merlons between myself and the entrance to Narkslump's east wing. Even if I ran this unknown thing would be there first, perhaps waiting for me. Neither was there any other route of entry—nor of escape—from my position on the outer face.

" 'Now, I am not a man to shrink from any normal darkness. Murky gloamings and the weird nebulosities of Sunside bogs had never frightened me. But this was no ordinary shadow. There was something sinister, knowing, *clever,* about it; it moved as on a mission, and in my heart I knew I couldn't stop it. Only let me try . . . it would certainly stop me! But as yet it didn't even know that I was there. Or at least, I hoped that was the case.

" 'And as quietly as possible I crept into my niche, drew as far back as I could go among the spiders and beetles— then farther yet until the sharp rock of the split scraped my chest and my back—and finally held still, so very still, there in the dark and the dust.

" 'And eventually something came.

" 'Do not ask me what it was, but it came and was a part of the darkness. And while I couldn't see it, I knew it was there. Then—

" ' "Indeed I *am* here!" A voice came to me like the rustle of leaves, so close I felt the breath of it! And it continued: "I see you are afraid, and that is good. *Be* afraid, my friend, and make no outcry. Stay here for long and long in this tight crevice, while I go about my business, and I won't harm you. But if you come out . . . ah, that would be a brief but very unfortunate affair. So then, do we have an understanding?"

" 'I could only nod, and though I saw nothing at all, still the shadow saw me. "Good," it husked, and spoke no more.

" 'Then I was alone again—and pleased to be alone—for long and long. . . .

" ' . . . How long I cannot say. But when I dared to come out I saw that my torches were expired, and looking closer

I saw they had been capped—put out—deliberately. And not only my torches but all the lights in Narkslump, till tip to toe the aerie stood in darkness most utter.

" 'Then when I went inside I found what I found, and discovered the hidy-holes of a handful of others with tales to tell much like my own. Following which . . . can you blame us that we fled that haunted place, and came with all dispatch here . . . ?'

"That was the thrall's story, and the other survivors with him agreed with everything he said. But survivors of what?"

Since the answer to Korath Mindsthrall's final question was obvious, a reply seemed unnecessary. But Harry Keogh answered him anyway, saying, *Survivors of Lord Szwart, of course.*

Harry's words—more definite, decisive in Jake Cutter's mind—startled him from the reverie induced by Korath's narrative; from what had seemed like a dream within a dream, where everything that the ex-vampire lieutenant described had seemed as real as if Jake himself had been there, in another time and another world. And:

"What? Where?" Jake gave himself a shake. And looking all about he saw debris: the buckled stanchions and shattered concrete slabs fallen from the ceiling, the partly-gleaming, scorch-scarred rim of the monitor conduit rising from the sullen swirl of dark waters. That was where this fragment of the history of a vampire world had its origin: that ugly pipe where Korath had died the true death, which still contained his bones, sloughed clean and washed white by the water. And Jake shuddered.

Harry sensed his unease, and asked, *Are you all right?*

"No," Jake answered. "And I don't think I'll ever be right again."

You will be, the other told him. *You have to be. Anyway, we still aren't through here. I want to know more about Szwart—what he is and how he came to be—and I think Korath knows it all. But I sense that he's slowing up, holding back.*

To which Korath immediately replied, *And you are correct! For it dawns on me that I do myself no good here. When you have learned your fill, what then of me? No forgiveness, shunned by the living and the dead alike, washed away to nothing and dispersed across an alien land? Hah! Surely I can do better.*

You are dead, said Harry. *These things are what happen to the dead, in circumstances such as yours.*

And Korath answered, *Ah, cold, cold!*

No, said Harry, *not entirely. Merely truthful. I won't lie to you that there's anything in this for you. Only our company, for however long it lasts.*

But Korath said: *Yet your dead converse! I know, for I have heard them whispering in their graves. When they sense me listening, then they keep quiet or exclude me. So why can't they converse with me?*

They don't like you, said Harry. *Can you blame them? Being dead, they hate death. And they know that you thrived on it!*

I did what vampires do. Is there no pity?

For you, none.

Then I have none for you! Korath sulked. *You dare to go up against Vavara, Szwart, Malinari? Without knowing all there is to know about them? Good luck to you. You are dead men and may think of me again some time, when you lie broken or drained, or minced into warrior feed. Then perhaps you'll wish we had spoken at greater length, but too late. Until that time you'll hear no more from me.* He fell silent. But:

You have no idea how weary I am of all your bluff and bluster, Harry told him. *What do you expect of me? What can I possibly do for you? You are dead, Korath!*

You, too, Korath answered. *And yet you have mobility, companionship . . . a future?*

My case is different, said Harry. *And as for the future: I never underestimate it.*

And Jake's case? His future?

There was a slyness in Korath's deadspeak voice, and

Harry didn't like it. He wondered if he detected some hidden innuendo, or more likely some kind of threat. *Jake is a dreamer,* he said. *Right now he is no more and no less. He's my apprentice, if you like, and for the moment knows very little about such things—but he will learn.*

"Huh!" Jake snorted. "Even if I don't want to, it seems!"

Yesssss, said Korath. *And I can feel your apprehension. But still Harry is right and you should . . . learn. If not from him, then perhaps from me?*

Harry was at once alarmed. *You know what we want from you. And that's all we want. So what's it to be?*

Szwart's origins?

(Harry's deadspeak nod.) *And more about Malinari's bloodwar—how you survived the Icelands, and how finally you came here.*

Korath sighed and said, *Very well. For I am forgiving, even if you are not.*

He was silent for a moment, then sighed again and said: *The rest of it, then . . .*

22

Survivors

"I CAN'T SWEAR TO SZWART'S ORIGIN," KORATH commenced the final chapter of his story. "I can only repeat what I heard of him in the service of my master, Malinari of Malstack, all those years ago. And of course I can report what I have *seen* of him, for he was after all Malinari's co-conspirator, along with Vavara, and shared with them in their banishment when they were whelmed by the forces of Dramal Doombody.

"As for Szwart's 'visit' to Lord Stakis's Narkslump: while that had occurred as a prelude to the actual hostilities, obviously it was an important factor in the heightening tension between the soon-to-be-warring parties. I recall that soon after Narkus's demise, as angry rumblings from the aeries grew louder, Malinari arranged the latest of several get-togethers with his future partners, Vavara and Szwart.

"By then, when they ventured abroad from their respective stacks, all three 'outsiders'—rejects, as it were, excluded or ostracized by the rest of the Wamphyri—were constantly on the alert for trouble: the imposition of restrictions over disputed air-space, skirmishes over boundaries, even ambushes were by no means unlikely. But since by chance their stacks formed a close triangle in the centre of the clump, and the space within that triangle was theirs, flights between were generally accomplished without threat or interruption. And of course the close proximity of their aeries was yet another good reason for forming their alliance: back to back, they presented a more formidable foe.

"Anyway, Szwart and Vavara came on flyers across the respective gulfs from Darkspire and Mazemanse, to meet with my master in Malstack. And that was the first time that I saw Szwart. For contrary to certain Szgany campfire tales of the time, Lord Szwart *was* visible when he so desired. In any reasonable degree of light, and when he chose to assume an acceptable form (which invariably cost, and indeed still costs him, no small effort of will) he could be seen, though he much preferred *not* to be. But in his condition . . . well, that was surely understandable.

"But I sense that I've whetted your curiosity; you are wondering what 'condition' I speak of, and what do I mean by 'acceptable form'? We shall get to these things.

"So then, Lord Szwart came from Darkspire, and I was sent to bid him welcome to Malstack and organize the stabling of his flyer, just as I had seen to Vavara's when a little earlier she had arrived from Mazemanse, her castle of vertiginous balconies and fretted, spindly spires.

"I remember the time was several hours past sundown, when only the last faint rays of a dying sun limned the peaks of the barrier mountains in gold. This vestigial glimmer posed no real threat to the Wamphyri in general (even at noon the deadly rays probed only the uppermost spires of Starside's tallest aeries), but it was a problem for Szwart, who dreaded to be seen.

"And there we have it:

"Lord Szwart's fear of light wasn't that it might destroy him but that it made him visible! This weird photophobia wasn't so much a physical as a mental disability. Which perhaps serves to explain his reclusive nature: his rumoured celibacy, and the fact that he so rarely went abroad from his aerie (and then only into Sunside, to hunt) and never mingled with other than his thralls or creatures of his own devise in lonely, shadow-cursed Darkspire.

"But it wasn't *only* in his mind, this ugliness that Szwart couldn't bear to display. It wasn't *merely* imaginary. Rather it was very real, and hereditary. . . .

"He arrived in a Malstack landing bay. His flyer was black as night; swooping across the gulf it had been clearly visible, but in the shadow of Malstack it simply disappeared. I stood in the gape of the landing bay, waiting—and suddenly Szwart was there! A black shape buffeted night-black air in my face as the shadows that were Szwart and his flyer alighted. Then, while he dismounted, I called for thralls to see to his beast. And looming close, Szwart said:

" 'You, lieutenant—take me to Malinari.'

"His voice was a gasp, a pant, a flurry of wind through a narrow crevice. And there he was, Szwart himself, all cloaked in black—a blot of a figure that showed neither features nor anything else of its once-humanity—standing before me in the flickering torchlight of the landing bay!

"But while Szwart himself was featureless, carved from jet, and his voice a flutter of bat-wings, his presence was awesome; as solid as the great rocks on Starside's barren boulder plains. And his *aura* in the night: that was such as to make even my vampire flesh creep—and I was a lieutenant! So that I could well understand how Narkslump's lowly thralls had felt when confronted by Lord Szwart.

"He gloomed at me through eyes like slits of fire, his only parts that weren't black. 'Well? And am I to be left to find my own way?' For I was so startled, I had made no effort to attend him!

" 'No, Lord,' I answered. 'I am your guide. But here in Malstack, protocol demanded that I stood silent until commanded by you.'

" 'Fool!' he said. 'I did so command you! And *now* take me to Malinari! Or perhaps I strike you as . . . *odd* in some weird way? Is it so?' With which he flowed closer, and his outline became less manlike, even more a blot or a shadow, like a lump drifted from the darkness in the unlit deeps of Malstack's basement.

" 'Not at all, Lord!' I backed off. 'I was simply in awe of my master's honoured guest—so much so that my tongue clove to . . . to the roof of my . . . of my mouth.' It was scarcely a lie!

" 'You must consider yourself fortunate that you still have a tongue,' Szwart whispered, withdrawing something that was not quite a hand from where it had been reaching for me. 'Also fortunate that *my* protocol forbids the killing of an ally's lieutenant on his home ground.'

" 'Yes, Lord!' I bowed, and before things could go even more awry turned and forced my numb legs to bear me in the direction of my master's chambers. Lord Szwart followed on behind me, and I could *feel* him there, silent, intense, and seething; though I fancied it wasn't his thoughts that seethed so much as his person! Perhaps it was so. I can't rightly say, for I never looked back. . . ."

"When Szwart left I was there to see him go, though on this occasion there was no contact. When the keeper of Malinari's pens handed him the reins of his flyer, I was situated in a window a little higher in the sheer wall of the aerie. From there I watched him mount, launch, and fly away.

"Aye, and I also saw his manlike outline melt to a liquid blot of a shape that hunched down and became one with the silhouette of his black flyer. And I saw the burning eyes— *but far too many eyes*—that gazed back on Malstack from that hideously humped shape, as if their owner suspected that someone watched!

"Then he was off, and flyer and rider both, black on black, disappeared into the yawning gulf like a scrap of burned cloth, or a tattered pennant slipped from its staff, fluttering on the winds that whine around the aeries of the Wamphyri. . . ."

"That same time:

"Having seen Szwart off from Malstack's lofty premises, I returned to my master and the luminous Vavara—the very opposite of Szwart—where they continued to talk in Malinari's private chambers. In his absence, Szwart had become the subject of their conversation. Hearing his name mentioned, and because my interest had been piqued, however morbidly, I slipped back into the shadows and listened.

" 'It was in his blood,' Malinari was saying (so that I knew what next he would say), 'and what is in the blood always comes out in the flesh—or in Szwart's case, what passes for flesh!' And he went on to explain:

" 'Seventy years ago—a little before your time, Vavara—Szwart was born to a Lord and Lady of the Wamphyri. That alone would make him an exception to the general rule. For as you are well aware, when the time is right the Wamphyri transfuse their eggs to make egg-sons or -daughters; or we take Szgany women—er, forgive me, or men—and so beget blood-children. But it's rare that a Lord will take a Lady to wife, or vice versa. Rarer still where Lord Szwart is concerned, whose father was also his mother's brother!

" 'Incest?—not so strange among the Wamphyri. But incestuous marriage, between twins?

" 'To find a reason you must look back in time, but not too far. Szwart's grandsire, his blood-grandsire, was cursed with a certain disorder which our kind don't care to mention. Oh, as a skill—a fearsome talent—we mention it with pride! But when it runs amok, then it becomes *un*mentionable. Metamorphism, aye. But note, my voice is hushed. Such matters are not to be spoken of lightly.

" 'Before he knew that this weirdest and most loathsome of diseases was upon him, Lord Szwart's grandsire got twins out of a Szgany girl. Brother and sister, they grew up in their sire's aerie—Mittelmanse as it was then, named for its proximity to the centre—and ascended. They were Wamphyri!

" 'By then their father's curse was known to all and sundry: he had practiced his metamorphic flux beyond reasonable bounds, putting too great a strain on a leech which finally rebelled or went insane. Whichever, his flesh was out of control. Once in a thousand years this will happen: that instead of remaining symbiont and host—two mutually dependant creatures in one body—the flesh of both mingles, and a resultant *Thing* emerges as a mindless, loathsome hybrid.

" 'But the process was a slow one; the Lord of Mittelmanse was not immediately a madman, and knew as well as his children what was happening to him. The horror of it played on his mind; as his flesh gradually succumbed, he would come shrieking awake from nightmares, to find his limbs like ropes draped all about his room! Or he would wander abroad in his sleep, to trap and convert his own loyal thralls by means of absorption and assimilation. Instead of the blood, whole bodies were the life! And he grew gross, when at times his flesh was soft as mud, and at others horny and corrugated. And even his colour was changed—no longer that of undead flesh but the mottled and leprous hue of the leech.

" 'And when he was lucid he made his children promise that they would not spread this thing abroad. Great Vampire that he was and malicious, still he would not wish this on another man or creature. For he knew what was in his blood, *and in theirs,* and that given the opportunity it would out. Wherefore it must not be given the opportunity. . . .

" 'The twins, grown up now, planned to put their father in a pit; for according to the lore or history of Starside— what little has ever been recorded—that was usually the best way. Or they could kill him out of hand, by trapping him in an inescapable place and setting fire to him, before he became totally ungovernable.

" 'But it didn't come to that. Fond of flying, he formed an airfoil and flew out upon the gulf one night. This involved, of course, a great effort of will—which he relaxed, perhaps deliberately, high over the boulder plains. And *Thing* that he was, his immediate devolution into something less than airworthy was instantly fatal. He fell like a stone, and even protoplasm will only stretch so far.

" 'So much for him.

" 'His sibling children made a pact: they would not go with others to spread the curse abroad but cleave to each other, and so keep the thing to house. And all the while, year after year, they lived in fear that it might be in them, too— which indeed it was. But because they kept their flux under strict rein, and used it sparingly, the curse skipped their generation—only to emerge in the next.

" 'It came out in the young Szwart, aye. Having been suppressed in his parents, the vampire essence they passed down to Szwart was of an entirely different order. How best to explain? When a man is born blind, his remaining senses may develop more fully in order to compensate for the loss. In Szwart's parents, the normal functions of their vampire leeches had been suppressed—which served only to *magnify* the essence that they passed down to Szwart!

" 'Szwart's will has kept him sane within limits, but he is a totally devolved creature. He sleeps alone, to ensure that no blood-son of his will carry this thing into the future. His ugliness is such that men might easily go insane if they saw him in the worst of his myriad . . . *designs.* Tonight he maintained something of a manlike outline in order to be here with us, but normally he can't bear to be seen, which is why he shuns light and companionship. This last is no great hardship; we Wamphyri were ever loners. But let any man speak out against him as a freak—or shrink from the horror of him—it's as if his phobias were reinforced. And despite that he knows his ugliness well enough, knows the truth of it, still he will kill the offender, if only because his action or reaction reminded him of his infirmity.'

"And Vavara said, 'Yet you say he's not mad?'

" 'Not yet,' Malinari told her, 'Though it must come eventually. Perhaps in a hundred years, or fifty, or maybe less. But he was here tonight; you saw him; he reasons.'

" 'I have seen him, yes,' Vavara answered. 'And his reasoning is as warped and fluctuating as his flesh! He looked like a mad thing to me, or close enough.'

" 'Have it your own way,' my master told her. 'But if he is a mad thing, then for the moment he's *our* mad thing. Also, he's the Lord of Darkspire, commander of men and monsters, and Darkspire guards our flanks. . . .'

"Then for a while they were silent, until Vavara inquired: 'What of his parents, the incestuous twins?'

" 'Szwart was born beautiful and seemed perfect,' Malinari answered. 'At seventeen he ascended. And at eighteen his father found him in Darkspire's *Desmodus* colony, hanging with the bats from the fretted ceiling—but hanging in flaps and folds, like a blob of dough such as the Szgany use when baking their bread! In his gluttony, he had absorbed a great many bats before falling asleep.

" 'Father and mother both, they tried to trap and burn him. He trapped and burned *them*—so the story goes. My advice: never treat Szwart with disdain because he is not pretty. And as for his quirks: we are Wamphyri and we all have quirks—even you, Vavara, or so I've heard it rumoured. But with the exception of our mutual enemies, no one takes us to task over our little . . . idiosyncrasies? As for Szwart, who is our ally: neither slight nor scorn him. And don't underestimate him, either.' . . ."

Korath had been silent for some little time. Perhaps he brooded on the past. Harry prodded him with a thought:

Korath? And he responded with a grunt:

Huh?

My time here grows short now, (Harry's deadspeak voice was faint and wavering,) *and Jake isn't far from waking.*

We've come a long way, in more senses than one, but we're by no means finished. When I go, your contact with Jake goes with me. Then you will be alone. If you ever want to hear from us again—for who knows? We might yet find some mutual benefit in renewed contact—then you'd best get on with your story. But make it as brief as possible. Here's how it goes:

Malinari and the others, they lost their bloodwar and were banished. Then for four hundred years you survived the Icelands and eventually returned to Starside. And finally you came here. That's the story, now fill in the details.

And Korath answered, *Ah, but the details may take a little longer!*

But not too long, said Harry.

As for Jake: this time he voiced no complaint. He was so "into" Starside now—Korath's story had so intrigued him—that he wanted to know the rest of it, no matter how ugly it might get. And:

Very well, said Korath. *Then let's be done with it. . . .*

"So then, Malinari, Vavara, and Szwart, they were made out to be the weird ones, the freaks, the outsiders. But in fact they were no more freakish than many of the Lords and Ladies in the camp of Dramal Doombody. Ah, but Lord Doombody had problems of his own. For the time being it seemed he had his leprosy under control, true, but what of the future? Even a man as mighty as Dramal has his limits, and likewise his vampire leech. He knew it was time to consolidate his position against a dubious future, when he might become weak and vulnerable.

"Since his aerie towered close to the centre of the clump, Dramal had resolved to annex all of the neighbouring stacks and so make them his own, or at least give them to allies with whom he had unbreakable pacts. This way—as he became less capable over however long a time—he would be surrounded by 'friends' as opposed to enemies. And there in a nutshell we have the real basis of what was falsely termed

'Malinari's bloodwar': in fact it was forced on The Mind and the other 'freaks' by Dramal himself.

"Anyway, my master and his allies were determined to make a good long fight of it, and they did. Briefly, then:

"Malinari, Vavara, and Szwart: they set to and strengthened their earthworks in Starside's bottoms, and manned them with every sort of vicious atrocity from their vats. The triangle of barren earth accommodating their aeries became their first line of defence. As for the stacks themselves: Malstack wasn't altogether impregnable, but still Malinari felt fairly secure. The Landing bays and walled ledges were few and well defended, and the gantlet approaches terrible in their severity. Over every possible avenue of invasion, corbels carved in the likeness of vomiting warrior-heads threatened boiling piss and flaming tar.

"Vavara's Mazemanse was more problematic. But it had good points as well as bad. In silhouette, the aerie looked like the roof of an ancient cave upended, with spindly stalactites going up instead of down. Causeways and buttresses stretched between, and various levels were roofed over with timbers out of Sunside and slate tiles from the scree slopes of the barrier mountains. Towards the centre the many rock spires were joined by massive, mortared walls to form the bulk of the aerie. Externally, radiating ribs of timber, the boles of Sunside ironwoods, supported slate rooves and timbered battlements, and boulder walls built by ancestral inhabitants protected the whole from attack up the sliding scree shambles of the bottoms.

"When the war came, Mazemanse suffered its greatest damage from aerial warriors driven to crash headlong into the delicate outer spires, thus bringing them down on the inner walls, causeways, barracks, and other habitations. Small-minded, such creatures as were crippled in these deliberately contrived collisions would then sacrifice themselves by smashing down on rooves to break them in. Sometimes this worked, but on many occasions the rooves were false and hid needle spires or stakes of mountain pine. Impaled warriors would then be set on fire and fried in the fiery jets of their own gas-bladders; their molten fats and noxious liquids would be drained off as ammunition for the castle's corbel chutes.

"Szwart's Darkspire proved the most obstinate of Dramal's targets, and Szwart's men the most furious fighters. For there was something of Szwart himself in all his creatures. His warriors in the stony rubble at Darkspire's foot were night-black things that could not be seen by footsoldiers until too late; his men manning the gantlets never retreated but fought to the death; others where they fed the corbel chutes—in the event that blazing fluids or white-hot-boulder ammunition should run low—would hurl themselves down on the invading hordes rather than quit the machicolation. Such dedication! . . . but a rather simple explanation. Men and monsters both, they had been given a choice: deal with the enemy, or be dealt with by Szwart.

"Well, there you go . . . the picture I paint is inadequate, but you require that I make a speedy end of it. We fought well, but a losing battle. Three stacks against the combined might of Starside? Still, I suppose it had to be. Avarice, bloodlust, and territorial expansion: such things are life itself, or undeath, or the true death, to the Wamphyri. But at least we were spared the true death. Had we died in battle, then that were something else. But we didn't. When the end was inevitable and we huddled in the blazing bulk of Malstack—Szwart blinded by the fires, Vavara smudged, bloodied, and wilting, and Malinari almost mindless from the sheer force of the telepathic demands he had made on his last few defenders—finally Dramal called for our surrender. What else could we do but accept? Following which, and in short order, we were spat upon, buffeted, generally humiliated, and banished.

"We were allowed one small warrior for escort, our flyers, and a handful of lieutenant and thrall survivors. That was all. Not much by way of a retinue, but beggars can't be choosers.

"And so we headed north for the Icelands, at first a distant shimmer, and then a hazy grey blanket that flickered on a horizon warped by weaving auroras and ice-chip stars. And from the moment of setting out, not one of us knew if we would make it or plummet into some frozen ocean and drown. But make it we did . . .

"Below us the landscape changed, however slowly:

"First the bitter, white-rimed earth; then the blue-grey lakes, whose cold and sluggish waves seemed to crawl to shore; finally the endless white drifts that went on and on as far as the eyes could see, sprawling ever northwards. The snow wasn't entirely strange to us; we had seen it before, however rarely, on the higher ridges of the barrier mountains—but never like this! No earth showed through; we could not know if we crossed land or iced-over ocean deeps. We fed ourselves and our beasts on the blood and flesh of great white bears—and only occasionally on thralls—and forged on. We had no other choice; if we tried to sneak back into Starside, that would mean the true death for all of us.

"It was hard. When there were no bears we sipped sparingly from the stoppered spines of our flyers. One of Vavara's lieutenants let his greed get the better of him; when his exhausted flyer spiralled down to an icy hummock, we followed him down to feed. We fed on him, too, for without his flyer he wasn't going anywhere.

"Another time, a blizzard came up. We could not afford the energy required to climb above it. Landing, we sheltered behind the bulk of the warrior, one of Malinari's. Then it was that my master took from me—took more than was good for me, so that I was weakened. But at the same time I received of his strong vampire essence, which helped in my survival—the tenacity of the Great Vampire, aye.

"Where the auroras soared highest, we came upon mountains; a lesser range than the barrier mountains of Sunside/Starside—and never a tree to be seen—but with crags, gulleys, and ice castles, even rivers of ice, frozen in position on the mountain slopes! And if nothing else, the endless boredom of our passage over this white wilderness was broken.

"But we were broken, too, and exhausted we put down.

Worst hit by the journey, Malinari's warrior was ready to give up the ghost. We saw to it that the beast didn't go to waste. Only its bones would be left, where for a while its rib cage would form the frame of an ice house that we would build. But before then, while still the warrior's shrivelled flesh provided sustenance, we had time and strength for exploration.

"To the south a crack of fuzzy light showed on the horizon: sunup on Sunside, so faint and distant that even Szwart made no complaint! And making use of what little warmth it brought, the four of us—Szwart and Vavara, Malinari and myself—flew off to investigate the range of ice-draped mountains. My master and I, we headed west, Vavara and Szwart went east. When total darkness crept in again and the writhing auroras returned, we would join up and make report at the carcass of the warrior. The rest of our men and beasts (four junior lieutenants and their flyers, for there were no more thralls left) would live off the carcass until we got back. In the bitter cold, the warrior's meat would keep for long and long. . . .

"We flew for many a mile, Malinari gaunt where he sat tall in his ornate saddle only a wingspan's distance from my own flyer. Gaunt and silent, aye, so that I wondered what he was thinking—perhaps that he was hungry, and that he had had enough of stinking warrior meat!

"And indeed The Mind was thinking, though mercifully his thoughts were not of me. No, for I could feel them, probing out and ahead of us, searching for other lives in this white waste.

And he pointed, and called out to me:

" 'That way: an ocean where mighty fishes cruise the deeps, only surfacing to break the thin ice and breathe. But these are great hot-blooded things, and never a Szgany hook and line that could pull them forth!' Then he shook his head, and said: 'This place—this land, these mountains at least—are cold and barren, and yet . . .' And he frowned.

" 'Master?' I said.

" 'Something . . .' he answered, still frowning. 'Something up ahead.'

"And in another mile or so . . . smoke, a distant puff! Several puffs, and a smudge, going up. And still we flitted across the wind-carved ice castles and frozen fangs of the mountains.

"But now Malinari's concentration was rapt on that column of fire-smoke rising ahead. I saw what he saw, or so I thought: a fire-mountain, black against white, where the snow had melted from its flanks.

"Then, suddenly, Malinari hauled on his reins, rose up and to one side and climbed in a spiral. I quickly joined him, but when I might have questioned him—or rather, as my mind framed its concern—he held up a hand to silence me. And now his mental probes were venting in such powerful bursts from Malinari's mind that I could 'hear' *his* questions, which he asked of some unseen other:

"*Who are you, in the mountain there? What do you here? Is this your territory, and if so by what right? By right of conquest, or simply because you are here?*

"And the answer came back with such force, in such a doomful cadence that we knew, my master and I, this was no middling intelligence or power which he had discovered:

"*It is my territory because it is mine. That is my right. If you dispute it, then come on by all means. I have creatures to shatter you in pieces. Or go away, and I shall perhaps leave you in peace—and in* one *piece. As to who I am: I am who I am. As to what I was: I was the first, even though I may not be the last. I have been here a thousand years, which is my sole right to this place and sufficient. So begone!*

"Then with a *hiss* Malinari ceased all telepathic sendings. And I felt his guards go up as he turned and gazed wide-eyed at me. 'I know him!' he said, his jaws agape. 'Something of him is in all of us!' And for a moment that was all he said. . . .

"Then I spied a pair of great white bears at the edge of a frozen lake. They had broken a hole in the ice and were fishing in the black water. I pointed them out to Malinari, and he took us down to hover over our prey. The bears, startled by our sudden arrival, took to the water and vanished under the ice. Malinari was quick to dismount; he waited at the hole until one of the bears lifted her head. Then my master struck—struck with the strength of three or four men—and his gantlet crushed in the bear's ear and the side of its head. Brained, the huge creature was dead in the water. We dragged it onto the ice in time to see the bear's mate surface. This time, in the moment before Malinari delivered his devastating blow, the great white beast roared its fury and raked his forearm. Containing his pain, my master wrapped his torn limb. Then, as we ate bear heart while our flyers sipped blood, he said:

" 'My wound is slight, and it will heal quickly. His won't ever. The strongest survive. You are a strong one, Korath, and quick-sighted. So you survive. If you had not seen these bears, perhaps you would not survive. For I wish to stay here awhile, to explore these ice castles, and blood and flesh are the fuels I burn. If not the flesh of bears, what then?' And his red eyes gloomed on me.

"Understanding him well enow, I deigned not to answer."

"And explore we did, but what we found . . . !

" 'Korath,' my master said, as we entered an ice-encased cavern. 'Before I sensed the Greater Power in yonder fire-mountain—if it is a *living* fire-mountain, for I fancy the smoke is of man's making rather than Nature's—I sensed lesser thoughts, dreamier thoughts, from this frozen cave. Aye, and from others near and far. Who sleeps, I wonder, in such places?'

"We soon found out.

"Locked in the ice where he had frozen himself solid—completely encased, indeed buried in the clear ice—we found the much-reduced body of what was once a Lord of the Wamphyri! Wrinkled he was; his skin as white as snow, whose deep corrugations were like some strange pale leech's. And so we knew that he had been here for long and long.

But strangely, his eyes were open, however glazed-over. And:

" 'Here we have one such dreamer,' said Malinari, and even his voice was hushed in this cold and echoing chamber. 'Except he doesn't so much dream as nightmare.'

" 'A dreamer, master?' I said. 'But surely he is dead?'

" 'Eh?' He raised a scornful eyebrow. 'Where is your faith, Korath? Is it likely that Nephran Malinari is mistaken? And for that matter, where is your faith in the Wamphyri, in their tenacity, their longevity? I heard this one's thoughts, I tell you—and I sensed his fear! No, he is not dead. Now look there.'

"I looked where he pointed.

"The ancient sat behind twelve or fifteen feet of ice. But level with his ribs, a row of holes some two to three inches in diameter had been drilled a third of the way through to him. On the floor, the accumulated ice chippings were heaped into small mounds directly beneath the holes.

"And Malinari said: 'I don't think we need puzzle over the look of horror on his face. Something has been busy here, doing its best to get at him! But this ice is centuries old and hard as iron, and he chose his niche well. When it is time to freeze ourselves—when our food is used up—we must do the same. . . .'

" 'Time to . . . to freeze ourselves?' I repeated him.

"He looked at me. 'In this cold place, only one way to survive the centuries. Like this one, we go down into the ice. But first we put some distance between.'

"And like a fool, I repeated him again: 'Between?'

"But he only nodded musingly, and said, 'Between ourselves and Shaitan, aye. A thousand years ago and more he was banished here, and now lives in that fire-mountain. Others like this one, who came before or since, have found their own ways to live out the years: they sleep in the ice. But Shaitan is awake! Can you doubt it was a creature of his did this drilling? Well, he has the mountain's warmth and shelter, and no doubt defends it with just such beasts as did this. And here we are starvelings, with just one dead warrior to sustain us. So it's the ice for us, be sure. But not here, not this close to Shaitan in his fire-mountain.'

"Following which we returned to the bears and loaded their drained carcasses aboard our flyers, then flew back to rendezvous with Vavara and Szwart. . . .

"Malinari told his colleagues what we had found. He convinced them that indeed Shaitan the Unborn held dominion in the west, and they agreed, however reluctantly, with his long-term plan of survival. As Vavara pointed out: 'We shall only know if we are successful when we wake up. And if we don't, we weren't.'

"The warrior lasted some little time, while we gradually stripped the flesh from its bones. Eventually its flensed ribs formed the framework of an ice house, which in the next blizzard became one with the landscape. But toward the end Malinari, Vavara, Szwart, and the others were weary of all this and ready for ice-encasement. Meanwhile they had explored the local terrain, discovering an ice-cavern that suited their purpose.

"There in a niche, broad at the front, narrowing to nothing in the rear, we positioned ourselves. In front, the three lieutenants (they were down to three now); then the flyers all in a huddle, and behind and beneath their shielding wings Malinari and his Wamphyri colleagues. Myself, I was positioned on a ledge overlooking the rear of the niche.

"So stationed, the lieutenants would be the first to feel any exploratory stab from outside the ice. With any luck their physical agonies would transfer mentally and be 'heard' by Malinari. He and the others might then be able to melt themselves free by will alone . . . if they retained sufficient strength.

"But the surest way to remain alive and intact down all the unknown and unguessable years to come would be to fashion such an ice-shield as could *not* be broken into and looted. To this end the Wamphyri trio willed a mist like none before. It swirled up from the ice-layered floor, down from the festoons of jagged icicles in the cavern's roof, out from the crystalized walls, but mainly from their own pores. And drawn down by their massed will to where we sat in our places, the mist solidified to form layer upon layer of ice, thick and thicker far than the sheath we had seen in the hidy-hole of the ancient.

"For long and long I watched it forming—until my eyes were frozen and I saw no more. . . .

"We woke up!

"The ice was melting, and the air . . . was warmer! Still cold, but warmer. Two lieutenants were dead—the true death, aye—and three flyers. Well, the third and last lieutenant, barring myself, was useless without a mount. He was Szwart's man, and though his blood was pale and slow, still it flowed . . . until Szwart stilled it forever.

"Then the three great Vampires drained him, and I had my fill of his shrivelled flesh. Shrivelled, desiccated, sunken in: such was the case with all of us, our flyers, too. But at least we lived.

"And the great cave dripped with running water, and outside—

"Such a transformation! Over the far southern horizon, a glow as was never before seen from the Icelands. It could only be the sun, but *visible* in the sky however low to the horizon. Malinari and Vavara felt its rays at once; not so much a burning as a severe irritation. It was the great distance, and the dimness of the glow through a mist over the ocean. But it must be said that Lord Szwart suffered, until he covered himself in his robe, averted his eyes and retreated into gloom. His suffering was more mental than physical, I fancy.

"There were bears in some profusion, many with cubs, and even a fox or two, snowy white where they scavenged for sprats at the water's rim. And great fishes as big as warriors spouting in the sea. 'More than sufficient of food,' said Malinari, 'to fuel us on our journey home.'

"And Szwart wanted to know: 'What has happened here?'

" 'A freak in the weather,' my master told him. 'It is the

only answer. And it is our freedom to return to Starside!'

" 'We were banished,' said Vavara, who had been a hag, but already was regaining much of her former beauty.

" 'Aye, long and long ago,' said Malinari. And he took her down to the ice house in the ribs of our long-extinct warrior.

Gnawed on by bears, wolves, foxes, whatever, its bones had collapsed to nothing and lay flat to the cold slurry. And: 'An hundred years,' said Malinari. 'Or two, or three—or maybe more! And our enemies in Starside? Killed off by now in their bloodwars. And that diseased old tyrant, Dramal Doombody: by now he is no more, sloughed away to rot and ruin. But we, the forgotten of Starside, go on. We are survivors, Vavara. And we *shall* return!'

"And we did. But before then we flew west to explore Shaitan the Unborn's fire-mountain. This was only made possible by his absence; Malinari no longer sensed his presence in the extinct volcano, and the smoke of his fires no longer rose up. We found mighty vats of plasma; once frozen, they were now rancid, crawling with maggots, and gave offence. These and other signs of fairly recent habitation told of a Being not long moved on.

" 'It seems that he, too, has returned into Starside,' was Lord Szwart's opinion.

"But be that as it may, we never found him there. . . ."

23
Nathan's War

IN THE SUMP OF THE ONCE-REFUGE (AND YET not really there, for in fact Jake Cutter was asleep and uneasily dreaming in a jet-copter speeding east towards Brisbane across the vastly sprawling Simpson Desert), Harry Keogh's deadspeak voice once again startled Jake from the weird reverie induced by Korath Mindsthrall's story:

You've done well, Korath, and we are almost finished now, Harry said.

Almost? The vampire answered gloomily, by now perhaps resignedly. *What more can you possibly want of me?*

Well, we know what you failed *to find when you returned to Starside,* the ex-Necroscope, or rather his revenant—or better still this facet of him—answered. *You didn't find Shaitan or any others of the Wamphyri, and you certainly didn't find their aeries! Instead you found the hollow stumps of those once-great stacks, which you, your master, and his colleagues were obliged to use as temporary dwelling places. Then, once again, you commenced raiding on Sunside's Szgany. You can take it from there.*

But it scarcely seems worthwhile, Korath protested. *For it appears you already know it all!*

Not all of it. (The shake of an incorporeal head.) *How did Malinari and the others fair on Sunside, for instance? We would like to know how the Szgany . . . welcomed them? Also, we want to know what made those three Great Vampires desert Starside, risk their necks by venturing into the ill-omened subterranean Gate, and come here. And since you were involved, who better to ask?*

Very well, Korath grated, his patience all but used up. *If it would please you—*

—It would, Harry told him. *And it would serve to keep us here a while longer at least.*

Then, with a sigh, Korath put the finishing touches to his tale:

"We flew home, to what had been our home. You are correct: the aeries were gone, like vast stone corpses fallen on the barren boulder plains. And arriving in the hour before sunup, we were obliged to find shelter in their shattered stumps.

"The *Desmodus* colonies were still there, and we found ourselves greeted by descendants of the descendants of our former familiars. At least they were the same! And like the bats themselves, we sheltered from the sun (which seemed to rise marginally higher in the sky) in their lowly crumbling caverns in the echoing basement levels of the shattered stacks.

"Night came, and with it the fear that perhaps the Szgany were no more: that they, too, might have succumbed to whatever disaster was befallen here. But when we flew to the higher ridges of the barrier mountains and looked down on Sunside—

"—Ah! But the Szgany were there, and in such numbers!

"Their campfires—and in many cases more permanent town or settlement fires—lit the night like so many glowworms in the dark of forests which, in our time, had not seen so much as a nightlight, but only the telltale smoke of cottage or caravan stoves! And here they were all joyous, juicy, and fearless, our beloved Szgany of Sunside. The sounds of their music drifted up to our keen vampire ears, and the smells of their cooking—and of *them*—to our wide, straining nostrils. Ah, that was a beautiful moment!

"And Malinari said: 'The Wamphyri are gone. We three alone of all the Great Vampires survive.' (He excluded me, of course.) 'Do you see, Vavara? We *are* survivors, the only survivors! And so I was right.'

" 'And now we go down,' whispered Szwart, 'to the feast!'

"But: 'Ah, no, not so,' said The Mind, holding up a cautionary hand. 'Those tribes down there, they do not know we are back. If we raid here, now, then they *will* know. And next time will be that much harder. But we have aeries to build and furnish, lieutenants and thralls to recruit, warrior creatures and flyers to breed in our vats—hah! When we have first discovered or dug vats, in the wreckage of those shattered stumps!

" 'Also, you must ask yourself what happened here. Did the Wamphyri destroy themselves or were they destroyed? And if the latter, by whom? The Szgany? Ah, no, Lord Szwart, having survived the Icelands, I am in no great hurry to show myself here. For my thoughts have gone out and found an odd sense of security and freedom in the Szgany.

Why, they are unafraid! Perhaps because they no longer have reason to be afraid. Which in turn might mean that we do. Wherefore we must be cautious and first discover the secret of these changes in the scheme of things.'

" 'So what would you suggest?' Szwart hissed. 'That we sit here all night and admire their fires?'

"Malinari shook his head. 'Those tribes down there, close-packed in this central area of Sunside. If we raid on one, then by morning all of them will know. And we need time to reestablish ourselves. So this is what we will do. Tonight we split up. Vavara raids in the far west, you in the east, but this side of the great pass. I shall raid beyond the pass. And we glut, aye, but mainly we recruit—we recruit *furiously,* taking as many as we can. We share our spoils equally, building together, allies by circumstance as we have always been. This way, gradually, we shall discover what's what here: how things stand, and why they seem so different now. Is it agreed?'

"After some small haggling it was so agreed, and as Malinari had decreed we recruited 'furiously.' We converted men into thralls, from whose ranks we chose lieutenants; these were soon able to make more thralls—and so on. And we stockpiled drink and foodstuffs (aye, and other good *stuff*) out of Sunside, and put a taskforce to work digging in the rubble-strewn stumps of the old fallen stacks, building walls around our chosen habitations and roofing them over.

"During all of this construction, occasionally our workers would uncover vats, gas-beast chambers, or cocooned *matter* from yesteryear. Of course, the greater mass of the once-living material was putrid, no longer useable; some of it, however, contained a spark and was digestible, assimilable by newer, fresher material out of Sunside. And so we progressed.

"But time passed, and word of our presence also passed—from tribe to tribe and clan to clan—until all the peoples of Sunside knew that the Wamphyri were back in Starside. It didn't take long, say ten or twelve sundowns.

"Meanwhile we had recruited some eight hundred men,

women, and children. Moreover, deep beneath the foundations of a toppled aerie, our workers had discovered a cache of well-preserved metamorphic liquids requiring little more than imprinting—an infusion of essence and a few nodes of rudimentary intelligence—to stimulate growth. And now we could fill the vats with vampiric life.

"First we made flyers, successfully! And later we tried for warriors, but that was when the trouble started. It was a tribe known for its aggressive nature in the olden times, and no less ferocious now: the Szgany Lidesci, whose territory lay mid-west of Sunside in fertile forests under cavern-riddled foothills.

"Apparently the Lidescis had found a hero, a youth or man called Nathan Kiklu, who had ventured into forbidden places and returned with awesome weapons. It was a story we heard over and over again from thralls recruited in Sunside: how this Nathan's brother had been Wamphyri—Lord Nestor, of an aerie so mighty it could only have been Dramstack, or whatever it was called in his time—and how he had contrived to hurl his Szgany sibling into the Hell-lands Gate.

"Well, the Gate was a legend; in our time it had been used as a punishment, and no man or creature who entered, 'banished' into the white glare of the Starside Gate, had ever returned to tell of his adventures. But that was then and this was now, and for a certainty this Nathan was extant; all too soon, we would begin to experience his works at firsthand.

"He was of the Szgany Lidesci. No longer nomadic, the Lidescis had built a sprawling town or fortification called Settlement. And the first time we raided on them—which was also the last time—ah, but *then* we discovered the meaning of 'awesome weapons!'

"Our warriors—which were far more complicated constructs than flyers—were not waxed as yet. We went in with a force of flyers and thrall riders, and a handful of lieutenants to guide the men into battle. Except it wasn't planned as a battle but a rout, when the Szgany would flee and we would pick off the hindmost. Vavara and Malinari between them made a mist (Szwart was above such devices when he could avoid them; since he could simply merge into the night, he deemed mists unsporting and indeed unnecessary deceptions). But be that as it may, the mist rolled down out of the foothills to swallow Settlement whole. We could see the fitful glow of the Lidescis' communal fires deep in its clammy heart.

"Then our flyers launched and settled towards the town . . . and flew straight into the teeth of hell!

"Fortunately, we leaders were not in the forefront of this offensive; instead, alerted by my master who was suspicious, we had held back to observe the initial Lidesci reaction. For when Malinari had sent his telepathic probes deep into the mist over Settlement, he had sensed something strange—a mental silence, an awareness, a threat. And he was right.

"The night came alive with deafening explosions, brilliant flashes of light and shrill screams—*not* Szgany screams! These were the shrieks of our thralls, and the hissing death-cries of stricken flyers. And echoing up to us from Settlement's wooden walls came sharp, spitting cracks of sound one after the other, like stones breaking in a fire or saplings snapping in an avalanche. And great, dazzling balls of fire came soaring up out of the mist into a body of flyers that was still descending. Wherever they hit, destruction followed: flyers bursting into flame and blazing thralls leaping from their saddles!

"And finally more aerial fireballs: this time aimed at us, where we looked on in utter disbelief from our 'safe' foothills ridge. Then:

"'Enough!' And uttering a curse, Szwart spurred his mount aloft and climbed into the night. A true fly-the-light, he had seen and suffered all he could bear; now he retreated from the blinding flares of man-made fireballs.

"Malinari and Vavara, they used Wamphyri mentalism to call off what handfuls remained of our forces, many of whom were too badly damaged to make it back across the barrier mountains into Starside. And as that sorry, scorched, and blistered rabble came limping through the mist—glad to escape from the roil and the reek—so we launched and rose on sulphur thermals, and headed for home. . . .

". . . *And* for the surprise of our lives!

"As we fell towards the triangle of rubble wherein we had commenced to build our new empire, we saw what could not be—such devastation! Our central gas-beast chambers, blown asunder, and their occupants in tatters all strewn about, exploded in the blast of their own gasses! And warrior vats ablaze with liquid fire that burned blue to melt the mewling monsters! And even as we circled overhead in stunned amaze, a thunderous explosion that tossed shattered vampire thralls and debris aloft over the battlement walls of one of Malinari's unfinished constructions (a warrior pen, which never would be finished now), bursting the walls themselves outwards with its force!

"We landed hurriedly, in unaccustomed disarray, and without ceremony my master and his colleagues hurled themselves in their fury upon those thralls who had been left behind to mind our works. But before a single question could be fired, a single thrall executed:

" 'Ho, there!' A strange voice from on high—but not the harsh tones, warning growl or threatening hiss of the Wamphyri. No, this was the voice of a young man, and entirely human.

"He stood on the ledge of a shattered stump, his back to the sheer rock wall. There was no way up from his position and none down, not without he encounter the Wamphyri or their lieutenants and thralls. And he was tall but slight, with nothing of the bulk of a vampire or the leaden look of a Lord. He was, quite literally, a man—Szgany.

" 'Who are you?' said Malinari. 'This Nathan, perhaps? And is this your work? If so you are a dead man!' I felt my master concentrating, the waves of animosity beating out from him, to enter the stranger's mind and befuddle it.

"But young as he was, and obviously mad (or perhaps not?) he only smiled a knowing smile, shook his head, and said, 'Ah, no, my mentalist friend—my mind is shielded. And if Maglore the Mage could not get to me, what chance have you? And you're right: I am Nathan, and this *is* my work. Nor have you seen the last of it.'

"Malinari gestured (with his mind); thralls crept towards the broken stairway that led to Nathan's position. He glanced at them, saw them coming, appeared to ignore them! Meanwhile, the voluptuous Vavara had stepped forward. She was almost physically aglow and issued her ultimate aura of feminine allure. Her mouth blew a kiss and a promise in Nathan's direction; she smiled up at him on his ledge—the knowing smile of a whore, yet one to cut into a man's soul, if he had one—and lit the night with the lustful heat of her jewel-green, crimson-cored eyes.

"Tipping back her hood and opening her collar, she shook out her raven hair, then let her long, bat-fur cloak fall open. Her blouse was a simple band of cloth crossing from shoulder to waist, cupping one breast and leaving the other bare. Her flesh was marble in moon and starlight, and that proud, naked, stiff-tipped breast shone with the oils she used. She twirled to send her skirt of ropes flying, then came to an abrupt halt. Tantalizing she stood, with her cloak poised on the air and the ropes of her skirt outflung. Her sturdy legs were spread wide, thighs like pillars, buttocks as round as an apple, dark-tufted in its dimple where the stem has been plucked and a leaf or two remain. And I stood there drooling my lust, for I had grown just such a stem as might replace it! Then Vavara's cloak floated back into position and she was covered. But the picture stayed printed on every eye.

"I felt my blood pounding; I might myself have rushed upon her—to my doom—but Malinari's hand was on my shoulder; he held me back. And this tall, pale Szgany whelp, this Nathan, he looked down on the priestess of lust, looked down on Vavara . . . *and curled his lip!*

"Vavara was astonished; she felt her aura repelled as this mere man scorned her, saying, 'As for you: you should know that I have been tempted by *real* Ladies! My mind is closed to you no less than to the mentalist there. And by the way, I know all of you. You Vavara, Malinari, and Szwart. You were legends and now you are reality, come back from the

Icelands. But if I were you I would return there, and now. There's nothing for you here but the true death. And like my father before me, who brought down these evil stacks to shatter into pieces on the boulder plains, so shall I bring you down. That is my vow, as a man of the Szgany Lidesci.'

"Through all of this, Szwart had melted himself to a dark shadow on the strewn rubble. Now, flowing like a black and sentient lichen—a living stain—he moved towards the crumbling stairway. By now, too, Malinari's thralls had climbed halfway up, which was as far as they would ever get.

" 'And you, Szwart,' said the youth from on high, perhaps fifty feet up the stony skeleton of that ancient stairway. 'Do you think to sweep over and devour me? As the legend goes, you are akin to the night and can disappear into it. But you and I know that men—and monsters—cannot simply disappear. It's true, Szwart, isn't it?' While he spoke he took something from his Szgany jerkin, twisted it in his hands, lobbed it down, to bounce from step to step. And he said, 'Well, perhaps it's true for you, at least. But as for me: I must be on my way. You may not see me, but you'll definitely be hearing from me.' So saying, he stepped back into the shadows where the wall angled.

"Lord Szwart flowed over the top of the wall where Nathan had stood, and onto the ledge from which he'd taunted all three of the Wamphyri. Szwart's darkness gathered there, shifting and seething, then rolled on into the selfsame shadows that hid the madman from view. And I knew that it was the end for Nathan Kiklu, whoever he had been. Lord Szwart's protoplasm would envelop him; its strange, metamorphic acids would work on him; he would shrink, devolve, and *dissolve* to become one with night's master. Or rather, his liquefied flesh would add to Szwart's bulk for a while, until it was converted into fuel.

"The egg-shaped item that Nathan had thrown bounced again, into the group of three climbing thralls. And there it exploded in a flash of light as bright and momentarily brighter than the sun itself! Light, heat, and a blast of alien energy that lacerated the flesh of the unfortunate thralls and blew them off the stone stairway, down into the rubble. They were in pieces, dead before they hit bottom. And Szwart hissing and shrieking, reeling on the high stairs where he tried to regain his man-shape, failed, and collapsed again to a slithering stain.

"All of this shocking, aye, but none so much as what Lord Szwart called out to us as finally he reformed, shaping himself into an airfoil and launching in search of some night-dark place in which to regain his composure:

" 'He was not there!' he shrilled. 'He *is* not here! No man, that one, but a ghost! Perhaps the spirit of all the Szgany we ever took in our lives, all combined in one vengeful ghost!'

"And Malinari turned to Vavara and said, 'Szwart is right. Not that Nathan is a ghost, but that he's no longer here. For a moment I touched his mind—*real* in the field of my probes, as real as the shields he raised against me—and in the next moment, gone! So if you think we have seen awesome weapons at work this night, well now we have seen a *real* weapon: the man Nathan himself. But all of this bears thinking about, and I shall give it my gravest consideration.'

"And despite that The Mind had chosen his words carefully, perhaps because he felt he must retain at least a measure of control, still his sprouting scythe teeth were awash in his own blood where he ground them deep into his lips and riven gums."

"And Malinari did give it his gravest consideration, as did we all; but no amount of thinking could compensate for our losses, or dream up a successful defense against future depredations by the demon Nathan. Thus that entire night was a disaster, and no guarantee that things were ever going to get any better.

"We went subterranean. Unthinkable, eh—that the Wamphyri should ever flee from a man? From the sun, aye, but not from a single man! Yet such was the case. If we could not build on high, then we must build below, where the stumps of the toppled stacks were riddled with tunnels, caverns, and places which, in the olden times, were only ever fit for bats and beetles.

"And despite that our work force was reduced—our flyers, too, and our warriors boiled in their vats—still we had several hundreds of thralls and provisions aplenty.

"The thralls were put to work; they cleared the debris from ancient diggings, moved our provisions to safety, and built defensive positions on the surface. New vats of metamorphosis were discovered or dug, into which we sacrificed a third of our manpower, the raw materials of our future flyers and warriors. And we commenced keeping a watch. . . . Can you believe it? The Wamphyri, vigilant against any further sabotage attempts by this mere man! Moreover, it was more rigidly enforced than any watch that our vanished ancestors had ever kept against each other.

"But this last was a necessity, for from then on, whenever we raided against the Szgany, we could be sure that retaliation would follow hot on our heels. And Nathan Kiklu—man or ghost or whatever he was—he was everywhere. If we raided in the far western reaches of Sunside, he would soon be there with a party of Lidesci fighters, with 'guns,' 'grenades,' and 'rockets,' setting fire to the wings of our flyers, blinding them with silver shot, and knocking our thralls out of their saddles before they could even touch down! Thus, for every man we recruited in Sunside, one of ours was killed by Nathan and his Szgany soldiers. And every forward step was followed by one to the rear.

"East, west, wherever we struck, Nathan and his men could be there in a trice. How? It was beyond us. Moreover, he would snipe on us from afar, and shoot our thralls dead in their defensive or watchtower positions. Until my master and his colleagues were obliged to devise a new strategy.

"Instead of inhabiting just one central area of Starside's olden ruins, now we spread out and stationed men in every shattered stump and heap of rubble. For one thing was certain: who or whatever Nathan was, and for all that he could appear almost magically, anywhere, in extremely short order, he couldn't possibly be everywhere at once! And so we maintained something of our equilibrium, despite that we made little progress. . . .

"One night my master flew out alone. Returning shortly, he complained bitterly that: 'This damned Szgany bastard—he has spies in the barrier mountains! *Hah!* That is how he knows where we will raid: they watch us fly up from the boulder plains, the direction we take, then make report to him. I tracked them with my mentalism—which is how I discovered theirs!'

" 'What? They are thought-thieves, these men?' Vavara found it hard to believe. 'Mentalists?'

"Malinari laughed like a madman, and answered, 'Even as we are mentalists, aye. So says Malinari the Mind, the greatest of them all. But . . . they are *not* men!'

" 'Not men?' And now Szwart was baffled. 'Not men, you say? Then what—trogs?'

"Malinari gave a wild shake of his head and waved his arms in consternation. 'Not trogs, no—but *dogs!*' he said. 'Wolves of the wild that *think* like men. Stranger still, they call this Nathan uncle! He is their kin!'

" 'Then he is a dog-Lord!' said Vavara. 'It's the only possible solution. This hated enemy of ours is Wamphyri! He dwells in the mountain heights, rules on Sunside, and keeps the Szgany for himself. His needs are so slight that the tribes suffer him for his protection. I must be right. Nathan is a changeling.'

"And Szwart said, 'But a dog-Lord? With powers such as he commands? And as for suffering him for his protection—against what? What was there before we came?'

"My master threw up his hands, crying, 'I don't know! I no longer know anything . . . except that I am sick to death of this Nathan, of this ruined place, and of all this endless work performed without reward. This work that gets us no-where . . .'"

"We took to raiding separately but simultaneously in locations far apart, and we covered our movements with great stealth. For again the principle applied: that Nathan couldn't be everywhere at once. And at last a small measure of success—which didn't last long. *He* couldn't be everywhere, but his weapons could.

"From thralls freshly converted we learned how he had disseminated his destructive devices—his guns and grenades, and so forth—among as many as possible of the tribes. And he had taught them how to use them. But these weapons and the 'ammunition' they used were not in unlimited supply. From time to time Nathan must replenish them by venturing into the Hell-lands.

"That in itself posed a question: how was it possible for Nathan to make these trips to the Hell-lands without using the Starside Gate? For the Gate was no longer accessible. Where in our time it had rested in the bottom of a crater in the lee of the foothills not far from the great pass, now it was raised up and stood in the centre of a lake! And that lake of white water had many small whirlpools to suck a swimmer down.

"Often in our forays across the barrier mountains into Sunside we had seen it there: that fountain of water, all lit from within, rising up high into the night and falling back into the lake.

"In order to solve that problem, we flew out one night; or rather, Malinari and Vavara flew out, and a few lieutenants and thralls in attendance. For Lord Szwart would not consider going anywhere near such a brilliant source of light, despite that it was cold.

"Ah, but that was indeed a fortunate trip—for the Wamphyri at least, if not (as it later turned out) for me; though of course I could not know that then. Anyway, during the long day previous, while we vampires slept or carried out our subterranean duties beneath the stumps of the old stacks, apparently the lake had run dry!

"And there stood the Gate, raised up in its crater socket, like the blind white eye of some fallen Cyclops shining up into the night. But as for the lake and its fountain of milky water: they were no more, not even a trickle! The earth was dry, caked, and wrinkled into channels that showed how the water had disappeared down circular boreholes that angled into the bedrock like conduits to hell. A weird thing, this Gate; weird as the tumbling moon or ice-chip stars, and just as inexplicable.

"Malinari, Vavara, and their men had left their flyers in the shadowy foothills between the Gate and the great pass, well away from the Gate itself. Facing downhill on a moderate slope, the flyers were positioned for immediate flight. It was a safety measure, to ensure a quick getaway should such become necessary. And so it may be seen that even among the Great Vampires the Hell-lands Gate was held in no small measure of respect.

"And separating into small, widespread groups, we applied the same caution to our method of approach—moving from boulder clump to boulder clump, and always sticking to the shadows—as we drew closer to the Gate. But we were still some distance away when suddenly my master threw up a warning hand, and issued a mental alarm that reached out to all of us:

"*Something is coming through the Gate!* his voice hissed in our minds as we melted back into darkest shadows.

"And he was correct, of course. He had sensed their alien minds, these men of the Hell-lands (of your world, that is), as they stepped forth onto the surface of our world. Far more importantly, however, Malinari had sensed their unpreparedness. Oh, they had weapons as devastating as Nathan's, but for protection as opposed to open aggression. Also, they had little or no idea what to expect in Starside, and to a man their minds were preoccupied with greed for the heavy, malleable yellow metal that you call gold, which in my world is common.

"They were thirty-two in number, half of them being soldiers who took up positions on the flanks as the rest formed into an unruly, excited, and chattering body. Then they marched for the great pass. Two of the soldiers rode noisy, wheeled engines that cut the darkness with beams of cold white light; they went ahead to pick a route through the many boulders that litter the area. Keeping still and silent in the shadows, we let them pass right through the various groups of our divided party.

"Then it was that Malinari apprised us, *These men are not like Nathan. They are like* infants, *with little or no knowledge of what they are about! Those on the outside—the soldiers—they have weapons. When we strike, we take them out first. Kill them with dispatch. They barely outnumber us and shouldn't be a problem; this time the advantage of surprise is on our side. As for the central body: these are the minds behind the muscle . . . puny things by my reckoning, and not a mentalist among them. So be it; they are weaklings and we must take them alive for questioning. Now make ready—in the next few seconds your destiny may change beyond all recognition!*

"Which of course it did.

"I cannot describe what next took place as 'a battle,' nor even a rout, for none of our victims had time to flee. Surprise was indeed on our side, and add to this our flowing, lightning-strike speed, and our vampire strength, equal in each of us to that of four or five strong men . . . the result was overwhelming. Hell-landers they were, but they had never seen hell such as we delivered that night.

"There was some gunfire, soon silenced. We lost a lieutenant and three thralls. The Hell-landers lost everything—their so-called 'fighting men,' anyway. As for the two on their 'motorcycles': they returned to see what was the trouble and, having seen it, didn't stop but headed out onto the barren boulder plains. We picked them off later.

"The freshly dead were carried back to fuel our vats, the living were taken for questioning by Malinari. I can't honestly say which group was least fortunate, the living or the dead . . . the living, I suspect. In the long run it would make no difference; the one group would join the other.

"What my master learned, however—ah, but *that* made a big difference! Sufficient to excite Malinari and his Wamphyri colleagues beyond measure. And for me, it was the beginning of the end. . . ."

*   *   *

Korath had fallen silent for a while. When next he spoke it was similar to a sigh in Jake Cutter's sleeping mind, and deadspeak in the metaphysical Harry Keogh's:

The rest you know. In a while, when Malinari had extracted and assimilated all he could of knowledge from the minds of the 'scientists' and their military leader, it was time to take our leave of Starside.

Before doing so, The Mind, Vavara, and Szwart made a great many lieutenants; they took them down into undeath, and brought them up again as burgeoning Wamphyri! And they divided between them all the remaining thralls, flyers and waxing warriors, and all territorial holdings, provisions, and so forth. It was done for spite, out of malice; if the three Great Vampires could not have Sunside/Starside for their own, then neither could Nathan and the Lidescis, nor the Szgany as a people—not without they fight for it for long and long, and pay for it in blood. And so you may be sure that even now there are new Lords in Starside, while in Sunside the blood flows as of yore. . . .

Finally Korath was done, and Harry said, *From all you have told us, your lot was not a happy one. And your end was unfair, to say the least.*

I am glad you finally agree! said the dead vampire. But:

—From what you have *told us, at least,* said Harry. *But I am more concerned with what you* haven't *told us, which is probably more important than all the rest put together. The Wamphyri have been here in our world for some time, but it would seem they've achieved very little. What are they up to, Korath? What is their plan? You were one of theirs, and so you must know.*

Ahhhh! said the other slyly, in a tone that suggested the shake of an incorporeal head. *And so to the crux of the matter. But no, what you ask is for me to know and for you to discover, or to guess at for a long, long time, until it is too late. For after all, it is my only remaining bargaining point— the last trick up a poor dead thing's sleeve. And when you have that, I shall have nothing at all.*

"Bargaining point?" said Jake, just a little surprised by his own voice, after keeping so long silent. "But you're a dead thing! What can you possibly bargain for—what can we give you—apart from a little companionship, a little cold comfort?"

Well, that might be a start. . . .

But the ex-Necroscope intervened and said: *You have already had that, companionship and cold comfort, and probably too much of both. It isn't a healthy thing to spend too much time in the company of vampires. No, there's no bargain you can strike here, Korath Mindsthrall. Also, I sense that your will is strong. You are dead, but your tenacity is very much alive! Jake, it's time we were leaving.*

"I thought you'd never get to it," Jake answered.

I only hope you remember some of this, said Harry.

"I'm still not a hundred percent sure I want to," Jake vacillated.

Well, get sure! said Harry, his fading deadspeak voice frustrated and angry. *Your entire world depends upon it. And if you can't remember anything else, do try to remember this:*

An incredible wall of numbers—like a computer screen run riot—evolved in the eye of Jake's mind, its symbols and equations marching and mutating until they reached a certain critical point . . . and formed a door. A Möbius door! And Jake knew without knowing how that all that remained of Harry was passing through it, moving on to another place, perhaps another time.

"I . . . I'm supposed to remember *that?*" he said, as the door collapsed and left him on his own in the dank and gurgling sump of the once-Refuge. On his own, but not quite alone. For:

Do not concern yourself, Jake Cutter, Korath Mindsthrall's leering deadspeak voice came to him out of the sudden inky darkness that enveloped him and the sump and everything, a darkness that was prelude to the light of the waking world. *No, for I am sure that we'll be able to work something out—*

—Er, between us?

Jake made no reply, or if he did it was left behind as he went spiralling up and up to the waiting light. . . .

24
Synchronicity

LIZ WAS LEANING OVER HIM AGAIN. "REMEMBER what?" she said.

"Eh?" Jake blinked sleep out of his eyes, groped to brush grit from their corners.

"You were rambling on about having to remember something," she told him. And while he was ordering his thoughts to frame a reply, she quickly went on: "And before you ask—no, I wasn't snooping on you. I came back here to give you a shake; you were mumbling, and I thought you were speaking to me."

Well, he hadn't been, but he had been speaking to someone. Harry? Korath? But who the hell was Korath? The name, so familiar one minute, was already meaningless, slipping from the edge of his mind. So that now, just a moment later, Jake wasn't sure it meant anything at all.

Well, get sure! . . . get sure . . . get sure (Like an echo, fading in his memory.) And numbers—a swirl of numbers, equations, symbols, like a mathematician's nightmare—all collapsing to a big Zero, nothing, where before they had meant something.

"Numbers!" Jake croaked, forcing the word out of his dehydrated throat. Liz handed him a can of Coke that she was drinking from, and he sat up and swilled his mouth out, then let the fizzing liquid burn and cool and sting all the way down.

"Numbers?" Liz repeated him. "What about them?"

Awake now, he frowned at her. "Are you sure you weren't in there with me?" Then seeing the look on her face: "Okay, okay! Just checking." He took another swig, climbed un-

347

steadily to his feet. "I think I was dreaming about—hell, I don't know—all sorts of stuff." He looked at his boots, then stooped to touch the bottoms of his jeans and wondered why he thought they might be wet. "I can't remember. A damp place? Voices? Numbers?"

But Liz only shrugged. "You tell me," she said, and turned away so that he wouldn't see the look she flashed at the others up front. And over her shoulder she told him, "We're on our way down. Brisbane next stop."

Ben Trask, Lardis, Goodly, and the others were looking at Jake while he worked the stiffness from his joints and followed Liz to her gunner's chair. As she strapped herself in, he indicated the gun ports and asked, "Is it okay to open one of these up? And which side is Brisbane?"

One of the technicians answered him. "Sure—you can open the doors. But you better hook yourself up first. Brisbane's to port." There were safety straps dangling from the ceiling. Jake pulled one down, hooked it to his belt, jerked on the port-side door's handle, and slid the door open. Air blasted in, the downdraft from the big fan, and immediately the *whup, whup, whup* of the rotors was a deafening throb.

Liz hooked up, joined him at the door. "Have you been here before?" she inquired, but her words were whipped away. It made no difference; he "heard" her anyway. And answered:

No, I haven't. And you're getting good at that.

She only looked at him and said, *But I'm not a natural— not at sending, not yet anyway—so maybe you're the one who's getting good at it.*

No. He shook his head to give his thoughts emphasis. *It's all you, Liz. It's your talent, getting stronger all the time. And maybe some kind of rapport we seem to be developing.* Which was the closest he had yet come to admitting any kind of serious involvement.

Their eyes met, locked just for a moment, and each of them knew that the same thought was in the other's mind: that out of the blue Jake was accepting telepathy that much more easily—as if he'd been getting some practice. And they both knew where he had been getting it. It was as he'd explained to Lardis: sleep, the subconscious mind, was a strange thing. And dreams could be stranger yet. Sometimes they could even be more than dreams.

Then they looked down on a small airfield six hundred feet directly below them, and, two or three miles to the east, central Brisbane.

Brisbane was big and sprawling, but it didn't lack order. On the contrary, if anything it was *too* symmetrical, ultramodern. Its streets were too broad, with too many parks, pools, green areas. It should have looked as cool and fresh as an oasis, which in all this heat, when even the downdraft of the rotors felt as hot as hell, would have seemed very welcoming. But the river, instead of being a fat, winding, silver eel, was more a thin, snakelike whiplash. Most of the pools were empty down to their liners, and all of the green places had yellow tints.

Jake frowned and might have commented, but the horizon was rapidly rising. As they watched, Brisbane came up level and finally disappeared behind the airport buildings. And just a moment or two later they bumped down.

When the rotors went into braking mode, their whine became unbearable. Grimacing, Jake slammed the door to shut it out. . . .

The small airport—more an airstrip, really—belonged to a private flying club for well-to-do members of Brisbane society. The chopper's pilot had been directed to it by air traffic control, who in turn had taken their orders from higher authority. It might look odd if a paramilitary jet-copter were to land at a main international airport . . . especially carrying the E-Branch contingent, whose members were by now beginning to look something less than reputable.

Trask had radioed ahead before decamping on the other side of the continent; discreet arrangements had been made while the chopper was still in the air; met by a pair of clean-cut, immaculately-uniformed "chauffeurs," the drivers of limos with one-way-glass windows, Trask and his people were soon on their way into the city.

As they left the airport heading for a main arterial road, they passed a small parking lot. Sitting on the hood of a battered, blue-grey, range-rover-styled vehicle, a tall, angular male figure in jeans, open-necked shirt, and broad-brimmed hat gazed intently into the sky over the airport through a pair of binoculars. With his hat shading his face, his features were blankly anonymous under the brilliance of the mid-afternoon sunlight.

There seemed nothing special about him—except to Liz. She'd seen how, at the last minute, before the car threw up a screen of dust in their wake, the man had turned his binoculars on the two vehicles. Now, with a frown, she tapped Trask on the shoulder where he sat in front of her.

"That man back there," she said, hurriedly. They were negotiating a bend and the parking lot was already disappearing in the driver's rearview. Trask turned his head, looked back where Liz was indicating; he saw nothing but a dust plume and a distant shimmer of heat haze.

"A man?" he said. "What about him?"

The intercom was on, and the chauffeur—a special agent—asked, "Something suspicious, miss? A man, did you say? Back there? What was he doing?"

"Sitting on a car," Liz answered. "He was watching the sky through binoculars."

"A plane-spotter?" Through the plate-glass screen that divided them, they saw the driver shrug. "A wannabe fly-boy member of the club. *Huh!* Some hope. Flying is for rich folks."

But Liz leaned forward and quietly, right in Trask's ear, said, "The last thing I saw, he was looking at us."

They were turning onto the main road and picking up speed. "Let it go," Trask told her. "It may have been nothing, and in any case it's too late now. If we've been made we've been made. But *if* we've been made, then obviously someone was sent to make us—sent *by* someone. Now all we have to do is find out who and where."

Liz nodded, said: "And . . . he was wondering about us."

"That's all you got?"

"Yes."

Trask shrugged, but not negligently. "Maybe he was simply curious. But by the same token maybe this wasn't as discreet as it might have been. Two chauffeur-driven limos, doing reception at a small, private airport? I mean, turn the situation around and I might be curious myself. Do you think you'd recognize him again?"

"Probably," she answered. "There was something unpleasant, spidery about him."

"Well, if you do see him let me know," said Trask. "Once is coincidence. Twice . . . this spider might need stepping on." And the cars sped for the near-distant city. . . .

Back at the parking lot, the long thin man got into his car and called a number on his portaphone. A disinterested female voice said, "Xanadu; reception."

"I want to speak to Milan," the thin man told her.

There was a pause and she said, "Your identification?" Now she was a little more animated.

"Mind your business," the thin man replied, with the emphasis on "mind," but with nothing of rebuke or unpleasantness in his voice. It was simply a code.

"Just a moment, sir," said the girl. And the phone played some indifferent Muzak.

While he waited, the thin man coughed to clear his throat, mopped sweat from his brow, got his thoughts in order. His employer—Mr. Milan, to whom he was about to make report—had a liking for ordered minds; he much preferred to hear and understand things clearly and precisely the first time around. And in a little while:

"Milan speaking," a deep, accented, seemingly cultured yet vaguely threatening male voice replaced the Muzak. "What do you want?"

And the thin man told his employer what he had seen of the jet-copter, gave him brief descriptions of the people he'd seen getting into limos outside the flying club's main building, and closed by saying: "They drove off towards Brisbane."

There was a brief pause before the other queried: "And you didn't follow them?"

"It was the chauffeurs," the thin man answered. "They were too good to be true. No one looks as neat, tidy, and as cool as they looked—not in this weather—without they're trying real hard. They looked like government men. And if they were, they'd be on me like flies on shit as soon as they spotted me in their rearviews."

"I see," said the foreign, Mediterranean-sounding voice of Mr. Milan. And in a moment: "Would you know these people again?"

"Sure."

"Good. I think this may be what I've been waiting for. You can call your other observers off, Mr. Santeson. Let them report to you in Xanadu. From now on I think you will find your duties more to your liking up here at the resort. Just be sure to come and see me as soon as you get in."

"I'm on it," the thin man said. And under his breath, when the phone went dead: "What are you—some kind of mindreader? But anyway, you're right—that's just *exactly* what I wanted to hear after a day spent sweltering in all this heat, sweating my balls off, watching, waiting, and trying not to look suspicious. Shitty work, in weather like this. But up there at the Pleasure Dome . . ."

. . . *Up at the Pleasure Dome,* he thought, putting the car in first and turning out of the parking lot, *life is sheer luxury! The pools, the broads in their bikinis, the good food and drink—even the casino, huh!—where I can spend my money almost as fast, or faster, than Mr. fucking Milan pays me!* And he grinned.

But on the other hand, no one could call Milan mean. Garth Santeson, a private investigator for twenty years and then some, had never had it so good. *What? Milan, mean?*

No way! Shady, definitely—how else would you describe a guy who only ever comes out at night? But never mean— hell, no! The way Aristotle Milan throws money around, it's like . . . like tomorrow there'll be no use for it!

Never knowing just how close he had come to the truth, and in more respects than one, Santeson headed his battered vehicle for the ring-road south around Brisbane. Then he would look for the signpost for the town of Beaudesert, which would put him on a heading for the Macpherson Range right on the border with New South Wales. Eighty miles of good road, and he'd be up into the mountains, yes.

And finally, Xanadu . . .

On the way into town, Jake said, "Now I remember!"

"What you were dreaming about?" said Lardis Lidesci.

"Eh?" Jake looked at him.

"On the plane, you were dreaming about something. When Liz woke you up you couldn't remember."

Jake shook his head. "No, not that," he said. "I'm talking about Brisbane—I'm remembering about this place. Looking down on the city from the chopper, I thought it looked too neat, too new. Well, that's because it *is* new."

Jake and Lardis were travelling in the first limo with the team's top technicians, a pair of young, whiz-kid computer and communications types who were fully-fledged members of E-Branch but not espers as such. One of these, Jimmy Harvey—a compact, prematurely bald man of perhaps twenty-six, with grey, watery eyes, lush red sideburns and bushy eyebrows that together were trying hard to make up for his baldness, and a genius for electronics—wanted to know: "Jake, where have you been hiding out these last three or four years? I mean, on the Richter scale of national disasters, Brisbane's Great Fire of 2007 ranks several notches higher than the sinking of the Titanic, and very nearly as high as Krakatoa!" There was little or nothing of sarcasm in Harvey's comment, just surprise.

Jake sighed, shrugged apologetically, and said, "Yes, that was what I remembered. As for where I've been: mainly I've been doing my own thing. My world has been—I don't know—kind of a small place. For a long time I've only had room for personal problems, things that I need to get sorted out."

"Aye," Lardis grunted. "Your vow! I can understand that."

"My vow?" Jake frowned at him. As usual, he found the old boy full of indecipherable statements. But now:

"In Sunside," Lardis deciphered, "when a man has something to do—a wrong that needs righting—he makes a vow, usually in public. And he holds to it until it's done. I made just such a vow one time, and it still isn't done. But if I can't be killing the bloodsucking bastards there, at least I'm helping to kill them here."

Jimmy Harvey, despite that he wasn't privy to Jake's past, believed he'd got the drift of it. "So how about you, Jake?" he said. "You mentioned things you 'need' to get sorted out: present tense. So like Lardis, you're not finished yet, right?"

"Not quite, no," Jake shook his head. "But there's plenty of time yet." And to change the subject: "Why don't you tell me about Brisbane, fill in whatever it is I've missed?"

The other wasn't about to start prying; the one thing he'd learned in his time with the Branch was that these people hated to talk about their private lives almost as much as their weird "talents." And as far as their powers were concerned: the majority didn't see them as bonuses at all, just extra baggage. Jake hadn't been around too long and was a new one on Harvey. Still, he was on the team and so must be an esper. Well, no one can be expert in everything. But . . . the Great Fire of Brisbane? Something like that had escaped his notice? Jake had to be pulling his leg. But he didn't look like he was. And so:

"It was about this time of year," Harvey started out. "And what do you know, 2007 was another El Niño year, just like this one—synchronicity or something. Anyway, these freaky weather years have been coming around far too often. 1997 to '98, and again in 2002, and finally in 2007. And this current one, of course.

"In an El Niño the currents in the Pacific go all to hell.

They circulate the wrong way, or something like that. The water gets warm where it should be cold, and vice versa. Since everything is connected to ocean temperatures—like, you know, the ecosystem?—the weather goes to hell in a bucket. Everywhere, everything, and everyone gets affected.

"Add to this the depletion of the rain forests, soil erosion, acid rains, holes in the ozone, the not-so-gradual melting of the ice caps, earthquakes, volcanoes blowing their tops left, right, and centre . . . the whole thing seems symptomatic of planetary and climatic upheaval. Or maybe I should say seemed, past tense, because these aren't just symptoms I'm talking about but the actual disease. In short, we're in it up to our necks! And finally people are beginning to sit up and pay attention to the ecologists and environmentalists, the guys who used to get tagged as sensationalists and doom-sayers.

"Back around 1997 or '98 was when it became really no-ticeable. Now hey, we're only talking a time span of maybe twelve or thirteen years here, but the speed at which things have changed you really wouldn't know it. Like, a thousand years worth of climatic damage packed into just a decade and a half?

"So, let's go back to the years leading up to and including 1997 and '98.

"The Antarctic pack ice had already started breaking into icebergs bigger than large English counties. There were grasses and mosses and flowers where before there'd only ever been ice. Similarly, in the Arctic, the sea ice was getting thinner every year, the so-called 'permanent' ice simply wasn't permanent any more, and the cap in general was shrinking. So, all that water had to go somewhere, right? My guess: into the air, the atmosphere, Jake. And as the old saying goes, what goes up must come down again—in pre-cipitation. And brother, did we get rain!

"The Netherlands: flooded to hell . . . so badly that for a while it looked like all the major dams would go. Germany, and Poland: all the rivers breaking their banks. Greece: un-seasonal hail, with hailstones as big as Ping-Pong balls that flattened the crops. The USA: *Jesus,* the Mississippi! All that water trying to get out of there, and God help anything that got in its way! And in '97, right here in Australia: first they had fires that scorched people out of their homes— destroying thousands of acres of prairie, woodlands, and national parks, and killing people, livestock, wildlife galore— and *then* monsoon rains to match anything the rest of the world had suffered. It was just crazy fucking weather!

"But the hell of it was, these were only warnings. The El Niños *are* warnings; the melting ice *is* a warning, and like-wise the ozone layer. Like planetwide alarms that have been sounding for a long, long time, all in vain because no one has been listening. Or rather, no one was listening to the ones who were listening. . . .

"In the Far East they wouldn't stop burning the rain for-ests. The Americans got annoyed when people said their car-bon dioxide emissions were off the scale. But they weren't so snooty in the summer of '98, when Texas turned into a desert! Heat-wave? They'd never seen anything like it! As for the Russians: well, as usual they hid or disguised or de-nied any and all wrongdoing whatsoever. *Huh!* But what else would you expect from the people who turned the Aral Sea into the Aral Pond? The folks with more toxic nuclear and chemical garbage per acre than most countries have per square mile! In E-Branch—during my three years with the Branch, anyway—we've been monitoring the hell out of the Russians. Ask Ben Trask about it sometime."

And Jake cut in, "Well, at least I know something about all that: the way they dump their clapped-out subs, et cetera."

"That's part of it," Harvey agreed, "but the rest of it is just as bad. Anyway, all that's away from the main subject, and in fact we were talking about . . . ?"

"The big fire," Jake reminded him. "Until you went a bit off track."

Harvey nodded. "Yeah, the Great Fire of Brisbane, 2007. It was around this time of year, and El Niño was up to its *un*usual tricks. The weather had been freakish everywhere, especially in the U.K., England. For fifteen years the various water boards had been moaning about declining water tables. It could rain all it wanted during the winter, but given just three days of good old heartwarming sunshine in July and these jokers would start leaping up and down, tearing their hair, and sticking in meters and standpipes and demanding that people should save water by cutting down on their bathing and putting bricks in their water closet cisterns . . . and so on, and so forth, ad infinitum. What a load of crap, *if* you could afford to take one! It was Nature all those years, warning us that the Big One was coming.

"Well, in 2007 in England it came, and that year we didn't have a summer."

"It was washed out?" Jake felt obliged to ask.

"It was drowned out!" Harvey told him.

"I seem to remember something about that," Jake said. "But I missed it. I was on the continent."

"But you must have read about it, seen it on TV?"

"I told you, I was doing my own thing. On the continent."

"Yeah," Harvey agreed. "About the only place in the world where the weather was moderately normal. You were lucky. In England it rained, and rained, and *rained*! And as for declining water tables: forget it. There's been no shortage of water ever since. Anywhere below sea-level turned into a swamp. The Thames Barrier failed, and high tides combined with a flooded river to drown the city six feet deep. Through July, August, and September—shit, there were gondolas in Oxford Street! Okay, so I'm exaggerating—maybe it wasn't quite as bad as all that, but it was bad enough. And I could go on and on. Except . . ." He paused again.

"Except that was U.K.," Jake helped him out. "And the people had plenty of warning, and there was little or no loss of life. Yes, I remember it now. But we were talking about Brisbane, not quite so close to home."

"Not *just* Brisbane," the other told him. "In 2007 it was Australia as a whole. Now, you've got to remember that in Australia the climate works backwards to how we'd expect back home. It's way hotter in January than in July: the difference between summer and winter, right? Oh, really? Well, in 2007 everything went wrong. From February on the summer weather held, there was no winter, and it didn't get any colder. Just like now, in fact exactly like now, they had the freakiest of freak weather."

Turning his head, Harvey gazed out through the limo's one-way windows at suburbs becoming city. "I mean, just take a look out there."

Jake looked, lifted an enquiring eyebrow. "Well?"

"Dry, brittle, parched. Those gardens that should be green are more like miniature deserts. The grass is withered to straw and the leaves are dead on the trees and bushes. Almost all the swimming pools are empty, and you won't see anyone watering any lawns. It should be a maximum of sixty, sixty-five degrees Fahrenheit out there, but it's well over eighty, and this is late afternoon. And naturally, it's an official drought. Perfect!"

"Perfect for what?" Now Jake was really puzzled . . . not to mention tired, of this circuitous route they were taking to the Great Fire.

"Earth Year!" said Harvey. "The big conference that starts tomorrow right here in Brisbane, billed as the ultimate ecological summit meeting. Synchronicity at work again, or maybe not. Naturally they chose this place, *because* of the fire."

"Well, you've lost me again," Jake told him. "And we still haven't got to the fire itself."

The other shrugged apologetically. "I'm sorry—it's this grasshopper mind of mine. Start me on a subject, it devours me. Okay, the fire:

"It was the weirdest thing ever—a one-of-a-kind sort of thing, or at least everyone hopes so. 2007, and we thought we'd seen it all: the worst tornadoes the USA had ever suffered, the worst floods, the strangest fluctuations and reversals of climate right across the world, with Australia taking the brunt of it. But no, we hadn't seen it all.

"Brisbane was like a tinderbox. The whole east coast from Rockhampton to Canberra—normally a green strip in the lee of the Great Dividing Range, with no water shortage and an

358

excellent annual rainfall—was bone dry from this drought that had lasted for eighteen months. Oh, they'd had rain, but all of it had fallen on the wrong side of the Great Divide! And daily the temperature was up in the hundreds.

"And it was then that it happened. It was like . . . what, a tornado? An almighty tornado, a whirlwind, yes. But a whirlwind of fire! Ma Nature, Jake, getting all hot under the collar. It started in the Gidgealpa and Moomba oil and gas fields, but how or why it started, no one knows. There are various theories but no one really knows. Though miles apart, suddenly the oil wells and gas installations became the epicentre of an enormous fireball. That in itself was a disaster, but nothing like what was to come.

"A fireball, vast, hot, rushing up on its own thermals, and sucking in the air to fuel itself; sucking the air into a self-perpetuating spiral, a superheated whirlwind. It swept east out of the Sturt Desert, its base widening out as it came, a column of fire five, and then ten miles across. At more than a hundred miles an hour it hit a place called Dirranbandi and burned the entire town, just took it out. And everything it burned fuelled the fire that got hotter and hotter. And on it came. The thing moved like a drunkard—never in a straight line but just exactly like a tornado—a pillar of fire reaching up through the clouds.

"Of course it was monitored; thousands of people reported seeing it. It came terrifyingly close to some towns, scorching them but leaving them intact; then again it seemed to swoop on others, tossed them into the sky in blazing rags. Firefighters tried to plot its course from the air; some airplanes flew too close and got sucked in, incinerated. And rotating ever faster, it rushed east to refuel itself on the Alton oil field. . . .

"So it goes, and I can't remember all of it. But who would want to? Anyway, the whole thing was on every TV channel. Every Aussie there ever was watched it happening, couldn't do a thing about it. The authorities thought the mountains would stop it—they were wrong. It blazed across the Divide, leaving a smoking track twelve miles wide in its wake, with secondary fires still ranging outwards. The latter would burn for weeks until torrential rains stopped them.

"And with only an hour's warning to the people of Brisbane—an indefinite warning at that, for no one could say for sure what this thing would do—finally it hit, this firestorm from hell, such as the world had never before seen. Never before and never since, thank God!

"Everything that could burn burned. If it couldn't burn it calcined. And if it couldn't calcine it melted. As for the Brisbane River: forget it. It was running at a trickle and had been for a nine-month. The firestorm took what was left of the river water, turned it to steam in a couple of seconds, and kept right on going.

"And that was in it: a one-hundred-miles-per-hour blast furnace had killed a city and everyone in it who couldn't or hadn't tried to get out following the warning. They hadn't all died by burning; a great many people, gone underground or into cellars, suffocated because the fire needed their air. All of it. Then:

"The thing hit the sea and sucked up a waterspout into its raging funnel. The water put the fire out, turned to steam, and formed clouds. The clouds drifted inland and rained on the raging inferno that had been Brisbane. Finally it was over. End of story. . . ."

. . . And after a while:

"Christ!" Jake said, under his breath. And a moment later: "That is some encyclopedic memory you've got there, Jimmy. What are you, an authority on world disasters?"

Harvey shrugged a little self-consciously—perhaps sheepishly?—and said, "Me? No—but I know a woman who is. Before we broke camp, I had to talk to HQ about a couple of communications problems. Millicent Cleary was on duty officer. She's our current affairs lady; she has that kind of memory, keeps a mental record of just about everything that's going or gone down. As Ian Goodly knows the future, she knows the recent past; but of course she has a big advantage: like, it's already happened. And unlike Ian's, her knowledge comes in amazing detail. So when I told her we'd be setting up next in Brisbane, she clued me in on the city, the fire, the Earth Year Conference. And there you have it: the fire's still fresh in my mind from my conversation with Millicent Cleary."

Harvey sat back and looked out of his window. After a moment's silence he said, "But actually, I wish it wasn't. . . ."

In the other limo, the episode of the tall, thin plane-spotter (if that was what he had been) had been forgotten by everyone except Liz Merrick. She, too, was trying to put it to the back of her mind, but knew she'd be able to recall it if or when it was required—

—His silhouette was etched on her memory: *his angular shape. And the tilt of his broad-brimmed hat that kept the sun out of his eyes. The way his binoculars were trained on . . . trained on what, a mainly empty sky? That was what had been bothering her! That, and the way those glasses had suddenly dipped, turning towards the limo.*

That was when Liz's mind had been closest to his, the moment when she'd sensed his interest in the vehicle and its occupants. . . .

"So how about it?" said Ben Trask, causing her to start as he reached over her and switched off the intercom connection to their driver.

"Eh?" she said. And: "Oh, I'm sorry, Ben. I must have been daydreaming. How about what?"

"Jake, on the chopper. What was going on? Did you get anything?"

And now the image of the thin man with the binoculars vanished completely from her mind as the other question arose, the one Liz had known she would have difficulty answering.

At first it had seemed simple, even exciting in a strange and morbid sort of way. The answer to not just one question but many. But after thinking it over she had seen the enormous hurt it might cause, so that now she had to find a way around it. If Trask would let her.

"But I thought we had an understanding on that," she said. "I don't like spying on Jake, and—"

"What?" He cut her off. "But on the chopper you seemed to indicate that you'd got something. So why are you holding back, Liz? What the hell is going on here?" The look on Trask's face was one of incredulity; he'd been sure they'd hammered this out and from now on it would be plain sailing. So what had happened to change her mind?

"I . . . I'm not sure *what* I got!" she blurted out, lying so unconvincingly that even without his talent Trask would have known. And she saw in his eyes that he knew, and in the way his lips tightened. "But . . . but he's my partner!" she quickly went on the defensive. "He's got to be able to trust me. He saved my life, and—"

"Oh, for Christ's sake, *spare* me!" Trask barked. But before he could say anything else:

"Damn you!" Liz snapped. And then more quietly, even desperately: "Can't you see? I'm *trying* to spare you, Ben!"

Which set him back a little, because he saw that that was the truth, too. And despite that Trask was still frowning, his tone was less severe when he said: "All right, so don't try so hard."

And after a moment, when she remained silent, he went on, "Look, whatever this is, there's only you, me, and Ian here to share it. So let's have it out in the open here and now, while we can still deal with it in private. For if it has to do with me—and if it's got anything at all to do with the Branch or the job in hand—then obviously I have to know."

"But it's so very little," she answered. "And his shields were up, like a blanket covering his mind, and—"

"Liz, I *have* to know!" Trask insisted. "It doesn't matter how small a thing it might seem to you, it could be all important to everyone else."

"In its way, I'm sure it is," Liz said. "It's just that I would have liked to find a way to tell you—I mean a different way to tell you—without this."

"This what?" said Trask. "And Liz, if you lie to me again I'll know."

She looked at him, looked at Ian Goodly, sighed, and shook her head. "I didn't want to lie, but I didn't want to hurt you either. You see, it's where Jake was—in his dream, I mean—and it's who he was speaking to."

"Go on," Trask nodded.

"He was down in the wrecked sump of the Romanian Refuge," she blurted it out. "But Ben, it had to be much more than just a dream because from what I saw of it—despite that it was so dark and shrouded—it was all so very real!"

"The Refuge?" Trask repeated her. "Jake dreamed he was in the wrecked sump? And he was . . . speaking to someone?"

"To more than one," Liz corrected him. And now that she'd got started, she quickly went on, "But you know how dreams are supposed to happen in the last few minutes before you wake up? Well, not this one. It started the moment he fell asleep, went on until he woke up. And it was more than just a dream, Ben."

The other's face was grey now, gaunt with the sudden, sure knowledge of what Liz was about to tell him. He knew, but asked her anyway. "Who was Jake talking to?"

"To Harry Keogh," she answered, "and to someone else who I don't know and don't want to know, ever. I couldn't read him—he was a complete blank—but I could sense his presence like a sick taste in my throat. And just the opposite to him, a little earlier there'd been a third presence like . . . like a breath of fresh air. She was someone I'd never known, who I wish I had."

"It was Zek!" Trask groaned. "He was talking to Zek. Jake was talking to Zek, through Harry." And clasping Liz's hands in his: "Liz, what was she saying? What did Zek say?"

"I don't know," she shook her head, wanted to put her arms round him but couldn't for fear it would crack him up. And anyway, they wouldn't be Zek's arms. "I got something of what Jake was saying—though very little, because he didn't say much—but nothing of what the others actually said. That was a void."

Ian Goodly said, "Of course it was. You heard Jake because he's alive. That was your telepathy working, Liz. But Harry and the others . . . they're a different category, and they were in a different mode."

"Deadspeak, yes," Trask murmured, gaunt and visibly shaken where he let his head flop back against the seat's headrest and closed his eyes. "And whether I like it or not, it looks like I now have to accept it. Jake is our new Necroscope, and Harry is introducing him to . . . to people who'll be able to help him. As for this numbers thing that Jake was talking about when he woke up—the difficulty he seemed to be having—I think that can mean only one thing."

Trask looked at the precog and Goodly nodded his confirmation. "Despite that Jake's future is beyond me, uncertain now," he said, "still I can only go along with you. It was the Necroscope's sidereal maths, his numbers, that gave him the edge. And now it looks like the old master is trying to teach his apprentice the tricks of the trade."

25
Synchronicity Again

THE SAFE HOUSE SET ASIDE FOR E-BRANCH USE was in the New Marchant Park district north of the city. An ugly two-storey affair, it had aluminium cladding designed and painted in a rather poor imitation of timber; Brisbane no longer favoured wooden structures of any kind.

The house was set back from the road up a short palm-lined drive; its gate was remote-controlled from inside the lead limo and opened into a featureless garden. Two medium-sized, innocuous-looking saloon cars stood on a gravel drive in front of the house. In fact they were fitted with bullet-proof windows, heavily plated bodywork, hidden roll bars and other anti-crash/antiterrorist devices. Short of a bomb blast or a head-on collision at speed, no one was going to come to harm driving one of these vehicles. They were for the use of Trask and his people.

Laid to lawn and enclosed within high stone walls, the garden was on a level and surrounded the house on all sides; every inch of grass (or straw as it was now) was clearly visible from the windows of both storeys. Of the house itself: it had bullet-proof, heavily curtained windows, and a security/intruder warning system second to none. In plan, the ground floor consisted of four long rooms, one on each side, each furnished and decorated in a slightly out-of-date style, with little or nothing to show that the place was anything other than a fairly expensive private dwelling house. The central room, however, which wasn't visible from the gardens, was an operational and communications nerve-centre of screens and computerized equipment.

The sleeping quarters (in fact a pair of cramped dormitories with beds for up to fourteen people, or maybe eighteen at a push, and a handful of curtained-off, cell-like units for VIPs) were upstairs. And overhead on the roof, a bank of "solar-heating panels" (tinted windows) concealed an array of hi-tech communications aerials and dishes.

The agent-chauffeurs showed Trask and his crew of six over the house, asked how they could help them settle in or if there was anything else they needed. Trask checked with Jimmy Harvey and Paul Arenson—in their elements where they switched on and got acquainted with the gadgets in the ops room—and Arenson told him, "We're fully compatible throughout. Give us ten minutes to hook our stuff up to this lot, and we'll have the HQ Duty Officer up there on that big screen so clear you'll think you're in London."

"Scrambled?" Trask wasn't that easily satisfied.

"As per SOPs, yes," said the other.

At which Trask thanked the Australian Special Intelligence men, who headed back to the airstrip to connect with incoming Chopper Two's military commanders and three more members of Branch ground staff. Once they were in, and until the slower backup squads of Australian SAS types had

365

arrived and taken up their tactical locations, the advance party was on its own. . . .

In fact, it took the technicians half an hour to complete their hookup. Meanwhile an uncharacteristically subdued Liz had brewed a pot of Earl Grey for Trask and herself, coffee for Jake and the others. Goodly had taken his coffee through into ops. Trask was enjoying his tea in one of the living rooms while poring over a small-scale map of the Queensland/New South Wales border areas. It was somewhere there, in the vicinity of the border, that the locator Chung had detected mindsmog, probably due to the mental activity of a master vampire, Wamphyri! Probably, but not definitely, not with 100-percent certainty; the Branch had long since discovered psychic "hotspots" where a proliferation of lesser, human ESP talents could produce the same result. It had been David Chung's "hunch," however, that this time it was the real thing, which the synchronous "coincidence" of vampire lieutenant Bruce Trennier's death had seemed to confirm.

Jake took his coffee over to where Trask worked, watched him use a red highlighter to plot a dotted line along the border from Stanthorpe to Coolangatta, then circle the whole area in a ring of pale red ink. As Trask looked up from what he was doing, Jake lifted an enquiring eyebrow.

"If our target is here," Trask explained, "and if he has established himself, then he's somewhere inside this ring. Personally, I fancy he is. I've known David Chung for a long time and he doesn't make too many mistakes. It was Chung who discovered Trennier. Once we had an approximate location, we checked with the local police and picked up on a handful of disappearances—Trennier's recruits, those creatures we killed at the Old Mine gas station. That one was fairly easy; in a region as thinly populated as the Gibson Desert, people are wont to take notice when their kith and kin cease to exist! But here in the east, on the coastal strip . . ." He paused, glanced again at the map, shook his head.

"Densely populated," Jake nodded. "And that circle

you've drawn covers what—maybe five, six thousand square miles?"

"Closer to eight," Trask corrected him glumly. "And folks disappear around here every other half hour, about the same as they do in similar areas of population all over the world."

Lardis Lidesci had been talking to Liz. Now he came over, put a gnarled finger on the map and growled, "These?"

"Mountains," Trask answered.

"Huh!" Lardis grunted. "Thought so. And the border follows the mountains, right?"

"In part," Trask nodded. "A natural boundary, yes."

"An *un*natural boundary, in Sunside/Starside!" Lardis said. "But there again, the Barrier Mountains are different entirely, and they never knew sunlight such as these mountains have seen. But beggers, and even the Wamphyri, can't be choosers. Not in a world like this. So there you are. And now maybe you can narrow it down."

Concentrating on the map, Trask was only half-listening to what Lardis was saying. But in another moment he looked up from where he sat at the table. "Eh?"

"Mountains," Lardis said. "I understand 'em. And so do the Wamphyri. If this one's a Lord, where do you think he'll be?"

"Where do I think—?" Trask frowned, looked again at the map, then came erect and snapped his fingers.

"In the mountains, aye," Lardis anticipated him, scowling in his fashion. "In his aerie, of course. That's a logical con—er, con*clusion?*—wouldn't you say? And here's another: if it *is* one of them, it *isn't* Szwart. What, in all this heat and light? No way—not a chance. It's too much for me, let alone for Lord Szwart. *Huh!* Darkness himself, that one!"

"Damn! You're probably right!" Trask husked.

At which point Ian Goodly returned from the ops room. "Up and running," he said. "And Ben, David Chung's on screen, wanting to speak to you. . . ."

"I have some hot-off-the-press news for you," Chung told Trask as he seated himself within the screen's viewing arc.

"Big deal," Trask answered wearily, with a touch of sarcasm but no real malice. "Just about *any* news fits that description! We've been busy, air-mobile, and only just got settled in here. So, what's going down in your neck of the woods that's such hot stuff?"

Chung shrugged. "In my neck of the woods? Not a lot. But in yours: an opportunity to speak to an old pal of ours, maybe, if that's of any interest?" And then, more seriously: "It's Gustav Turchin. He's going to be there at the Earth Year Conference in Brisbane. The time in the City is now—" he glanced off-screen "—a little after eight A.M. But just an hour ago Turchin himself was on-screen, unscrambled, from Moscow. He was interested to know if you'd be attending the conference. He was *very* careful, oh-so-polite, and diplomatic as usual, but John Grieve was doing duty officer and read him like a book. Premier Turchin is eager to see you, Ben. It was a last minute call, probably monitored, before he boarded an Aeroflot VTOL Atmozkim to Brisbane. And John says Turchin stressed the fact that he would be accompanied by 'several members of his staff.' "

"That's very interesting," Trask answered. "His bodyguards will be special police, KGB lookalikes—watchdogs for the *real* leaders, all the military types like Mikhail Suvorov—who will be making sure he doesn't step out of line. So maybe Turchin is on his way out, his days of power at an end. But of course I'll see him. I have a few questions for him, and while he still has some pull there's a favour I need to ask of him." Trask glanced at Jake, perhaps musingly, then turned back to the screen.

"So, thanks for the information, David," he continued, "and you can be sure I'll act on it. But now I'd like you to tell me something about our main problem. How is the search going? Have you picked up anything new to corroborate your original lead?"

Chung pulled a wry face. "There's something there, I would swear to that. But it's too distant, too shielded, literally on the other side of the world! *Your* side of the world, Ben. Which is where I have to be if you want any kind of accuracy. I mean, how can I be expected to locate someone or thing through eight thousand miles of solid rock and white hot magma?"

"You want in on this?" Trask's face was a blank.

"Absolutely!"

"And you wouldn't be playing on your talent simply so you can come swanning around out here?"

Chung's face showed his confusion. For the truth was that he would dearly love to go "swanning around" in Australia with his E-Branch colleagues—and if he denied it Trask would know he was lying! So after letting his face work its way through a number of mutually contradictory expressions, finally he said, "But isn't that the wrong question? What you should have asked is do I think I'll be better placed to find what we're searching for if I'm out there with you . . . to which I would have to answer, yes."

At which Trask's stony expression broke and he grinned. "I know," he said. "I'm good at asking awkward questions, right?"

"Too true!" Chung rubbed his chin and looked hurt—until a moment later, when Trask said:

"Okay, so how soon can you be out here? The fact is you'll come in useful apprising Premier Turchin firsthand of all that you've discovered about the Russian navy's illegal pollution of the world's oceans . . . and in Earth Year at that! Which in turn will afford me a little more leverage on what I would like from him. That's if leverage is required, which I doubt. For in fact Gustav Turchin isn't a bad sort of bloke."

Watching Chung's face come alive with anticipation on the wall screen, Jake thought: *Synchronicity again! Like some kind of weird word-association. E-Branch: Gustav Turchin: the down-at-heel Russian military's systematic pollution of the oceans: the Earth Year eco-summit. And all of it coming together right here and now, in Brisbane—along with a whole bunch of other shit, possibly.*

And meanwhile, with a smile as broad as his face, the locator was saying, "I, er, already mentioned the possibility that I *might* be needed to John Grieve. He's happy to take over here, and there'll be no shortage of staff in support. So . . . when is the next flight out?"

Trask nodded knowingly. "I'm sure you'll be able to check that out for yourself," he said. "Er, *if* you haven't already."

And Chung laughed and said, "I have an hour and forty minutes to make Heathrow!"

"I thought so," Trask said. "Very well, Ian Goodly can get his head down now and pick you up in the wee small hours at the airport. You'll travel under an assumed identity, of course."

"Of course." And Chung was still grinning his delight when Trask broke the connection.

Chung wasn't the only one who was met at the airport in the wee small hours. Premier Gustav Turchin was there first, along with his minder entourage. No one paid them much attention.

Russia was no longer a world superpower—in fact she was rapidly crumbling, held in siege not by the world community but from within her own borders by political and ideological intractability, corruption, organized crime, and desperate poverty—but still Turchin was recognized as a world leader of sorts, if only a figurehead without any real power. In any case the Earth Year Conference wasn't diplomacy-conscious; it wasn't that kind of venue; the eco-summit's organizers were not so much standing on ceremony as requiring action.

Australia, now a Republic and a very powerful nation in its own right, was still viewed as a "clean" country and was determined to stay that way. While the all-too-frequent El Niños and other ecological disasters were not caused by Australians, Australians were suffering their consequences. Now they and other like-minded—indeed *right*-minded— countries were considering real action, political, legal, and economical, against nations with bad to criminal ecological records. Since Russia was reckoned more than merely "suspect" in this regard, and since Premier Turchin's attendance had been an eleventh-hour decision, no red-carpet arrangements had been made for him and his party.

370

A limo and driver *had* been arranged—which was literally the least that the organizers could do without being seen to be rude—but Trask had seen to it that these had been called off. This hadn't been the easiest thing in the world to arrange, but Trask's connections were second to none.

Diplomatic immunity saw the Russian Premier and his poker-faced party of four clone-like minders through the international airport's red-tape entry procedures without too much fuss, each man carrying his own spartan to modest luggage, until they were met in the arrivals lounge by a pair of "chauffeurs" who introduced themselves as "Mr. Smith" and "Mr. Brown."

Swiftly escorted to the carport by Smith and Brown, Turchin was bundled into the back of the first limo . . . the doors of which immediately clicked shut and locked, all except the driver's door, which stood open. And before the jet-lagged, travel-disorientated quartet of grey suits could even begin to object, Mr. Smith slid into the driver's seat and drove away.

As the minders got into the second limo, one of them growled a concerned, heavily accented: "Who was that man sitting in the front of the first car?"

"Er, that was Mr. Smith," said Mr. Brown. "I believe he's an important convention official. It seemed only right that a person of stature should welcome your Premier personally."

"Oh, indeed, yes!" said the other, gruffly. And then, with a frown: "But, er . . . wasn't the driver also Mr. Smith?"

"That's correct," said Brown, quickly recovering from his gaffe. "We have an awful lot of Smiths, you know—and Browns, too, for that matter. Why, we even had a Prime Minister called Smith once over! And anyway, what's wrong with that? I imagine it's much the same with Ivans and Ivanovs in your country."

"Yes, certainly. I understand. Pardon me. *Ahem!*" To cover his embarrassment, the minder coughed into a handkerchief.

Over the intercom Mr. Brown chuckled and said, "Let's face it, this *is* Australia! I mean, who did you think would be meeting you—Marx and Engels?"

"Oh, ha ha ha ha!" The minders laughed woodenly, almost

in unison. "No, not at all. Indeed, no!" But when they'd quietened down, their head man cautiously enquired, "Er, how long will it be before we get to the hotel?"

"Eh?" said Mr. Brown, grinning. "Well, I don't really know, mate. All I know is I have orders to tail the car in front, and that's it. About an hour, at a guess—maybe more, maybe less. But now, if you'll excuse me, I have to concentrate on my driving."

"Yes, of course. Just as long as you stay right behind the car in front." But the car in front was already out of sight.

"Oh, don't worry, I won't lose him. No fear of that. But I do understand your concern. It must be very daunting, having to keep an eye on someone like Gustav Turchin. What, dodgy is he?"

But now Mr. Brown's familiarity was getting to be too much. "What's that?" the leading grey suit said stiffly. "Did you say dodgy? Something about keeping an eye on him? Now you listen to me, Mr.—"

"Well, that's what you are, aren't you?" Brown cut him off. "I mean, just how long have you lot been special policemen anyway—or KGB as was—or whatever you call yourselves now?"

But suddenly the four were very tight-lipped, scowling at each other. And with his mouth twitching in one corner, and his eyes like black marbles, their leader slowly answered, "We have been—ah, shall we say, specialists?—a lot longer, I fancy, than you have been a chauffeur, Mr. Brown!"

At which Brown looked back, grinned, and then switched off the intercom. . . .

Out on the airport service road, Trask got out of the front of the limo and into the back with Turchin. Then they shook hands, and Turchin hugged him in a typically Russian greeting. "Funny, but we've never met person to person," Turchin said then. "Yet it seems I know you."

"A meeting of minds, perhaps?" said Trask. And, "Listen, I apologize for the subterfuge back there, but your friends—"

"No friends of mine!" Turchin cut him short. "Indeed, they

are only here to make sure I don't talk out of turn. But before you ask . . . yes, I do know about the despicable and destructive activities of our armed forces. They are like dogs fouling someone else's garden. But Trask, understand this: I am not the one who let those dogs off the leash. In today's Russia, my friend, they roam wild. Indeed, I've been lucky to hold onto what small degree of power still remains to me. But if I were to tell this conference everything I know, then even that would be lost, and our currently uneasy east-west relationship would slip a little bit farther downhill."

Trask nodded. "I understand, and it's much as I suspected. But Premier, you don't have to explain to me, not about that at least. And I know that you won't be able—won't be allowed—to explain it to the conference. So, why are you here?" He fell silent, wanting to let the other do the talking. Maybe he would learn more that way.

"How long do we have?" Turchin inquired.

"The drivers are taking the scenic route," Trask told him. "I've asked for half an hour at least, an hour at most. In fact we could be at your hotel in twenty minutes, but I wasn't quite sure what degree of privacy you'd have later."

"Half an hour?" Turchin nodded. "Good. I'm sure it's going to be enough, but we'll need to get on. As for privacy later—*huh!*"

"My fault," said Trask. "I should have been more subtle. I didn't want to compromise you, but I simply didn't have time to make any other arrangements."

"No," Turchin shook his head. "It's just how things are. I have made myself unpopular with certain people. If a country is rich and strong and its people are well fed, then maybe the man in charge can afford to be unpopular and do things his own way. Me, I can't afford to do *anything* my own way! The only reason I hold on is in the hope that things will change. But change is a long time coming."

Trask had been studying him. The Russian Premier wasn't by any means the same man he'd known previously. Even though Trask had only ever seen him in television broadcasts or on-screen at E-Branch HQ, still he had radiated a lot more power than he did now. And Trask's mind took him back to a time all of five years ago, when he had negotiated a course of action on the Perchorsk Gate with this selfsame man:

Then, Gustav Turchin had seemed unshakable. He had been a rock of a man. Blockily built, square of face and short in the neck—with a shock of black hair, bushy black eyebrows, dark, glinting eyes over a blunt nose, and an unemotional mouth—he had been a veritable bulldog. But even then the Premier had had problems. Coinciding with Trask's, they had served to bring the two together in a mutually beneficial understanding.

Now . . . there had been changes. Turchin was a lot thinner, grey-streaked where his hair was brushed back from his temples, less bright and sharp of eye; even his voice had lost something of its former authority. The intellect was still there—still lethal, Trask supposed—but the drive was failing. Seven years of political power, and nothing to show for it, had taken their toll of him.

But the way the Russian Premier was studying Trask . . . the head of E-Branch couldn't suppress a snort of self-derision. If he found Turchin changed, what must Turchin think of him?

As if reading his mind, the other said, "The years haven't been kind to us."

And Trask smiled wrily and answered, "It's not so much the years as the mileage." Then he stopped smiling and said, "We've not long had definite evidence about what your navy is doing. I certainly won't be saying anything about it here in Brisbane. I wouldn't embarrass you like that. In fact, I'm not here on Earth Year business at all, and I doubt if I'll attend a single session. But you should know that sooner or later—probably sooner—I'll have to bring it to the attention of our Minister Responsible, and that he has obligations, too."

"I appreciate that, er, Benjamin?"

"Ben."

"Then by all means call me Gustav. But you are not the only one whose purpose here is other than it seems. Indeed

374

I am here simply because *you* are here! Oh, they have been badgering me to attend these things all over the world, but so far I've managed to hold them off. The admirals, generals, despoilers, et cetera, requiring me to lie for them—*huh!* Well, and now that I'm here I shall lie for them, telling Brisbane and all the world of the marvelous efforts Russia is making to clean up her act. But you and I, we know the truth. And, as you have pointed out, so will everyone else in the not too distant future. Unfortunately that is the least of my worries—or if not the least, it is not my major concern. No, for that is something else entirely."

Trask nodded. He remained silent and thoughtful for a few moments, then said, "Perhaps I can anticipate you? I think it's only fair to tell you that I'm also aware that Mikhail Suvorov has led an alleged 'expeditionary' party of soldiers and scientists through the Perchorsk Gate into Sunside/Starside, Nathan Keogh's world."

Now it was Gustav Turchin's turn to smile wrily. "Ah!" he said. "The Opposition! And sharp as ever. Yes, and you are correct: that is my problem. But alas, it's also yours."

"Probably more than you suspect," said Trask. "But perhaps I should hear your side of the story first."

"My side is simple," said the other. "Five years ago, when Turkur Tzonov escaped justice in Perchorsk by fleeing into Starside, some of his dupes were taken prisoner. That was a mistake on my part; I should have had them shot for mutiny, conspiracy, desertion of duty, sabotage . . . oh, half a dozen charges. But I didn't, and one of them talked to Mikhail Suvorov. Not the best possible move, for *he* had them shot! Or rather, he saw to their disposal. There were several very unfortunate accidents."

Trask understood and said, "Which left General Suvorov as the sole heir to whatever he could steal from Sunside/Starside. He knew that the Gate would lead him into an alien world, knew about the gold, and wanted it for himself."

"The gold and whatever else he could find there," Turchin answered. "A whole new world, which he would annex and rape for its riches. And he would have control of the Gate.

Why, in retrospect it seems perfectly obvious: if Suvorov had wanted these things for the good of his country, for Russia—which was what he told me—then surely he would have explained his purpose to everyone; to his military colleagues and the whole country, and not just . . . not *just* to me." He turned his face away.

"He told you he was going through the Gate? And you didn't try to stop him?" Trask believed he understood something of the predicament Turchin must have faced, but wanted to hear it from the horse's mouth.

"How could I stop him?" Turchin threw up his hands. "After the Perchorsk Complex was flooded, a task force of military engineers was sent in to strip and salvage lead from the shielding in the ravine. That was what I was led to believe, though later it turned out that wasn't all they were there for. Anyway, many of these men were long-term criminals from the punishment garrisons at Beresov and Ukhta. Hand-picked by Mikhail Suvorov, they had been given the choice of serving out their sentences or serving him: his first step towards securing Perchorsk. In return, and after the job was done and everyone else had moved out, Suvorov let them stay on and turn the dry upper levels into living quarters serviced by hydroelectric power from the dam. They had vehicles, and documentation that allowed them to resupply themselves from Beresov. From then on they were the 'official' team of engineers, responsible for servicing and running the dam. As for the dam's continued existence: that was easily justified in that the bulk of its electrical power had been rerouted to the service of local logging camps and other communities. . . ."

"And you were in the dark about all this?" Despite Trask's respect for the other—and the fact that so far the Premier's every word had been the truth—still he was relentless in his pursuit of all the answers.

"I was *kept* in the dark about it!" Turchin told him. "Ben, I don't control the armed forces and I never have. If they want me to know something, then they tell me. And if I require their services, I tell them. And that's it."

"Bringing a democracy to life isn't easy," Trask said.

"Neither is killing communism!" said the other, then went on to explain: "Oh, they are still there, the hard-liners. And so we're—how do you say it—between a rock and a hard place? The old guard on the one hand, and all the greedy opportunists, like Suvorov, on the other. Do you know what happens to a Russian bank if it runs out of money?"

Trask shrugged. "It goes bankrupt?"

"No, they turn it into a pizza house! *Huh!* Among the Muscovites, that is currently a 'joke.' Here's another that's not so funny: what does a general do when there's no money to fund his parades or pay his troops, and his pension's only good for cheap vodka and cabbage soup?"

Trask nodded. "He goes gold-prospecting. But you know, no one lives forever. Not me and not you. Somewhere there must be documentation on the Perchorsk Project, the Gate, the complex, and everything that happened there. While we're alive, of course we'll do our best to protect such records, such secrets. But when we're dead or no longer in office—what then? If not Suvorov, sooner or later someone else would have tried it."

"I thought of that a long time ago," said Turchin. "Also, I liked Nathan and I'm sure I would like his people. There was something about him that was very Russian, you know? And in my way, well, I'm a humanitarian, too . . . you'll just have to take my word for that. So, I took what precautions I could."

"Precautions?"

"Long before Mikhail Suvorov found out about Perchorsk, I was destroying everything I could find on that place. Every bit of documentation, records, reports, you name it. Not the experiment, you understand, not the Projekt itself—for it's better that men should learn from their mistakes—but the horror that came after it, the very knowledge of a vampire world. And I was quite successful, perhaps even too successful. For now . . . why, even the so-called Opposition knows a lot more about it than I do, and certainly more than anyone else!"

"We always did," said Trask.

"Of course you did, yes—and of course you *do*—for you have even been there, to Nathan Keogh's world in an alien, parallel dimension. But isn't that a peculiar circumstance in itself, since Perchorsk and the Gate lie deep inside *my* homeland? And if you were me, wouldn't you feel . . . left out?"

"Not really," Trask shook his head. "No one who saw what I saw, experienced what I experienced, would ever want to go back there. Believe me, you must consider yourself fortunate. And as for General Mikhail Suvorov: well, you can consider him unfortunate. He's dead, Gustav."

"Oh?" And Turchin lifted a great bush of an eyebrow. "Does that explain it, then? The accident or vandalism or whatever it was at the Romanian Refuge? Was that Suvorov?"

"You know about the Refuge?"

"I have my sources." Turchin shrugged.

For the moment at least Trask let that one slide and said, "No, it wasn't Mikhail Suvorov—but it *was* as a direct result of his 'invasion' of Sunside/Starside. That was what brought it about." And he quickly told the Russian Premier everything that had happened, including the fact that three Great Vampires were now at large in the world, and that he and E-Branch were trying to hunt them down.

"And that is why you're here?"

"We believe that one of them is here in Australia, yes."

And Turchin said, "Ah! Then that would explain why initially you were on the other side of the continent, and not here in Brisbane. And so it's a pure coincidence that the trail has led you here: you think that he—your 'man,' shall we say?—is close by."

"He's not far away, that's for sure," said Trask. "And now I have a question for you."

"Go ahead."

"If you knew we were in the west, in the Gibson Desert on the other side of Australia, why did you ask my headquarters if I'd be attending the conference? Also, how did you know we were in Western Australia in the first place?"

"That's two questions," Turchin smiled.

Trask nodded. "Yes, but please don't spoil things by lying to me on either one of them."

"To you?" Turchin raised that eyebrow again. "Do you think that's likely, Ben?"

"No, because I know it isn't possible," said the other. "I was reminding *you* of that fact, that's all."

"I don't need reminding," the Premier told him. "And I say again, I'm not here to lie to you but to ask for your help. And now you ask how I know so much. Very well, then listen:

"When our Russian equivalent of your E-Branch failed— and failed so very spectacularly at the hands of Harry Keogh—ESP as a weapon was largely discredited and the Russian organization disbanded. Or at least it was 'officially' disbanded. For our military commanders, down-to-earth fellows who would rather put their faith in conventional spying techniques, wanted nothing more to do with it. Which made it an ideal tool for a Premier who—"

"Who was pretty much powerless but desperate to keep an eye on things," Trask finished it for him. "You yourself, Gustav. You are now in charge of the Opposition!"

"Covertly, yes. What's left of it." Turchin nodded.

"And you've been using your mind-spies to watch us?"

"Don't look so hurt, Ben! Haven't you been watching me and mine?"

Trask thought about it and grinned . . . and was serious in a moment. "But you still haven't told me why you asked my HQ if I was attending the conference."

The other smiled. "It was my way of telling you that *I* was attending, without spelling out a request to meet with you."

"Still sharp as a tack," Trask said. And: "Okay, so as you now know, I too have a problem . . . shit, I mean the whole world has a problem! Three of them, and big ones. But yours has to be urgent, too, and probably personal, else you wouldn't be taking chances talking to me. Obviously we need to make a deal, and we will, a mutually beneficial arrangement. But I can't do or promise anything until I know what your problem is."

"Urgent, yes, definitely," said Turchin. "But personal? Not any longer, not after what you have told me. For it seems to me our problems mesh, becoming one and the same. Very well, I know one of yours—or ours, as it now appears—and the worst of them at that: that there are vampires in our world. But somehow I think there's a lot more than that to it. Am I right?"

"A tangled skein, yes," Trask nodded. "But synchronous, all coming together at the same time. And meanwhile *our* time is flying. So okay, you first. Just what is your problem, comrade?"

26
Dilemmas, Dreams, and Deadspeak

"MY PROBLEMS, PLURAL, ARE NOT SO SIMPLE," said Gustav Turchin. "Suvorov told a handful of his military cronies that he was onto something big; also that he'd probably be out of touch for a while, but in the event he was gone for too long they should come to me for answers. Well, some eighteen months ago they started to ask questions, not too many, for with Suvorov out of the way they had been playing their own hands. These are people with small armies of their own, funded by the drugs trade, I suspect, for they certainly can't be getting it through official channels. Why not? Because the bank is broke! Anyway, sooner or later they'll become more insistent, and I'm the one who they'll squeeze for information. Obviously I don't want to tell them anything about Perchorsk, so what *can* I tell them?

"Next problem: The Perchorsk Complex is still dry, the Gate stands open, and the Wamphyri are back in Sunside/Starside. Which means, of course, that the Gate has to be closed. But how, since Mikhail Suvorov's gang of criminal 'engineers' are still in control up there, standing guard on the place and waiting for his return? Which brings up another question: how long before some of them decide to follow him through the Gate?

"Well, despite that the complex is isolated, remote—still, I can't attack it. Even if I had the military muscle I wouldn't dare use it for fear of attracting the rest of Suvorov's 'colleagues' to Perchorsk. There you have it: it's a vicious circle, and frankly I can't see any easy way to break out of it."

"Me neither," said Trask, frowning. "But that doesn't mean it's hopeless. In E-Branch I have a good many first-class problem-solvers, and I promise I'll do what I can. But first let me get it straight. No one else knows about Sunside/ Starside's mineral riches?"

"Now that Suvorov is dead, no. Not that I'm aware of."

"And there are no documents to lead anyone in that direction?"

"None that I know of." Turchin shook his head.

"Then what it boils down to is this: you've got to find a way to tell Mikhail Suvorov's cronies he's dead, while simultaneously ensuring that they don't go looking for him."

"What?" Turchin was at once alarmed. "*And* without telling them how or where he died, surely—that is, if you would save Nathan's world from uttermost destruction! For if you think for a moment they wouldn't go searching for Suvorov, you're wrong. They would. And they would see what they would see, and having seen it . . . *then* they would turn a whole world into a nuclear, chemical, and biological wasteland!"

"*If* they managed to get back here to tell about it," said Trask. "But in any case you're right: eventually we'll have to get into Perchorsk and close the Gate, for good this time."

"Precisely. Until which time the problems remain. . . ."

Trask was silent for a moment, then said, "As for the one we've just formulated, how to get into Perchorsk and close the Gate: I may soon have the answer to that one, at least. But not right now. It's something I'm working on."

"Harry Keogh could have done it," said Turchin knowingly, perhaps wistfully.

"Harry's dead," said Trask.

"But Nathan isn't," said Turchin. "And he owes me."

Trask shook his head. "No, Nathan can't help us. Not right now. He has problems of his own in Sunside/Starside. And there isn't any way we can contact him."

"But didn't you say you were working on something?"

"Something, someone, yes. Don't ask me any more about it."

Turchin nodded. "I see. . . ."

"But don't lose hope," Trask told him. "Like I said, we'll do what we can. Meanwhile you'll have to sit tight, play dumb."

"Play dumb?" Turchin snorted. "I may be the Premier, but I can't hold these people off forever! Suvorov and a good many men, scientist and soldier both, have gone missing and they believe I have the answers. And when I won't supply them, then they'll think I'm involved."

"Then keep out of their way for as long as you can."

"I intend to," said Turchin. "That is the other reason I'm here in Brisbane. Because it keeps me out of Russia. And that's why those 'friends' of mine in the other car, those—"

"Those goons?"

"—Why those goons are here, yes." Turchin tried to smile but it was a futile effort. "To make sure I'll find my way back home again. *Huh!*"

"You could seek political asylum."

"Which might solve my problem, but it wouldn't solve ours, yours, Russia's, or the world's."

"So what will you do?"

"These conferences look like they'll go on forever. Certainly for the rest of this year. Here, and in London, Brussels, Rio de Janeiro, Calcutta, you name it. I shall attend them all, one after the other if that's at all feasible. And of course I shall sweat and worry, and wait for you to come up with an answer."

"And at the same time do something for me," said Trask.

"Ah, yes! Your problems," said Turchin. "I had almost forgotten that this isn't a one-sided affair. So then, what can I do for you?"

"It's all part of the same problem," Trask told him. "Remember that and it might give you an incentive. First, call off your mind-spies. If we're to work together—or at least on the same wavelength—you don't need to be watching me. But on the other hand I do need them to be watching out for me. Or rather, for vampires. But there's more than one kind of bloodsucker involved here. You mentioned the illicit drugs trade. It's no big secret how the so-called Russian Mafia are flushing your people and your country down the toilet. But in another way, a different way, they're also connected with our problem in general. So here's what I want you to do. . . ."

And he quickly explained what he wanted: information from Turchin's side on the Moscow Mafia's connection with Marseille, with specific reference to Luigi Castellano's organization and its operation in the northern Mediterranean. And:

"This man Castellano is of particular interest to us," he finished up. "He's a dark horse indeed. My people in the Branch haven't so far been able to pin him down, and Interpol has next to nothing on him. I mean, it's not unusual for a drugs boss to keep a low profile, but this one's near-invisible. And frankly, I want his backside in a sling."

Turchin looked doubtful. "But doesn't this smack of common or garden police work? How does it fit into the big picture?"

"I'm trying to help someone who may soon be in a very good position to help me—or us," Trask answered. "If I scratch his back, with a bit of luck he'll scratch ours."

And Turchin nodded. "I'll see what I can do. Is there anything else?"

"You can try to find out just exactly what we'll be going up against if or when we do try to take Perchorsk," Trask said.

The Russian Premier looked at him; indeed his dark, glinting eyes bored into him, as he inquired, "With a British force, do you mean? In which case you might require a route of access. Not to mention one of egress, an escape route."

"Good idea," said Trask. "You can look into that, too, by all means. And you can think how to give us cover in the event of political flak,—that is, if we were seen to be involved. But at the moment I don't see it as a problem. It's like you said: Perchorsk is remote, isolated."

"Oh? And you can come and go into foreign lands and alien places at will, can you?" And now Turchin's gaze was even more intense.

But Trask only said, "We've talked enough, and our time's up." Then he switched on the intercom and said: "Mr. Smith, the hotel, if you please."

In a little while, Turchin said, "Well, it seems our business is done for now. But if that's all you want, and if things eventually work out, it would appear I get the best of the bargain."

Trask looked at him and shook his head. "I understand what you're saying, Gustav, but I think it's a very narrow viewpoint. The way I see it, the whole world gets the best of the bargain. Which is to say, we all come out of it alive . . . and as men."

Turchin shrugged and answered, "Yes, yes, of course you're right. Still, on a moment-to-moment basis, one's skin is oddly precious."

But Trask only said, "How about one's soul?"

And a little later while Turchin thought about that, if he thought about it, the limo arrived at his hotel. . . .

. . . And Trask was long gone before the second limo drew up where Turchin stamped "angrily" to and fro, waiting for his minders.

"Huh!" He grunted as they got out of the car. "Couldn't at least one of you have made an effort to stay with me?"

"But Premier—" the senior man began to protest.

"No buts!" Turchin snapped. "I shall report your inefficiency back in Moscow. And I'll also be making a strong complaint here."

"A complaint?" The other's jaw dropped.

"Of course, fool! No, no, not about you, but my driver and this bloody conference official, this Mr., er—"

"Smith?"

"Indeed, yes!"

"Both the driver *and* the official were Smiths?"

"Eh? Yes, I know that, you idiot! Please try not to inform me of what I already know. But, damn! You'd think that at least *one* of them would know the way to the hotel, wouldn't you . . . ?"

By the time the precog Ian Goodly picked up locator David Chung from Brisbane's international airport, Trask was in bed asleep. But he had left a message not to be disturbed, with a note that said:

> *David, welcome—*
>
> *But I'm afraid you will have to start "swanning" in the morning. Right now we're all badly in need of a few hours' sleep. I imagine it must be pretty much the same for you, what with jetlag and all.*
>
> *Ian: make sure the D.O. knows to wake me if anything important comes in during the night. Other than that, give me a shake when the sun's up and there's a pot of coffee on the go. Thanks . . .*

Jake Cutter had had his fill of sleep en route; so he thought. He sat up downstairs and played a quiet game of poker with the warrant officer commanders of the military contingent from the second jet-copter. By three in the morning, however, they were all yawning; then, deciding to call it a night (or a new day), each of them went off to his cramped sleeping quarters.

Jake didn't know it, but on the other side of his bunk's thin, plasterboard panelling Liz Merrick had taken the cubicle next to his. Acting on Trask's instructions, she was intent on getting into his mind and following his progress through whatever esoteric activities might take place in his—and whoever else's—head or heads. Still not keen on what she was doing, Liz had nevertheless come to realize its importance.

Frustrated when Jake stayed up, she had tried to wait him out and failed. But as finally he went to his bunk, and tossed and turned a while before settling down, she was disturbed and came awake. Following which it became a matter of establishing telepathic rapport. As Jake grew still and his breathing deepened, so Liz concentrated on strengthening her now instinctive connection with his subconscious mind, inviting his "detached" thoughts to mingle with her own.

Then for a while there was nothing, just a vague uneasiness of psyche as Jake's shields relaxed and his thoughts automatically sought to rearrange themselves into typical dream-patterns, or perhaps into something else. And before too long Liz found herself nodding again. . . .

. . . Until she came starting awake to an unnatural psychic *stillness* or pent awareness which had its origin in Jake. Next door, he was motionless and physically asleep; but *psychically* his mind was something else. It, too, was still—breathlessly still—like a cat watching a mouse emerge nervously from its hole; or, more probably (Liz decided), like someone in an empty house, suddenly aware of an unusual sound in the night.

He was *listening* to something—but so intently!—and for a moment Liz thought he had detected her presence. But no, while Jake's attention was definitely rapt upon a subconscious something, it wasn't focussed on Liz at all. On what, then?

And so for an hour Liz "listened" to Jake as attentively as he was listening to some sensed but unheard other or others, but with little or no result, except on occasion he would come alive and ask, "Who are you?" Or he would say: "I *know* you are there—I hear you whispering—so why not talk *to* me instead of *about* me?"

But even though Liz was given to understand something

of this, she sensed rather than "heard" what he said, because (a) Jake wasn't speaking to her directly, and (b) his recently discovered shields, while they weren't fully engaged, were nevertheless shrouding his thoughts.

Until, unable to bear the not-knowing any longer, she tried to break in on him and ask, "Who is it, Jake? Do you know them? What are they talking about?" At which the doors of Jake's mind at once slammed shut and she found herself locked out entirely. For a while, at least.

But lying there on her bed, Liz believed she knew who he had been trying to talk to. And that was knowledge that sent a shudder down her spine, so that even in the oppressive heat of this El Niño night, still she felt cold. And she also knew how he had detected her and shut her out. It was the difference.

For the precog Ian Goodly had had it right when he'd said: "When you heard Jake speaking, or thinking, that was your telepathy working. You heard him because he's alive. But the others . . . they were in a different category, using a different mode."

Deadspeak, yes. The difference between a live conversation and a dead one. . . .

They were talking—arguing among themselves—about him, Jake Cutter. And Jake knew it. More than that, he knew or suspected who or what they were, which was something he had yet to remember and admit in his waking hours, perhaps because no sane man would ever *want* to admit such a thing. Well, with the possible exception of a handful of dubious psychic mediums.

The dead in their graves were talking about him, and Jake could hear them like the buzzing of bees in a clover field, or more properly the rustle of dry leaves on a wintry garden path. For bees and flowering clover are redolent of burgeoning life, while the rustle of fallen leaves . . . isn't.

All of the voices belonged to strangers; he didn't know—or hadn't known—a single one of them. And while it was quite obvious that they heard him, no one bothered to answer

Jake on the few occasions when he felt galvanized to break in on their conversation; but his brief bursts of eager questioning invariably found long-drawn-out silences following in their wake.

And the worst of it was that these voices seemed afraid to talk out loud: they whispered, so that he found it difficult to follow what they were saying. But they seemed to be arguing the pros and cons, Jake's merits against his drawbacks, to what end he couldn't rightly say.

We don't—we daren't—let them in among us! one of the voices said quite clearly. While another mumbled:

But he isn't one of them. See, his light burns like a lantern in the dark, and we feel its warmth. Only the Necroscope— only Harry Keogh and his sons were ever like this—beacons in our everlasting night, or places to warm ourselves in the presence of the living; our only contact with the world and all the loved ones we left behind.

And another voice said, *But in the end even the Necroscope succumbed. Is that what you would have us do? Befriend this one and give him access to the dead? And if he, too, were seduced—what then? A vampire in our midst, and one who knows our every thought and secret? But the difference between a Necroscope and a necromancer . . . is vast.*

And monstrous! said yet another, whose voice shuddered. *We can't risk giving such a gift to anyone who would misuse it.*

But he already has the gift! said the voice, or its owner, who spoke in Jake's defence. *And given to him by Harry himself, if we can believe what she has said.*

Ah, but she's not long cold. Naive in the ways of the long night, what can she know?

She knew Harry.

And what good did that do her? Like so many others before her, and like Harry himself, she too became a victim. No, she's no guarantee. And as for Harry: don't speak of him. The teeming dead know all about him.

But Harry never harmed us! He was our friend and cham-

pion, right to . . . to the end. But here the defending voice grew very quiet and uncertain.

And what an end, said another small voice, *when the Necroscope must flee his own world in order to keep faith!*

She was the last of the living who Harry spoke to, the one who was unafraid came back. *She says he made promises—* and *he kept them.*

True, said another, more doleful voice. *But Harry isolated himself for the sake of the living, not for the dead.*

I say we should trust the woman, the other insisted.

No, said the doleful one. *For in the end she brought down a DOOM upon herself. Why, she was fortunate that she only died! And now—if we trust this one on her word—perhaps she will bring a DOOM on all of us.*

At which point:

"Zek?" Jake tried again to cut in. "Is it Zek you're talking about? Zek Föener?"

And again a long, cold silence. Until out of nowhere:

I presented your case, Jake, and now we must let them talk it through. (Zek's voice, which he recognized at once.)

"Talk what through? I'm not with you."

If the Great Majority, the teeming dead, decide that they don't want you to have or to use deadspeak, Zek explained, *then you can talk all you like and they won't listen. They'll simply ignore you. Oh, they're drawn to you—we're all drawn to your warmth, Jake—but at the same time they're afraid of you. They were afraid of Nathan, too, once upon a time, but Nathan proved himself, showed them they were mistaken. If he was here now . . . well, he could far better plead your case than I can.*

"And what about Harry?" Jake said. "Where is he? Couldn't the Necroscope, er, 'plead my case'—whatever that's supposed to mean—even better?"

Not any longer, Zek answered.

"He did something to upset them?"

Something . . . happened to him, she answered carefully.

"So," Jake tried to reason it out, "Harry is dead, but the Great Majority won't have any truck with him. Yet you get along okay with him, and that thing in the sump was positively clinging to him. All very weird."

If E-Branch, or Harry himself, had wanted you to know certain things, then I'm sure they would have told you, said Zek.

But Jake was still puzzling it out. "Trask, Ian Goodly, and Lardis—yes, and Liz, too—they've all had a go at hinting at something without being specific. They seem concerned that once I know the whole thing, or when I can see the big picture, then that I'll run from it. But surely it would have to be something terrible to scare the Great Majority, who have absolutely nothing to lose! Yet even the dead won't spit it out up front. They speak in whispers, as if afraid to even talk about it. Not only that but Harry Keogh, a once-powerful metaphysical mind, is now an outcast among his own kind. So what in hell did he do?"

Jake sensed that he must be close now. But so did Zek, who was anxious to divert him. And:

Jake, she cut in, *you'll have an explanation. All of this will be explained eventually—or you'll work it out for yourself—but for now let it go, and let the teeming dead deliberate. The wisdom of the ages is down in the earth, Jake. I can't see that they'll make a mistake on your account. I know they'll let you in . . . eventually.*

"Huh!" he snorted. "In a way they're just like Trask; even like you, Zek! Everyone seems to think I should *want* to be 'in'—that I should consider it a privilege—but all of these E-Branch types will tell you their talents are a curse. So why is it different for me? Why should I accept a curse? And just what sort of a curse is it, anyway? I mean, that *is* what this is all about isn't it? The stuff that Trask isn't telling me? The bottom line? The downside?"

Then for a while there was silence in the psychic aether, until Zek said, *I can't ask you to trust me, can't promise you anything, for the dangers are enormous. But one thing is certain: you can be the new Necroscope. You* are *the Necroscope, if only you'll accept it.*

"I would accept it," he told her then. "I *have* accepted it in a way. For how can I deny what is? But if there's a short-cut to my—well, to my being—then why can't I take it now? And as for the drawbacks . . . surely it's my right to know what they are? I mean, what's the big mystery?"

Jake, Zek answered, *Harry Keogh was born with his skills, or with some of them at least, but you've had them thrust upon you. What came naturally to Harry is coming unnaturally to you. But some things are so unnatural—and the very possibility of others is so frightening—as to make deadspeak and the Möbius Continuum seem mundane by comparison.*

"Now, if that was intended to give me confidence—" Jake started to say, only to be cut off as Zek broke in:

Personally, you wouldn't have been my choice. (He sensed the sad, reluctant shake of an incorporeal head.) *But you were Harry Keogh's choice, which has to be good enough, for he must have had good reasons. And now there are others I have to talk to, others to convince—on your behalf, yes—on the far side of the world. Before I go, however, it seems only fair to tell you: you're not making it easy, Jake. . . .*

"That seems to be one of my big problems—" he started to say, then realized that she was gone.

But I am here, Jake, always, said another voice, phlegmy, lustful and darkly sinister, close and even too close to hand. The voice of Korath Mindsthrall, fading to a distant, bubbling chuckle.

And in a little while, coming to Jake as if from far, far away, the whispering of the teeming dead started up again. But it was now more fearful than ever. . . .

Morning found Jake in an introspective mood. But before he was up and about Liz took the opportunity to have a word in private with Trask about her experience of the previous night.

They were out in the grounds, walking under the high wall, breathing easy while still the sun hung low in the east. It was early, and the dawn chorus of various parrot species clattered in the still air. Another hour or two and the air would be dry, "sub-tropical" Brisbane baking in furnace heat.

Trask heard Liz out, was silent a while, thinking it over. Then he asked her, "He was definitely using deadspeak?"

"I don't think so . . . but does it matter? I mean, the way I understand it, as a Necroscope—or the Necroscope—his very thoughts are deadspeak. Unless he's shielding his thoughts, the dead will hear him thinking. And they will always know where he is. It's like an extra sense, their only sense. They can't see, hear, feel, taste, or smell, but they'll know when he's near."

Trask shook his head defeatedly. "I probably know as much about deadspeak as anyone else," he sighed. "Indeed, more than anyone else. But I still don't *know* about it. I talk about it, yes—I know it exists—but sometimes it's hard to believe in it. So don't ask me about it, because I don't know. Hell, Liz! You're the telepath!"

"It *was* deadspeak," she said. "Or at least, he was listening to deadspeak. Listening to—my God!—to dead people, conversing in their graves. And they were talking about him. That was all I got: the fact that he could hear them and was trying to join in their conversation, but they wouldn't let him."

"Huh!" Trask grunted. "Who can blame them? Neither would I 'let him in' if I could help it. His bloody attitude . . ."

"But to mature, to be the Necroscope, he has to be able to talk to them, right?"

"That's part of it, yes. Well, let's just hope it comes to him, as everything else will have to come to him—the good and the bad. And meanwhile you keep an eye, or an ear, on him."

"You're still not sure of Jake, are you?" Liz said.

Trask shrugged. "I'm not sure he's sure of us! And despite what he has said, I know he still has his own agenda. Anyway, I spoke to Premier Turchin about that, and I'm hoping he can come up with some answers. If we can just find a way to lay that one ghost—kill off the one thing that's burning a hole in Jake's brain, this revenge thing, this course he's set on—maybe it will leave him with an open mind."

"You mean with Castellano out of the way, Jake would more easily be able to concentrate on the job in hand?"

"Right. So Turchin will try to dig some dirt on this fellow, see if he can get something solid on him. If we could lock him away it would be a start. But Ian doesn't think that would be enough, not for Jake. And the hell of it is: I understand. I know how Jake feels. Think yourself lucky, Liz, that you don't know the kind of hatred we're all capable of. What if I should tell you that I would gladly give my right arm at the shoulder just to see Nephran Malinari writhing, burning on a cross, and to revel in the stink of his smoke? Well, now I'm telling you. And I mean it."

"And Jake's no different," she said with a small shiver.

"Neither was the Necroscope Harry Keogh," Trask told her. "And neither am I. Few men are, when the crime and the pain it brings is nasty enough. An eye for an eye, Liz."

"But in fact, Jake hardly knew that girl."

"He knows that she was raped and tormented and died horrribly, because of him. He knows it was fixed so that he'd take the blame, and that Castellano tried to have him killed in the jail in Turin. That's enough. It would be enough for me, too."

"Yet you're still hard on him. You *think* hard on him."

But the other shook his head. "He's hard on himself. Anyway, let it go now. And let's hope Turchin comes up with something."

Hearing footsteps on the gravel drive, they looked toward the house.

It was the precog, Ian Goodly. He came in his accustomed, long-legged lope—with a long face, too—for all the world a cadaverous mortician. "Fresh coffee's on the go," he said in his piping fashion. And: "Did I hear someone mention Turchin?"

"What about him?" said Trask.

"It was on the early news," the precog answered. "He'll be attending a couple of conference sessions this morning, but tonight or tomorrow he's out of here and back to Moscow."

393

"What?" Trask frowned. "Moscow is the last place he'd want to be right now. What happened?"

"A fistfight, apparently," Goodly answered. "In Turchin's hotel bar last night. An Australian delegate got drunk, accused the Premier point-blank of lying about Russia's soft ecological policy, went on to call him a puppet mouthpiece for his industrial and military masters back home."

"Which right now is true as far as it goes," Trask nodded. "Mainly because he has no other choice. So what else?"

"Turchin got a drink thrown in his face before his minders stepped in and started throwing their weight around. The upshot is that he'll speak today—state Russia's case, protest about his treatment and what have you—and take the first plane out tomorrow. Tonight if he can get one."

Turning it over in his mind, Trask stroked his chin. "That doesn't sound like Gustav Turchin to me," he said. "Long before he made Premier he was a diplomat, could talk his way through a minefield. Something like this happens . . . I just can't see him *letting* it happen." He shook his head. "Not unless he wanted it to happen. In which case . . . it has to be a ploy."

"A ploy?" Goodly looked surprised.

"An excuse to get him out of here," Trask said. "He has a couple of things to organize in Moscow. I made a deal with him, gave him one or two problems to solve on our behalf. It's possible that the only place he could work on it is back in Russia. And isn't there another Earth Year Conference starting in Oslo in just a few days' time? Acid rain or some such? I'll give you odds that's his next stop. He's something of a fox, Gustav Turchin. I'm betting he'll go home, set a few wheels turning, then head for Oslo. And of course, with the rest of the world baying at his heels, it will make him something of a hero with his own people. A temporary thing, but it ought to distract his enemies awhile. Anyway, and whatever's going on, wish him luck. Gustav has come through for us in the past and he probably will again. I'll brief you on our conversation later."

"Gustav?" said Goodly. "First name terms?"

"Right," said Trask. "It's called *detente*, my friend. And with the Opposition, as it happens. Well, it won't be the first time." -

"Tell me more," said Goodly, wide-eyed.

"Later," Trask said again, as they headed back toward the house.

27
Mindsmog!

IN GENERAL, TRASK'S BRIEFING WOULD BE THE very simplest thing. As yet he wasn't speaking to a full team—and he wasn't about to mention his private arrangement with Premier Gustav Turchin to any others but core members of E-Branch—but in the current lull he knew that he needed to keep his people sharp, keep them in the picture, and give them some sort of incentive. Thus, while he intended to stick to a loose broad-screen scenario or overview, still he would remind them of what they were dealing with here, emphasizing the extreme dangers of the job in hand.

His audience included everyone available, which left only the technician Jimmy Harvey doing duty officer in the ops room; but in fact Trask's words were directed mainly at the Australian Military contingent. Dressed in casual, lightweight summer "civvies," and while for the moment they didn't much look like soldiers, in fact these young special-forces officers were the best that their vast country had to offer. Which is to say (in their own down-to-earth terms, and as members of an elite Australian regiment) they were "bloody useful in a scrap, mate."

"I know we've been over some of this before," Trask began, "but I just want to make it plain what we're dealing with. That job we did in the Gibson desert—Bruce Trennier and his creatures—it wasn't big stuff. Trennier was a lieutenant, a right-hand man, but he wasn't the boss by any means. Just what he and those others were doing out there in the middle of nowhere, we still aren't sure. Maybe that entire setup was just a bolthole, somewhere that the big chief could run to if things went wrong. But as for the boss himself—who incidentally could as easily be *her*self—he or she is here, not far away from us even as I speak. At least, that's our belief. It's what our experts are telling us.

"Now, that night when we camped out in the Gibson desert. After the fireworks were over, one of you—no names, no pack drill—asked me a question. Normally it would be a perfectly reasonable question: why couldn't we take a lesser creature, a thrall, captive in order to talk to him, study him, and try to see what makes him tick? Which as I've said would seem reasonable . . . *if* we were dealing with an entirely human enemy. But circumstances being what they are, and our enemy being what he is, your question told me that you were either poorly informed, or you hadn't understood your original briefing, or you really didn't appreciate what you'd been dealing with that night. And for all I know, it mightn't be just one man I'm speaking about here, but all of you could have the same problem.

"So, despite that I've had experience of these things in the past—or maybe because I have—and you people are newcomers to the game, I tried to put myself in your shoes. Maybe it had seemed too easy. Unpleasant, yes, but not really difficult. And I began to see what the problem was. You've probably seen yourselves as men with a nasty job to do . . . but someone has to do it, right? I mean, maybe it seemed to you that these *people* you were killing were like, what—escapees from an isolation ward somewhere?—and you were putting them down simply to ensure they didn't pass on the infection. A pretty effective preventative measure, certainly, but perhaps a bit drastic to your way of thinking.

"So, let's go back to that perfectly reasonable question: why *don't* we just immobilize these things, lock them away, and study them? And wouldn't that be a far less drastic solution?

"Well, let me tell you again—let me remind you—about vampires:

"Oh, they can be downed. Shoot at them with bullets, especially silver bullets, and you can knock them down . . . even if they don't always stay down. Burn them—burn them entirely—and they die. Lock them up in silver cages, and keep their systems topped up with garlic so that they can't work up a head of steam, and you might even manage to confine them—for a little while. But as for studying them . . .

"Only make a mistake—your first mistake, just one—and *you* become the prisoner. And you don't get a second chance.

"Think of it this way. Men have devised chemical and biological weapons, toxins and living viruses, that could wipe us all out—destroy humankind itself—if they were to get loose. We keep these things in secure laboratories where we study and even develop them. Well, when I say 'we,' I mean humans: 'scientists,' in outlawed lands mainly, dabbling in a mainly outlawed science. For happily a majority of governments have long since banned all such agents; they deem them simply too terrible for study or development, and they're right.

"But the unpleasant fact is that because some people continue to experiment with this stuff, *our* people are obliged to follow suit in order to find vaccines and antidotes. They don't want us to be caught with our immune systems down, as it were. So yes, these terrible poisons still exist in just about every country that's capable of handling them. But by God, you'd better believe they take damn good care not to spill this stuff!

"So then, why am I bothering to tell you what you probably already know, and what does it have to do with vampires and the Wamphyri? Well, it's this simple:

"If you think of the Wamphyri and their works in just such terms of reference you won't go far wrong. That is, you have to think of them as something that must be destroyed. But whatever you do, *don't* think of them on the same scale of danger! I mean, we all know that the Richter scale is a yard-stick for the power of earthquakes. But if it was a scale for *all* potential disasters, then to cover man-made biological weapons it would have to stretch from the current nine to ninety, and to cover the Wamphyri it would need to carry on from ninety to infinity! That's by *my* personal scale of reckoning, and I am not wrong.

"And remember: our man-made toxins and viruses aren't bent on escaping; *they can't think!* But only imprison a vampire, and from that moment on he's thinking of ways to get free. He *wants* to be free, like you, and wants you to be a prisoner, like him. The prisoner of something growing inside you, that will gradually make you someone—some*thing*—else. Something other.

"So then, now maybe you can see why we can't suffer a vampire to live. The point being, we really *won't* suffer a vampire to live. Be sure of this: if you get infected, there's no cure. Which means we'll kill you. Oh, it'll be clean, but it will happen.

"So remember, a moment or so after one of us—I include myself—shows up positive, he also shows up dead.

"And on that point, enough said.

"Now let's move on:

"We think it's likely that our quarry has a hideout some-where in the mountains. Where they come from, the Wam-phyri are very fond of their aeries—the places where they live—and the higher the better. Unfortunately that doesn't tell us very much, doesn't narrow down his or her location. For as you know as well or better than I do, there are moun-tains galore around here. But there's also a paradox in that the Wamphyri don't go much on sunlight. And right now we've rather a surfeit of that, too! Weird, wouldn't you say, that our alien friend has chosen to set up shop here? Well, maybe not.

"You see, he's not dumb. He knows that we know his habits, and that we've known about his 'invasion' from square one. That means he also knows that normally this would be one of the last places we'd expect to find him. So where better to hide himself away and do his thing, whatever that thing is? The only problem is, he might also know that we found and dealt with Bruce Trennier, and by now he could well be expecting us to come looking for him here.

"Indeed, he could already know that we've arrived. And if so he'll be doubly dangerous, because there'll be little or no element of surprise.

"Okay, we have a couple of days before our backup squads and the big ops vehicle are in situ. And that has to be one of our first priorities: to find suitable and preferably unobtrusive sites, with access to principal mountain approach roads, where we can harbour these men and vehicles as they arrive. So as of noon today we'll be air-mobile again, but not in the jet-copters that you've grown used to. They may have been great in the desert, but to Brisbane's civilian population—not to mention our quarry—aircraft that look like they do are bound to attract attention. So for the time being they'll be on standby in hangars at the airfield where we came in.

"So, there's a firm in town that does aerial sightseeing trips by helicopter, north along the Coastal Range to Gladstone, and south over the Macphersons and along the Richmond Range as far as Grafton. Which is ideal for our purposes in that it covers the ground we're interested in, and the pilots know all the routes by heart and have first-class local knowledge. Alas that we can't simply commandeer this firm, its men and machines; but no, that would be to give the show away, and so we'll be paying our way. But I will try to get us a bit more clout than the average tourist. Obviously we have to have the final say on where we fly and what we look at. So later this morning I'll speak to Prime Minister Lance Blackmore and see if he can sort something out for us.

"Very well, so assuming we're airborne again, what will we be looking for? Military commanders, you'll be looking for naturally concealed campsites for your contingents, harbour areas, and access routes. And you'll also be checking your maps, doing an aerial reconnaissance of the entire area. As for my people:

"We'll be scanning the mountain heights for our quarry.

In truth, we don't really know what we're looking for; we can only hope we'll know it when we see it. But it isn't all blind luck. Two of my men, Lardis Lidesci and David Chung, are specialists in this regard. One of them will travel in each chopper.

"Okay, that's it. From midday or soon after we should have these planes at our disposal. Get your maps, cameras, and whatever else you'll need sorted out now. As for myself: well, much as I'd like to be going with you, my duty for the time being is right here. Someone has to watch the shop.

"A final reminder. This is a covert operation. Try not to give anything away to these civilian pilots. Have a set of answers ready to hand. For instance, you could be fire chiefs carrying out preliminary aerial surveys, ensuring there won't be a second Great Fire of Brisbane. Something along those lines. I'm sure you'll think of something.

"That's it, and I hope I didn't bore you too much. Ladies, gentlemen, thanks for your time and attention."

Brisbane's Skytours helicopters were small, conventional pleasure machines custom-built for the job. Capable of carrying four passengers, they had wraparound, Plexiglas side windows which allowed for superb viewing, but would prove a shade vertiginous for people with height problems. As the Old Lidesci would later describe it, it was "like flying in a bubble!"—and he didn't much like it. The only other problem was their range. Two hundred and eighty miles was their safety limit without refuelling; which meant that a chopper on the northern route must land at a small airport in Gladstone, and on the southern route in Grafton. The good side of that was that it gave the passengers time to take on food and water to see them through the return trip.

The pilots were isolated up front behind see-through bulkheads, and they communicated with their passengers on headsets. But since in the main their commentaries consisted of monologues learned parrot-fashion over years of flying the same routes, pretty soon the drone of their voices became one with the whirring of rotors and ceased to have meaning.

If passengers didn't want to listen they removed their headsets; when they wished to converse or ask questions, they replaced them. A simple system.

In the early afternoon, Jake flew south toward the Macpherson Range with Ian Goodly, the Old Lidesci, and an Australian major whose rank was never on display or used to unfair advantage; he had his job to do and was simply another member of the team. But truth be told, it was a strange team. The precog was there in the uncertain hope that should they fly over an "aerie"—in whatever shape or form—he might catch a glimpse of some significant future event and recognize it for what it was. The SAS major had his own tasks to perform; he understood that Jake, Goodly, and the old man were "specialists" in their own right, but in what specific areas he neither knew nor cared.

As for Jake: ostensibly he had been sent along so that he could "get a good look at the lie of the land," but he assumed that in fact it was to keep him out of Trask's way. And he was partly right: Trask hadn't wanted him around cluttering up the place, asking awkward questions, generally being an obstacle. But that wasn't the whole story. Mainly Jake had been sent out with Lardis and Ian Goodly in the hope that something of their team spirit might rub off on him.

And truth to tell, Jake was actually developing a strong feeling of kinship with the Old Lidesci, and he already acknowledged a growing measure of respect for Goodly ... this despite that the precog seemed as enigmatic as ever. As for the Australian major: Jake wasn't about to mention (or invite questions about) his own brief "career" as a member of the original British Special Air Service. For after all, he had been "required to leave" in rather short order, and compared to this professional would seem the veriest amateur. But at least he had remembered some of his training ... the useful, more deadly bits, anyway.

And there they sat, scanning the beautiful, sun-bleached coastal strip far below, the valleys and hills, but especially the rearing mountains, as the Skytours helicopter whirled them south, and their pilot/tour-guide's monologue droned on and on in their headsets.

Flying north along the Coastal Range, the locator David Chung shared a second Skytours helicopter with two SAS warrant officers and Liz Merrick. It said a lot for their personal discipline and commitment that these fit young Australians were able to concentrate on their work with Liz along. For her part, she was aware of the occasional appreciative glance at her curvaceous figure in tight-fitting jeans and loose shirt. But while the SAS men found this British "Sheila" easy to talk to, frank and friendly, they also knew that she was a member of E-Branch and so must be special in ways other than the purely physical. She was treated accordingly, and with the utmost courtesy.

Liz was part of this second team in her capacity as a telepath. Not that her talent was in any way specific to vampires, but if David Chung were to detect mindsmog, that might provide her with a target area, a "direction" in which to cast her mental net if only to corroborate the locator's find. Before letting her go, however, Ben Trask had cautioned her that that was as much as she could do, and warned:

"Liz, you'd better know what you could be up against. That stuff with Bruce Trennier? Child's play by comparison with what you could expect from a 'real' Lord of the Wamphyri! I remember once over—oh, it seems like a million years ago—how Harry Keogh wouldn't hear of Zek using her talent anywhere near Janos Ferenczy. Janos was a powerful mentalist, too, but according to what Lardis has said about Malinari, Janos couldn't have held a candle to him! And it might well turn out that Nephran Malinari is our man, that he's the one we're dealing with here. It's unlikely to be Szwart, we're fairly certain of that, so it has to be either Vavara or Malinari. But if it's the latter, and if he really is better than Janos . . .

"Listen, twenty-odd years ago I had a friend called Trevor Jordan. He was E-Branch, and a telepath. Janos Ferenczy caught Trevor spying on him and got into his head—I mean *literally!* And later, at a distance of some seven hundred miles, Janos was able to invade and even inhabit Jordan's mind. And just to show us how good he was, he made Jordan put a gun to his own ear and pull the trigger! Now *that* . . . is mentalism.

"But this Nephran Malinari isn't just another telepath. In his own world, in Starside four hundred years ago, his own kind, the Wamphyri, called him Malinari the Mind. Doesn't that say it all? Anyway, we've learned the legends from Lardis, and the Old Lidesci's word is good enough for me. And even if it wasn't . . . well, I know I'll never forget the things that Zek showed me on the night she died. That bastard vampire *thing,* trying its best to leech on her mind.

"So I'm asking you, Liz. Please be careful. You . . . you're very special, and in my time I've lost too many special people. I just need to be sure you fully appreciate the danger. I don't want you locking on to something—and perhaps receiving something—that you don't want and can't get rid of."

That had been some three hours ago, and now . . .

. . . Trask's words were still echoing in Liz's mind when the pilot's voice climbed a notch in her headset to declare, "We're going down now, folks. Gladstone next stop. So if yer'll excuse me, I'll just radio a pal o' mine on the ground, tell him to get the beer out o' the cooler, and slice up a fresh batch o' sarnies. By the time yer've all freshened up, I'll be done refuelling and we'll start back. A slightly different route this time, if yer'd like. We can stick more closely to the coast and—"

"No," Liz interrupted him. "I'm sorry, but we're especially interested in mountains. On the way back, it would suit us just fine if you'd show us some mountains that we haven't seen yet." And then, perhaps a little self-consciously, "Er, sorry to be a nuisance."

The pilot glanced back through his window, looked from face to face, shrugged his shoulders and said, "Suit yerself,

Miss, fellers. I'm to accommodate yer as best I can, so whatever yer say is okay with me."

At which Liz craned her neck and looked for confirmation from David Chung where he sat behind her . . . only to find that the locator's attention, indeed his concentration, seemed rapt on something that no one else could see. With his jaw hanging slack, he gazed as if transfixed eastward, out across the open sea. It lasted for a single moment only, then Chung started as he became aware of Liz's eyes upon him, the unspoken question that was written in them.

His gaze met hers and he half-nodded, half-shrugged, then said, "I . . . I don't know. I can't be sure. It was so faint."

They were settling fast towards a small airport. The locator snapped out of it, put his headset on, and asked the pilot, "What's out there? I mean east—er, the sea?"

"Exactly, mate," the other's tinny voice came back, seeming to vibrate as the pitch of the rotor vanes changed to landing mode. "The sea, a handful o' little rocks, and stretching a thousand miles to the north, the Great Barrier Reef." And then a laugh. "Sorry, but all that's way out o' our itinerary. . . ."

They freshened up, drank ice-cold beer out of glasses dripping with condensation, ate prawn sandwiches and barbecued chicken, and talked while they waited for their pilot to call for them.

They were in a private Skytours suite that overlooked the small airport through a soundproof panoramic window. While eating they had watched a handful of planes coming and going, not said too much, been glad of the overhead fan that struggled to waft a stream of warm, sluggish air around the room.

But eventually curiosity had got the better of the military men. Liz was aware of it but didn't find it intrusive, and anyway they were all members of a loose-knit team.

And the fact was that, apart from Trask's briefings—and that these men had been ordered to accept all Branch members as voices of authority here—there hadn't been and could never be a great deal of understanding of E-Branch's role. Not to disparage the military, but it would have proved extremely difficult for entirely military minds to grasp the concepts, motivations, and operating practices of an ESP-oriented intelligence agency. And indeed, they weren't required to. But now, here in the intimacy of a much smaller grouping, these young soldiers had been presented with an opportunity to dig just a little deeper.

On the other hand and on behalf of E-Branch, both Liz and Chung were sworn to a modified version of the Official Secrets Act, and so had to be circumspect in what they revealed.

"You're a psychic, right?" one of the warrant officers, a slim, well-muscled, crewcut redhead in his early thirties asked of David Chung. "I mean, don't take offence, but isn't it a bit strange, using—what do you call it? parapsychology?—against bloody awful things such as that nest we burned out in the desert?"

"No offence taken," said Chung. "But you'd do well to remember that I'm the one who *found* those bloody things out in the desert! And I've been dealing with such things on and off—but mercifully more off than on—for some twenty years. Currently, however, we're definitely on again, and like most of the others in E-Branch I'm getting past my sell-by date. Oh, we're recruiting young blood all right, such as Liz here, but the years take their toll. So on a job like this we're obliged to call in different kinds of 'experts.' We like to be sure there's plenty of muscle behind the mind."

"Like us?" said the other.

And Chung nodded, smiled, raised an eyebrow and said, "No offence?"

"But a psychic? I mean, how can you simply *think* the location of these creatures? Like, you read their thoughts or something?"

And though he was polite up front in his talking to Chung, Liz couldn't help reading that he was more than a little skeptical. She read one or two other things, too, such as: *Never kid a kidder, Mr. Chinaman. Old Red isn't buying it!* Red:

a nickname no one had used since his teens, and one which he wouldn't accept from anyone else despite that it fitted him so well and was how he continued to think of himself.

So before Chung could answer Liz told herself, *to hell with the rules,* and said, "Whether you're buying it or not, my friend Mr. Chung here—who is in fact a fourth generation Brit, despite that his roots are Asian—*isn't* kidding, Red!"

The young soldier jerked in his seat, instinctively touched a hand to his crewcut, and stuttered: "Er, my hair, right?"

But Liz shook her head. "Your thoughts," she replied. "And Red, the next time I walk into a place ahead of you, please try to remember I can't help how I walk, and find somewhere else to look . . . okay?"

Fuck me!!! thought the other.

And Liz said, "No thanks. I'm spoken for."

"J-Jesus, I'm s-s-sorry!" the other gasped.

"It's okay," Liz told him. "But maybe we should change the subject now? And yes, you're safe: I promise not to peek."

"What's going on?" asked the other soldier, genuinely puzzled.

"Nothing much," Liz told him. "I was reading your friend's thoughts, that's all. Yours, too, if you like."

"Oh, really?" The second W.O. was older and less inquisitive. But he did have something on his mind.

"In the chopper," Liz said, "just as we were landing. You were wondering what was wrong with David. Like me, you noticed the way he was looking out over the sea, his expression."

"You saw that?" the W.O. said.

"No," said Liz, "I overheard it, 'Joe'—in your head."

And Joe accepted that she had, because they had only ever been introduced as Warrant Officers Bygraves and Davis!

"Let me have one of your maps," Chung said, deciding that Liz had gone far enough. "This area, and small scale. Covering as much ground as possible."

"Red" Bygraves spread a map on the table, and Chung

began poring over it. While he searched he explained:

"I'm a kind of bloodhound. It's nothing weird" (though in fact it was), "just a knack, sort of instinctive. But sometimes I can sense where these things are hanging out. In the helicopter, I got a feeling that there just might be something . . . out there!"

He stabbed his index finger at the map, their current location, then drew it in a straight line east and a little north. "In that direction, anyway. And you know, it's still there, but so very faint. . . ." Chung shook his head, narrowed his eyes in a frown. "What we could use, really, is a little triangulation."

"Now *that* I understand," said Red. "Let me see the map."

They let him jostle into position, watched him point out a location: Sandy Cape on the northern tip of Fraser Island. And: "We can't ask the pilot to fly us east and out to sea," he went on, "because that will add air-miles and run him low on fuel to get us back to Brisbane. But there's no reason why he can't fly us over Fraser Island, which lies south of here. He did suggest a coastal route, right?"

"Good!" said Chung. "And as soon as we get over the northern tip of the island, I can—well, do my thing, take a bearing north—and see if we come up with something."

Red looked at Liz. "And you'll do what? Or does this part include you out?"

Now Liz saw the error of saying anything at all. But since it was too late now: "If David senses anything, I'll try to, well, hitch a ride on his probe," she said. "But since this looks like a long-distance thing, I really can't be sure I'll get a reading."

And Joe asked Chung: "Did this talent of yours really lead your people to that Gibson Desert nest? I mean, we haven't seen you around until today—and you weren't out there—so . . . ?"

"Bruce Trennier had a very powerful aura," Chung answered. "But as a comparative newcomer among these creatures—even as a lieutenant—he wasn't too good at hiding himself away. When he slipped up, myself and some other E-Branch people, we picked him up from London. Since when the rest of them seem to be masking their presence—a kind of mental camouflage, you know? So I came out here to get a little closer to the action. Well, and now we might have found some."

"You picked Trennier up from London?" Joe said.

The locator nodded, and thought, *Yes, like a dense bank of fog on a sunny day. Fog that's there one minute, gone the next. Mindsmog!* But out loud he only said, "Yes, we did."

To which there was no answer, and the two W.O.s could only look at each other and shake their heads in wonder.

In the other helicopter an hour later, Jake Cutter was lost in his own thoughts, somewhat moodily enjoying the mountain scenery, when Lardis Lidesci reached across the narrow aisle, jogged his elbow, and said something.

"Um?" Jake murmured a response. He had long since removed his headset, and so had Lardis.

"I said, what's that?" the Old Lidesci said again, pointing out of the window on his own side of the aircraft.

"Why not ask the pilot?" Jake grumbled. "How am I to know what something is?" But loosening his belt, he stood up, leaned across, and looked anyway.

Ian Goodly was seated in front of Lardis. Feeling the movements, he looked back, saw where the others were looking.

They were on the return trip, covering different mountains than on the outward-bound leg. A thousand feet below, a massive geological "wrinkle" in the Macpherson Range had left a tightly angled dog-leg fold. In the west-facing lee of the fold, a saddle or roughly oblong-shaped false plateau maybe two and a half by four acres in extent stood out in stark contrast to the surrounding heights. For it wasn't naked rock. Anything but.

At an elevation of almost three thousand feet, someone had built . . . a small town? No, not a town but a complex of sorts: with gardens, pools, fountains, a monorail, tennis courts, bowling greens, even a small ski-slope up against the mountainside, and terraced chalets to house the guests. The walkways between concentric rows of red-tiled chalet accommodations radiated out from a roughly central location: a circular garden surrounding a great, silver-shining bubble of a structure, with windows on three levels and a smaller dome on top.

Lardis was lost for words; he found it too fantastic. But Jake only grunted and said, "You should see Las Vegas!" While in his own mind he wondered: *A holiday camp? A fantastic hotel complex for the jet-setters and beautiful people? Or maybe—*

"An aerie!" sighed Lardis. "Now wouldn't that make a wonderful aerie? Er, without all this sunlight, of course."

The precog was still wearing his headset, and he had been conversing with the pilot. Now he put a hand over the mike and said, "Xanadu, and the centrepiece there . . . why, that can only be Kubla Khan's pleasure dome! Put on your headsets. The pilot knows some stuff."

Jake and Lardis complied, heard the pilot tail off:

". . . There were some private homes here, hence the road up the mountain. But after the fire some kind of tycoon bought up the land and built this place. He's a philanthropist, uses the money from this for other 'good works,' allegedly. *Huh!* A typical tax gimmick, if you ask me. All of these fat-cat rich bastards are the same. Xanadu, yeah, that's what it's called. The dome's a casino, all three floors of it."

"The fire?" said Goodly. "You mean the Brisbane Fire?"

"Nah, not the Great Fire," said the other. "This was back in '97, an earlier El Niño. The place was a tinderbox, and the fire must have started in one of the weekend homes. They were simple timber cabins, holiday homes, you know? Went up like so much kindling."

"Take her lower, can you?" The precog was plainly interested.

"So what's on your mind, boss?" With a chuckle, the pilot leaned his machine into a descending spiral. "You want to wave at the girlies around those pools?"

"Er, something like that," said Goodly.

And certainly the girlies were there, and sun-bronzed fellows, too. There were three pools situated equidistant from the central dome; they glittered like dazzling blue jewels in Mediterranean settings, and were surrounded by low windbreak walls and mosaic-paved sundecks. The sundecks were dotted with chairs and sunbeds. And sure enough, as the chopper circled lower, the girls were sitting up, tilting their mirror-shades at the furnace sky, waving lazy arms at their imagined aerial "admirers."

"That's low enough," Lardis muttered, nervously. "The next thing you know, I'll be swimming!"

And the major said, "Mightn't we attract a little too much attention?" He was on the headset and the pilot heard him.

"So what's the problem?" he inquired. "Are you worried the people who run the place will complain? Nah! It's good free advertising, and we do this all the time. Tourists who can afford it sometimes take time out after they've seen it to come up for a few days' relaxation—though how anyone with red blood in his veins could relax up here is beyond me!"

Then the precog said, "That . . . that's enough. We'd better get on our way now." And there was a certain edge to his voice that had Jake looking at him across the aisle.

He saw that Goodly's face was suddenly drawn, and noticed how his hands gripped the armrests of his seat.

Part Four
The Hell of It

28
Here Be Vampires

THAT EVENING AT THE SAFE HOUSE, WHEN Trask's people had eaten, he got them together in the ops room to debrief them and start them working on the correlation of their findings. For he knew by then that they had been partially successful—or at least that they'd detected something out of the ordinary—and that a lot might soon depend on their observations.

For instance, the military contingent: it was most likely that the siting of the SAS backup teams would be based on the as yet unproven suspicions or "hunches" of Trask's espers. And in just two days' time those men and vehicles would start arriving and moving into harbour areas whose locations were as yet undecided. Time was of the essence.

After Trask had settled his people down, David Chung described his temporary contact with something during the landing at Gladstone, and went on to talk about the system of triangulation that they had devised.

"Taking Gladstone as the centre of a clock face," the locator said, "the first reading would see the minute hand at some thirteen minutes past the hour, or a few degrees north of east. As for the second reading, over Sandy Cape, that would be about twelve and a half minutes before the hour, or north-west."

Chung stood before an illuminated wall map of the area and used his index finger to point out the coordinates, then traced the directional lines to their junction some sixty miles out in the open sea. "Which puts it—whatever it is—right there," he said. But staring at the map, he could only offer a baffled shrug. "The last place on Earth that we'd expect to find a vampire or vampires. Right in the middle of an ocean,

413

with nothing but water and lots, I mean *lots* of sunlight, for miles around!"

"But you got readings," said Trask. "You got mindsmog. So, how do you explain it?"

The locator looked at him, frowned and said. "Explain it? But if it wasn't for Liz here I'd probably simply ignore it! A glitch, something out of kilter in my head . . . a headache? The evidence of the map, the location, it's all against us. I mean, what would a vampire be doing out there? Also, we know that in the past we've puzzled over similar effects from other espers, from talents outside E-Branch giving off vibes they don't even know they've got! So but for Liz I'd probably settle for someone on a ship out there—maybe a cruise liner?—using precognition to place bets in the casino, or maybe telekinesis to drop the ball on his numbers at roulette. Someone who's extraordinarily 'lucky,' who doesn't even know he has a skill—who thinks he has a 'system'—but who's nevertheless been banned from half a dozen mainland casinos. That's what I'd be tempted to think, except . . ." He paused and looked at Liz. "Liz doesn't think so. But there again, no matter what *anyone* thinks, nothing can change the fact that it's sixty miles out to sea."

Trask said, "But so were those Russian nuclear submarines, and you haven't been wrong about those. And I remember the time when a certain Jianni Lazarides had just such a ship, *The Lazarus,* out on the Mediterranean. Yes, but his real name was Janos Ferenczy! He was Wamphyri, too, one of the very worst. And remember: just because there's a lot of sunlight, it doesn't mean our man has to go out in it."

He turned to Liz. "David says it might be nothing. But he also says you don't think so. So what *do* you think?"

Liz looked anxiously from face to face, bit her lip, and said, "Ben, are we right to place this much faith in my talent right now? I mean, at that kind of range, riding David's probe . . . I could easily be mistaken. I'm not really sure that—"

"No, no, *no!*" Trask cut in, waving his hand dismissively, impatiently. "Just tell us what you got and let us try to figure it out. It isn't the first time we've done this, Liz. And it isn't as if we're vying with one another to see who will be first to find these damned things! But while no shame attaches to being in error, still we do have to find them. Which means anything is better than nothing. So whatever it was you sensed out there, let's have it."

Liz, Trask, and Chung were on their feet; the rest of the team was seated. And now Liz sat down, too, and thought about it for a moment. Casting her mind back, she asked herself exactly what it was that she had experienced when the locator took his second reading from the helicopter as it circled high over Sandy Cape.

Chung's face—his slightly damp skin gleaming a pale yellow, his nostrils pinched, eyes slanted more than usual in deep concentration—gazing out of his window, northwest at the distant curve of the world, the horizon, the sea's wide expanse.

Then his gaze becoming a vacant stare, and his eyes almost glazing over as his mind . . . as his mind went out!

No, not his mind but a probe. And Liz Merrick a part of it—riding it like a carrier wave—sharing telepathically in the emptiness of the locator's search, his far-flung probing of the psychic void . . . or what should be a void!

But there was something there—faint, so very faint, but definitely there—and she felt it like . . . like an emotion as opposed to a conversation. Like something spiritual, or lacking in spirit. For it was shivery cold, this thing, where it walked on her spine with icy feet. And now she knew its name.

"Well?" Trask was leaning over her. And:

"Fear!" Liz blurted it out. "I felt fear!"

The look on her face; her great green eyes wide in sudden knowledge where they stared into his . . . and Trask took a pace back from her. "You were afraid?"

"Not me, no," Liz shook her head. "He, they—whoever they were—were afraid. That's what it was, Ben: terror, gnawing at them, eating their hearts out."

"Them?"

"More than one, I'm sure."

"Uncertain a moment ago, and now you're sure?"

She shook her head. "I just wasn't willing to believe that there could ever be such hopelessness, such utterly black despair. I suppose I thought it was the emptiness, the psychic void before David's probe found—well, whoever they are—and that the fear was in fact mine. But now . . ."

"Yes?"

Again she shook her head, searched for words. "I know that I, personally, have never been that afraid—that I couldn't *be* that afraid—unless something happened to cause me to lose all hope, all faith."

Trask nodded grimly. "In short, unless you'd been vampirized!"

"I . . . I don't know. I imagine so."

But now Trask took a different tack. "Or could it possibly have been fear of discovery? Had someone detected David's probe and reacted to it?"

Liz shook her head. "No, I don't think so. It was simply—or not so simply—an aura of overwhelming doom."

"Good!" Trask grunted. "And on both counts. One, that you weren't detected. And two, that therefore whoever it was couldn't have been afraid of you. But they were afraid, and I think we can all imagine of what."

He looked up from Liz, from face to face around the room, and paused at Lardis Lidesci.

And Lardis said, "Thralls. These were thralls, and fairly recent. Thralls who don't have much contact with their master, but who know he's there nevertheless. Aye, and they have every right to fear him!"

"Another nest," Trask nodded. "Why not? It's entirely possible." Then he frowned. "But out at sea?"

"My point exactly," said Chung.

"Maps," Trask said, turning to Jimmy Harvey where he sat at a keyboard. "Jimmy, see if the computer has an even smaller-scale map of that area, and blow it up on the wall there."

"I've been working on it," said the other, tapping a key. "Consider it done."

The wall screen turned blue, if not entirely blue. For in the specified area they now saw the dotted outlines of reefs and other irregular shapes: islands or islets, and a legend identifying them as Heron Island and the Bunker and Capricorn groups, the latter because they lay on or close to the Tropic of Capricorn. Other lettering at the top of the map said that this was The Capricornia Section of the Great Barrier Reef Marine Park.

And very quietly, Trask said, "So, not necessarily a ship after all."

But looking sick, the locator David Chung could only shake his head and remark, "What a fool he is who has no faith in his own God-given skills!"

Trask might have denied it, but Ian Goodly beat him to it. "Not at all," the precog said. "When we use talents like these, it's against nature. I mean, even we appreciate that what we're doing isn't, well, mundane. Is it any wonder we're skeptical of our results? Or that we occasionally fail to see their significance?"

And then Trask said, "You're right, Ian, and I was on the point of making much the same remark. But as I've already said, this isn't a skills contest. How we get there doesn't matter a damn, only that we get there. Where these monsters are concerned, the end always justifies the means. *Any* means."

"Huh!" said Lardis. "And in Starside, whenever a man ascends to a vampire Lord and becomes Wamphyri, they have much the same saying—it's not the route but the getting there. In that respect, and except that their evil has been made ten times as great, these monsters are much like men, you know."

"Because they *were* men," said Trask. "And God knows we're none of us pure. Very well, now let's get on—but as soon as we're done here I want the duty officer to contact our aide in Prime Minister Blackmore's office. We need authority for liaison with someone high in the administration of the reef marine park. We need to know who or what is out there on those islets in the Bunker and Capricorn groups. . . ." A moment's pause and he turned to Goodly: "Ian, you and Lardis were in the other chopper party. And just like David here I know you, too, have a concern. Time now to have it out in the open."

The precog stood up, tossed a pamphlet attached to a tourist map onto the table. "I picked this up at the Skytours helipad," he said. "It's a freebie: a give-away route map into the Macpherson Mountains, and a colour brochure describing the wonders and benefits of the Xanadu health and pleasure resort. But that's not all I picked up. There was—or I should say there may have been—something else, when we flew over the place."

Sitting at the table (feeling more than a little useless, and wondering what he was doing here), Jake remembered the odd, strained look on the precog's face—the way his hands gripped his seat's armrests—after they'd descended to have a closer look at the resort. And now his interest focussed more definitely on Goodly as he saw once again the same nervous tension in the man's face and attitude.

"The thing is," Goodly went on, "I have precisely the same problem as David. The location: all that unhampered sunlight. I just can't see how the kind of creature we're looking for could exist up there . . . *if* that's what it was about." Seeing Trask's face, he held up a hand placatingly. "Yes, all right, I promise I will get on with it. But there are complications. . . .

"First: as we were descending toward the place so that we could get a better look at it, our pilot/tour-guide mentioned a fire that occurred during the El Niño back in 1997. And I found some of his descriptions vivid and perhaps evocative: the place was like a tinderbox . . . it went up like so much kindling, et cetera.

"Also, while we've been here I've heard quite a lot of talk about the Great Fire of Brisbane, and what with this awful heat and all—"

"You saw a fire?" Trask cut in.

Goodly nodded. "But I didn't see its cause, and I couldn't tell when it was happening. I mean, it could have been a mental response to what the pilot had said. For example, when someone says, 'do you remember' this or that other thing, you are made automatically to see it, relive it, in your mind's eye. Do you see? It could be that our pilot had evoked just such a response in me. And Ben, if this *was* one of my things, then it was only the very briefest glimpse. Smoke, and leaping flames . . . gouts of yellow fire roiling to a night sky, and a full moon hanging there . . . and someone shouting, 'To me, to me!' "

Listening to him, Trask displayed a kind of amazement, as if he'd only just realized something that should have been obvious for a long time. "How long have I known you?" he said. "It sometimes seems that I've known you forever. And yet I've never thought to ask you—do you sometimes see the past?"

The precog raised an eyebrow, said, "I *remember* the past, just like anyone else." And then a wry chuckle. "It's just that I sometimes remember the future, too!" But he was serious again in a moment. "That's what we have to consider, Ben. The future. And we know just how devious that can be—or is it perhaps my talent that's devious? I've never been able to figure it out."

"Okay," said the other, "so you don't know whether it was the past or the future. It's just one of those times when your talent leaves you in doubt. But there's one clue, at least."

"Oh?" Again Goodly's eyebrow.

"You said it was night time when Xanadu went up in flames, and—"

"Not Xanadu," Goodly stopped him. "Just a handful of weekend or holiday homes, on the false plateau where Xanadu stands now."

"Whatever," Trask waved a hand. "But you did say there was a full moon?"

"Yes."

"Well *that* . . . is one hell of a clue!" He turned to Harvey where he sat at the computer keyboard. "Jimmy, can you get into the local libraries on that thing?"

Harvey looked up from where he was working and smiled. But before he could say anything Trask said, "I know, don't say it: you're way ahead of me. The newspapers? For the fires of '97?"

Harvey nodded toward the wall screen. "On the screen, just about any time . . . now!"

Gadgets and ghosts! thought Jake, as headlines sprang into life on the big screen, and Harvey brought the small print into focus. The location, date, and time—everything was there, written into the report. And Trask said, "Good! Now then, Jimmy, can you cross-reference that date with phases of the moon?"

It took but a moment, but then Trask's shoulders sagged as he slumped into a seat and said, "Damn it all to hell! The last thing I wanted: A bloody full moon!" And looking at the precog: "So maybe you *can* see the past and not just remember it, after all."

"And maybe he can't," said Jake. It was the first time he had spoken, and now everyone looked at him. And after a while:

"Well, go on then," said Trask.

"Shouldn't we take the next step?" Jake said. "The same as we did with David Chung? I seem to have been hearing about synchronicity, coincidence, and what have you ever since I collided with this outfit. So couldn't this be exactly the same thing? I mean, just because there was a full moon on the night in question back in '97, that doesn't mean the precog wasn't seeing the future up there at Xanadu. Or aren't there going to be any more full moons? Me, I'm wondering when the *next* one is due."

Trask frowned, stared at Jake, then turned again to Jimmy Harvey. "Do it," he said.

And in a very short time the answer was up on the screen.

"Three days' time!" Trask husked then, open-mouthed, staring at the date and full-moon symbol. And Goodly cautioned:

"But does it mean what we're thinking? Are we going to do it, or is it our old friend El Niño again? Will it result from us attacking the place and burning out a nest, or from a freak of nature, a terrible disaster? I still can't see how it's possible for our quarry to exist up there."

And Jake said, "Neither could the locator see how a vampire could live out on the ocean. And maybe I'm stupid, or a lot less bright than you people, but *I* can't see there being a fire up at Xanadu without our being the cause. Surely the first thing we do if Xanadu isn't what we're looking for is to warn whoever's responsible about the fire. *And* we'll be able to tell him when, so there'll be no loss of life."

The precog shook his head. "You're not at all stupid, Jake. In the dark it's always the blind who see best. But believe me, you don't understand the future. *I* don't understand the future! And I say again: it's not knowing what will happen that counts, but *how* it's going to happen. The only sure thing is, once it's foreseen, it *will* happen. As for loss of life: I did hear that voice calling, 'To me! To me!' "

"Rescuers?" said Liz.

"Or one of us, pulling the teams out," said Trask. "Didn't you recognize the voice?"

Goodly shook his head. "Not over the roaring of the flames, the shattering of glass."

"Glass?" said Jake. "Did I miss something, or is that something you didn't mention before?"

"I just this minute remembered it!" said the precog.

"There was plenty of glass in that topmost dome," Jake said, "In the pleasure dome itself. Black glass, from the look of it, covering everything but the windows."

"No," said the precog. "Not black glass but solar panels— a sort of glass, I suppose. The upper dome was covered in them: a very startling effect. But the windows themselves, they were glass, certainly, and they circled all three lower floors."

Trask was looking at the colour brochure. "You think that the casino's going to burn?"

But Goodly could only shrug his defeat. "It's all speculation. Don't ask me what I think. I still don't know for sure if the fire was in the past or the future. And I'm damned if I can see how any kind of vampire could live up there!"

"But I can," said Jake, watching Harvey searching for Xanadu, and finally putting that area of the Macpherson Range onto the screen. And as before Jake was suddenly the centre of attention. "It was something Lardis said that got me thinking about it," he explained.

"Me?" said Lardis, looking surprised.

"When you said, 'Now wouldn't this make a wonderful aerie, without all this sunlight, of course.'"

"That's right," said Lardis. "I said that."

"Look at the map," Jake told them. "That dog-leg fold and the false plateau sitting in the middle. The mountains are much higher, and steep-sided. The fold goes north to south, and then backtracks. Certainly Xanadu gets plenty of sunlight, from, say nine-thirty A.M. to four-thirty in the evening. But the rest of the time it's in the shade, and during the night the darkness must be utter—except for electric lighting, of course."

"Artificial lighting can't harm them," said Trask. "Szwart doesn't like it but it can't kill him. Only natural light, sunlight itself, can do that."

"Not quite true," Lardis barked. "The Dweller, Harry Hell-lander's son, used artif—er, arti*ficial* light, yes, in the form of ultra, er, ultra*violet* lamps, when he battled the Wamphyri in his garden in the mountains west of Starside."

"But that's sunlight, Lardis," Trask told him. "Artificial, I'll grant you, but sunlight nevertheless." And to Jake: "Maybe you're right. For sixteen or more hours a day, the sun isn't in fact shining directly onto that place. When it *is* shining, however, it's doing it *very* brightly."

And Jake answered, "But don't they sleep during the day?"

And again Lardis: "In Starside, when the sun's rim came up over the Barrier Mountains, the Lords and Ladies usually ran to their northernmost apartments. There they slept—and even there with drapes at their windows! If they were caught out in the open Sunside of the mountains, as occasionally happened, then they must find caves or deep holes in the earth till nightfall."

Jake nodded, and said to Trask, "So, do you think there are no 'deep holes in the earth' in Xanadu? But that brochure says it all. Fancy fountains, swimming pools, saunas, and gymnasiums. An aerial monorail and a casino. I mean, do you think that all of that stuff is *above* ground? No, a complex like that is like an iceberg: you only see its tip. All the cellars and conduits; the pipelines, tunnels, sewerage, and water systems; the reservoirs, pump-, boiler-, and storage-rooms; refrigerators—they're all underground—or rather, they're on the old bed of the plateau, while the resort has been built above them. That's why the place looks so clean and uncluttered."

Trask blinked, shook his head as if to clear it, and said, "Do you know, I believe you could be right? This creature we're looking for could be right there in or under Xanadu!" He tossed the brochure onto the table. "A place like that, where we would least expect to find him!" Then once more he said, "Three days, and we have a lot to do . . . not least to prove our point, clear the way before we can take any real action."

"Prove our point?" Liz looked at him.

"Make sure we're on the right track," Trask nodded. "So we can be certain when we go in that what we want is there. And as for clearing the way: well, the Gibson Desert job was one thing but Xanadu is quite another. All of those people; we'll have to find a way to get them out of there before we go in—and without arousing anyone's suspicion." Then, offering another curt nod: "Right, so let's get to it. This night is still young, but there may be only three of them left."

Heading for a door leading to an outer room where the SAS commanders were poring over their maps, Trask's heart was a little lighter; for now at least he had something to tell them. But before leaving, he turned and said, "Ian, David, Liz—and you, too, Jake—I'm very grateful. You've all worked well, despite initial doubts. But today was only your first time out and you're not finished yet. I want you all back in those Skytours choppers again tomorrow. So, maybe we have struck it lucky this first time, but who knows what else could be hiding out there?" Then he looked at his technicians: the gnomish Harvey and the gangling Paul Arenson.

"But there are more skills than this freaky stuff that we espers use—or that use us, whichever," he said. "Our ghost-talents may serve us well, but without your gadgets for backup they wouldn't be nearly as effective. So well done, all of you. And now get your thinking-caps on and try to look ahead. Jimmy: dig up some plans of Xanadu, its sub-surface systems, et cetera. Ian: please draft a comprehensive record of this meeting. Paul: it's late now, but first thing tomorrow ensure I have access to Prime Minister Black-more's office so that I can organize a liaison with someone on this marine park thing."

Turning away, he offered one of his rare smiles and said, "And that, I think, is that. Now I have to speak to our Australian friends. I'll see you all in the morning. . . ."

The next day, a Saturday, they split the teams up. Lardis, Jake, and Liz were together on the northern routes (Trask didn't want Liz anywhere near Xanadu); Goodly and Chung flew south, each of them hoping to complement the other's strange talent.

The trips were mainly uneventful; the precog's mind was a frustrating blank—at least where the future was concerned—and the locator dared not get too close to Xanadu in case someone, or thing, should locate him. But in any case and as per Trask's orders, they were looking at different mountains this time out.

As for Trask himself: he had a very satisfying day, and when the teams returned to the safe house he was waiting to speak to them. This time he brought the SAS in on it—at least for the first stage of his briefing. For while it wasn't his intention to explain his findings in their entirety (the way E-Branch had used its combined paranormal talents to discover their targets), still, he did have to display those targets, and advise these people as best possible on what they would be up against.

This was done with the aid of the wall screen; Trask supplied the narrative:

"This island in the Capricorn Group—its grid reference is shown alongside—is our secondary target. Now, I've called it an island, but in fact it's little more than a rock or coral reef. It has a few trees, some other tough vegetation; nothing much to mention. It was a marine park conservation station some years ago, but that moved to Heron Island forty miles away. All that's there now is the reef, a shallow lagoon, a private villa on the island, and, we presume, our enemies. But I have to emphasize that they are *probably* lesser enemies, which is to say we don't think they're of the order of unpleasantness that we were obliged to deal with in the Gibson Desert. However, and having said that, you should remember that they will be vampires.

"How many of them? No more than five or six, which is six too many. But with a chopper, a hired vessel, and half a dozen or so of your men—along with Jake Cutter here and Lardis Lidesci from our side—that should be sufficient. You, which is to say the military, will have command; but you'll listen very carefully to Lardis, and you'll take his advice in the . . . the *handling* of whatever you find on that island. Take my word for it, Lardis is the foremost authority in these matters.

"Very well, what can you expect to find in the villa? The master of the house for one, a man of some fifty-eight years of age. Easy? But he'll be a vampire, and as strong as any four or five of your men! Then there'll be his married daughter and her husband, also his son and possibly a woman friend. The worst of them will be a fourth man, not family, who we think will be acting in the role of their keeper. And *he* will be dangerous, much more so than the others.

"Now, the problem is this: some if not all of these people will look and act perfectly normal. A bit edgy, perhaps. But if you were to strand your boat on the beach there, they'd probably help out; they might even call the coastguard for assistance. That's because they want to appear normal, because they *daren't* be discovered for what they really are—not until their master decides they're no longer of any use to him, or her. So, assuming it's a 'him' for the time being, what use *are* they to him?

"Well, for one, the island is a bolthole: it's a place for the Vampire Lord to hide in the event he gets driven out of his aerie. So in fact it's much similar to the Old Mine gas station in the desert. You must plan to take it out accordingly and, if necessary, in exactly the same way. With an air strike, yes, if it comes down to that—though of course we'd vastly prefer the kind of hit at which you people so excel: seek and destroy, and as quickly and quietly as possible.

"And that's about it, all you need to know about this secondary target for the time being. But I would like to take this opportunity to remind you: you *won't* be taking any prisoners.

"Which leads me to your main target. Xanadu, the so-called 'health and pleasure resort' high in the Macphersons. And so it *is* a resort, but only as a front for the ugly Thing that's runing the show.

"And here's another problem: this time we don't know—we have no idea—how many people he's vampirized. The only thing we can say for sure is that when they know they're being hit, then they'll protect their master with all that's left of their miserable lives.

"Oh yes, and one other thing. When the Wamphyri came into our world, they brought thralls or 'lieutenants' with them. Now an original lieutenant out of Starside is a very dangerous creature, much more so than our old friend Bruce Trennier, and you know what he was like. So I'm just reminding you, it's possible that one of these things is up there, too."

The map on the big wall screen had changed. Trask pointed to it again, said, "Here's Xanadu; you know where it is, for of course you've all flown over it and seen it for yourselves. And anyway the bloody place is signposted! A resort, as we've seen. The perfect cover, yes. Which also

426

makes it difficult for us to deal with the creature or creatures that we'll find there. Why? Because this time the master vampire is hiding in a crowd!

"That's my next job: finding a way to get the people—I mean the *ordinary* people—out of there before Monday night.

"And so, gentlemen, that's it for now. Now you can go work out your harbour areas, decide where you'll locate your men and vehicles as they start to come in. The one good thing about it: they won't have much spare time on their hands, won't lose their edge or get bored. They'll no sooner be in situ than they'll be in a firefight. And I think I can promise you that where Xanadu is concerned, that last is guaranteed. Take it as a foregone—or at least a foreseen—conclusion."

The SAS commanders left the ops room, and Trask was alone with his own people.

"So as you can see," he said. "The techs and I have had a busy day. But fruitful? Judge for yourselves."

He gave Jimmy Harvey the nod, and the big wall screen displayed the group of islets again. And Trask continued:

"This island in the Capricorn Group—it's such a rock it doesn't even have a name—is the home of wealthy philanthropist, Jethro Manchester. Like many another rich do-gooder before him, he's something of a recluse. Five years ago, in return for his patronage and a whole lot of money, the Barrier Reef's Marine Park Commission gave him the island to live on. He owns it, or as good as. But that's not all he owns. . . ."

Trask paused and glanced at Harvey, whose fingers tapped at his keyboard. And now the big wall screen was divided centrally between the islands and a map of the dog-leg fold in the Machpherson Range. Trask glanced at the screen and nodded his curt nod. "Hands up who knows what I'm talking about."

And Liz said, "He owns Xanadu, too?"

Trask looked at her. "Used to," he said. "But now he has a partner. Two years ago Manchester signed documents that

427

transferred fifty percent of Xanadu to one Aristotle Milan, an alleged 'shipping magnate' of mixed Greek and Italian descent. We might perhaps assume—or rather, I believe we're *supposed* to assume—that his surname derives from the city of his origins in the old Italian fashion. But I don't think so. The coincidence is just too great, not to mention the rest of the story.

. "First: there is no record of any Aristotle Milan as being the owner of *any* ships! Ergo: the man isn't a tycoon—though I can easily understand how the *idea* of being one would appeal to such as him—and as for his name—"

"Not *Milan* but *Malin*," Jake came in. "Instead of using *ari* as a suffix, to denote 'son of,' he's using it as a prefix, denoting 'first of.' Meaning that on this world, he's the first or highest of his kind. And so for Aristotle Milan, read Malin-ari. Malinari the Mind!"

"Exactly," said Trask. "What's in a name, eh? So, how did Malinari make his connection with Jethro Manchester? Ah, well, here's another name for you: Martin Trennier. Bruce Trennier's brother, a marine biologist employed by the Marine Park Commission until Manchester—our philanthropist, conservationist, recluse, and latter-day Jacques Cousteau—stole him away from them to be his very well-paid odd-jobs man, skin-diving companion, and general dog's-body. This happened about the same time that Manchester and his family got away from it all and retired to the island. Bruce Trennier would have known all of this when Malinari vampirized him at the Romanian Refuge, the said knowledge going secondhand to The Mind himself. Which leaves us with the same question we've all worried about before: What else did Malinari learn on that . . . on that terrible night?"

Trask's face was grey now, and all of his people knew why: that his concern wasn't alone for Zek—who was gone now—but also for them. For Zek Föener had known as much as anyone about E-Branch and its workings.

And Malinari?

Ian Goodly determined to change the subject, take Trask's mind away from it. "What if we're wrong and it's all coin-

428

cidental, circumstantial? This pseudonymous names business, our various hunches and observations, and everything else we've come up with?"

"A hell of a lot of coincidences, I'd say!" Trask frowned at him.

"But what if?"

Trask shuffled notes he'd made earlier, and said, "Well, there is one more thing. In Xanadu, the pleasure dome or casino has a smaller, uppermost dome like a blister on top of the main structure. It sits on a spindle and revolves like certain fancy restaurants on their high towers. But in the nine months since Mr. Milan moved in half of its windows have been painted black, both inside and out. Oh, and incidentally, the dome's rotation was originally designed to track the sun, letting in the light that the higher solar-panelled surfaces necessarily exclude. So it would appear that our Mr. Milan has an aversion to strong sunlight." Pausing, Trask looked at Goodly.

The precog was quiet now, saying nothing, but his alleged "concerns" hadn't fooled Trask one bit. For in its way Goodly's subterfuge had been a lie, a diversion to take Trask's mind off his lost Zek and get it back on track, and of course Trask knew it. A lie, yes, but a white one. And:

"So thanks, anyway," he finally continued, looking directly into the precog's eyes, "but I think we can safely conclude that here . . ." he pointed a steady, resolute finger at the locations displayed on the wall screen, ". . . that here be vampires!"

When no one had anything further to say, Trask finished up with: "Very well, and now we have plans to make."

Later that evening, Jake was sitting on a bench in the cool of the garden, lost in his own strange, meditative thoughts, when Lardis found him and sat down beside him. After he had sniffed at the air for a while, the old man said, "Carypsu?"

Oddly enough, Jake understood. "Eucalyptus?" he answered. "It's a tree, growing outside the wall."

"Yes," Lardis nodded. "Carypsu. We have them on Sunside." And, after a moment or two's thought: "May I ask a question?"

"What's on your mind?" said Jake.

At which Lardis smiled. "But I might ask you the selfsame thing! What's on, or what's in, *your* mind?"

Jake frowned. "Some kind of word game?"

"No," Lardis shook his head. "No word game. But I have to admit, I'm curious."

"About what?"

"About you. About how you knew that in Starside in the old days a Lord of the Wamphyri might occasionally add ari to his father's name, denoting that he was his father's son."

"You mean like Lord Malin was Malinari's father?"

"Indeed. And now that you mention it . . . how you knew *that*, too?"

Jake frowned again, deeper this time. But then he relaxed, and shrugged. "You must have told me," he said. "Or maybe I've read of it somewhere. In Ben Trask's files, perhaps?" But:

"No," Lardis shook his head, smiling in that knowing way of his. "No, I haven't told you. I've had no reason to mention it to anyone. And as far as I know it isn't written anywhere."

Then, creaking to his feet, the old man yawned and said, "Well, goodnight, Jake. And pleasant dreams. . . ."

29
A Dream and A Word-Game

BUT IN FACT JAKE'S DREAMS WERE ANYTHING but pleasant. . . .

It wasn't so much what had happened, though that was bad enough, but that he had been made to watch it happening. More than anything else, that was what had preyed on his mind . . . until he'd made it up to put things right. Perhaps he'd hoped that by killing the cause he might kill the memories, too.

But such a lot of memories, burning like acid in his head, until he'd thought they would burn his brain out.

Memories, yes.

That fat, pallid, slimy-looking bastard—the second one of these pigs that Jake had got back at—the way he had taken Natasha in the classical or orthodox position, but scarcely an act of love. Rape, yes, and his long, slender grey dick in her rectum according to his taste.

Memories, those God-awful memories . . .

They'd piled pillows under her, raising her hips, and two of the others had held her legs under her knees, to allow this fat slug standing at the side of the bed to get into her. That had made it easy for him, because unconscious as she was— or between bouts of conscio:ness and unconsciousness— she'd been likely to flop and eject him. But holding her like that, Natasha had been a lot more accessible; accessible to viewing, too, for Jake had been tied to a chair where he could see all of the action. Of course, he could have closed his eyes, and from time to time he did just that, but he could still hear it even if he couldn't see it.

That grunting pig! His dick like a long finger poking into her, in and out with the heaving and clenching of his fat backside. And this sweaty, grunting, slug-like slob—this giggling queer—oh, it was obvious why he liked it like this. With any normal woman in any natural act of intercourse he'd be lucky if that pencil penis of his touched the sides. But this way . . . at least he would get some satisfaction, however minimal. At least he would know he'd had it into something.

And Jake had to watch, he had to, because long before that too-long night was over he'd known that if it was the very last thing he did he would avenge her.

But the worst thing was when it was over, and the fat bastard zipped his fly and waddled over to Jake, saying, "A shame she wasn't awake, eh, English? It would have been so sweet to know she'd felt that last big bang, and to feel

*her guts spasm as I greased her dirt chute! Ah well, there's
time yet. Oh, ha, ha, ha!"*

*He had a strong German accent, and when he laughed he
put his face close enough to Jake's to cause him to recoil
from the stench of cigar smoke and* senf, *hot German mus-
tard. . . .*

But Jake didn't even know the pig's name—didn't know
any of their names—except Castellano's and Jean Daniel's.

Well, Jean Daniel was dead now, of an unequal argument
between his soft guts and the alloy core of a plastique-
propelled steering column.

And the fat faggot had been number two. . . .

Jake had known the route the fat man took from Castellano's
place on the northern outskirts of Marseille to a gay bar on
the Rue de Carpiagne which he visited regularly on Friday
nights. He knew, too, that the fat swine was a little shy to
admit openly of his predilections (that it didn't sit too well
with him that he was both a hoodlum *and* a pervert), which
was why he invariably approached *Le Jockey Club* down a
narrow side street.

It was raining on the night in question, and Jake had
parked his car so as to block off one side of the rain-slick,
cobbled alley on the fat man's approach route. The other side
was liberally sprinkled with inch-and-a-half spikes which
Jake had laid down with malice aforethought and in great
deliberation.

Jake was waiting in a recessed doorway when the fat
man's fat tyres blew, and he was quickly into the alley as
the expensive Fiat slewed to a halt and its cursing driver
slammed open his door, got out, and creased his belly as he
bent to hear the front nearside's last gasp. A moment more
and Jake was standing over him.

The fat man was suddenly aware of him; he had time to
say, *"Uh? Bitte? Was ist?"* before Jake sapped him behind
the ear. . . .

*   *   *

In a deserted copse on a wooded hillside over the motorway near St. Antoine, Jake wafted a small bottle of smelling salts under his victim's nose until he twitched, moaned, and came out of it with a series of useless, spastic jerks. Useless because he was tied up—literally tied *up*—and spastic because he was tied by his ankles and wrists, so that all he could do was shake and shiver like a great, globular white spider in its web.

Jake had woken him up because in his position, upside down, the fat Kraut might easily die without ever regaining consciousness of his own accord. And that was the last thing Jake wanted . . . that he should die easily.

The man's legs were spread wide; at a height of about seven feet, his ankles were roped to a pair of springy saplings which were just strong enough to hold him in position. His wrists were likewise tied to the bases of the twin trees, which formed his body into a fat, totally naked X. He was gagged with his own underpants, tied off at the back of his neck, and the rest of his clothing lay in a neat pile close by.

At first the fat man struggled a little, but since that was pointless he quickly gave up and hung still, watching Jake pour a hip flask of fiery Asbach Uralt brandy over his heaped clothing.

"A waste of good German liquor, eh?" Jake said. "But that's not the only German *thing* I'll be wasting tonight." Then, stepping closer: "You don't remember me, do you?"

The fat white spider had begun to shake its web again, however hopelessly, but now it paused to say, *"Umph? Uh-umph?"*

"But I'll bet you remember the girl. That night at Castellano's place? The Russian girl, Natasha?" Hearing that name, and finally recognizing his tormentor, the fat man commenced yanking on his ropes with a vengeance, his eyes blinking rapidly in a face as round as the moon, all bloated with pooling blood.

"Oh, sure, you remember her," Jake said, as he got to work.

Though it had stopped raining, he was still wearing a light-

weight raincoat. From one side pocket he took out a small
paper parcel, and from the other several indeterminate items.
The fat man, being inverted, couldn't make out what they
were; but perhaps he recognized a certain marzipan smell
when Jake unwrapped the stained paper parcel and weighed
a blob of grey, dough-like stuff in his hand. At any rate he
began shaking the trees furiously, and did a lot more serious
umph-umphing.

But Jake wasn't listening; he wasn't the least bit interested
in his victim's complaints. Stretching a pair of thin surgical
gloves onto his hands, he stepped closer and began molding
plastic explosive into the fat man's anal cavity. And:

"I might have expected it," he said, finishing the job as
quickly as possible, "that a fat, ugly *thing* like you would
have a hole like a horse's collar. You've done your fair share
of time in the barrel, right? But this time—I mean this *last*
time—it's a little different, eh?"

He showed the fat man a small brass cylinder the size of
a pencil-slim torch battery with copper wires protruding from
one end, said, "Detonator," and rammed it home. And con-
necting the wires to a miniature timer, he said, "Which gives
you maybe, oh, fifty seconds? As of right . . . now!" And he
pressed a tiny button.

Then, in no special hurry, he stepped to the neatly piled
clothing, stooped and applied the flame of his cigarette
lighter. The pile caught with a small *whoosh!* and blue flames
flickered on the hillside.

And starting to count, "Five, six, seven . . ." Jake set off
through the damp undergrowth, down the uneven, wooded
slope to where his car was parked on a rutted farm track.

"Twenty, twenty-one, twenty-two . . ." He looked back up
the slope. Thirty or thirty-five yards away, the fat white
spider-thing vibrated in its web, looking luminous in the
darkness of the wooded hillside. And Jake—who had fairly
danced down the slope, his face fixed in a mad grin as he
counted off the seconds through clenched teeth—suddenly
Jake felt nauseated.

But at a count of thirty-two he realized he was probably

too close and couldn't afford to be sick. It had been his intention to stand there and shout back up the slope, remind that poor fat sod of what he'd said that night: something about Natasha feeling the last big bang? And her guts going into spasm? But there wasn't enough time left—and maybe not enough hatred left—for any of that now. Or could it be simply that he didn't want his car covered with . . . with whatever?

Feeling his gorge rising, but still counting, he started up the car and nosed off down the track. "Thirty-eight, thirty-nine, forty . . ." And when he was on the level, heading for the motorway, he applied the brakes and looked back—felt obliged to look back—like the night when he had looked without wanting to at something else. Looked back because this was what he thought was needed to burn that memory out of him.

"Forty-six, forty-seven, forty—" But that was as far as he got. Obviously he'd been counting just a little too slowly.

Jake saw the ball of fire leap up and out from the trees on the hillside, pictured in his mind's eye a hideous rending, and then heard the bang. The only mercy was that the fat queer himself couldn't possibly have heard it, and there had been no time at all for a spasm. . . .

Then for a time Jake just sat there in his car, until the sweat began to turn cold on him. But damn it to hell, the horror and the hatred were already creeping back, sated for a while but by no means done with. And Jake knew that they always would be there, until he tracked down the rest of those bastards and finished what they had started.

He gave himself a shake, put the car back in gear, and made for the motorway. But—

—something was obscuring his interior mirror, something that had got itself stuck to the rear window.

Something round, that once was fat but now was flat, dripping scarlet from its ripped rim. And its eyes hanging out, and its mouth still stuffed with its own underpants!

A face. But just *a face!*

Jesus God!
Jesus—

"—God!"

Jake came awake with a small cry and a massive start, the sweat still dripping, and that mask of a face still printed on the darkness but fading as he realized it was only that awful nightmare again—and that while the rest of it was all too horrifyingly real, the last part had never happened *except* in the dream. It always happened in the dream. Every time.

But then, while he sat there trembling, his heart hammering in his chest, utterly alone in the darkness of his cubicle, someone very close quite clearly said:

Ahhhhh! What stuff you are made of, Jake! And what a host you would make! But together *we'll make a very fine pair, you and I . . . .*

Jake recognized the voice at once—only this time he was awake, had been shocked awake—and the knowledge saw him fumbling for his bedside light switch with rubbery fingers as the damp short hairs at the back of his neck stiffened into spikes.

But as the light came on so that evil, chuckling deadspeak voice was already receding, was being *driven* away. Because acting instinctively—almost without knowing he had done it, and certainly without knowing how—Jake had erected mental shields against intruders, blocking them from his mind. For as well as Korath Mindsthrall, he had sensed someone else there, and possibly many someones, listening to his thoughts.

Or was it *all* a bad dream? For now that they were gone, he couldn't even be sure that his intruders had ever been there in the first place. And Jake flopped panting, back onto his pillow, wondering if perhaps it had only been a part of his dream after all. One of those dreams that crashes the barrier of consciousness, however momentarily, to cross over into the waking world.

He wondered about it, but was by no means certain. . . .

*   *   *

. . . While just a few feet away, trying desperately hard to keep still· as a mouse, Liz Merrick crouched shivering and shuddering on her bed, in the farthest corner of her cubicle, with a sheet drawn up under her chin. She hung on tightly to that sheet, and even more so to her thoughts (so as to *keep* them to herself, but in any case as far away from Jake as possible), and tried to forget what she had seen. But much like Jake himself that night at Castellano's place, gripped by some kind of morbid fascination, voyeurism of a sort, she'd found herself unable to "look away" . . . until now.

Damn Ben Trask that he had ordered this surveillance! But it wasn't only Trask, for Liz, too, had "had" to know.

Well, and now she knew. She had seen—she'd even "experienced" Jake's passion, his hatred, and the resultant nightmare—and knew how far he would go in his vendetta, and exactly what he was capable of (literally *anything*), in his craving for justice. Or for a kind of justice, at least.

But *such* justice!

On the other hand, perhaps that was why Harry had chosen him: because an eye for an eye had always been the Necroscope's motto. The eye, yes: that most vital and vulnerable part of the body. *An eye for an eye.* Why, the thought itself was horrific! But now, as Liz was witness—and as it had been brought forcefully home·to her—she realized that other parts of the body could be just as vulnerable, and their use or misuse even more horrific. . . .

Jake hadn't thought he would sleep again, but after tossing and turning for an hour—and *listening,* though for what he wasn't quite sure—he did in fact sleep.

And as he relaxed his shields—a natural, necessary relaxation borne of mental fatigue, from listening so intently for an unidentified something—so Korath Mindsthrall was alert and waiting for him. Jake felt the ex-vampire's gradual insinuation like a slimy, creeping mist, or a damp shroud settling over his mind. But at the same time he also sensed something of urgency, a desire to speak, to communicate with him. And if for no other reason than his own curiosity, he allowed it.

"I know you're there," Jake said, as the other's hesitancy, his too-cautious approach began to irritate him. "So why do you hold back? If you've got something to say, get it said."

For answer there came a sensed "sigh" of relief, and: *But I thought that you would shut me out, send me away. I thought you would reject me,* Korath said.

"That didn't stop you the last time," Jake said. "When you spoke to me after my nightmare? You seemed to have enjoyed spying on me, as if you approved of what you had seen, of what I'd done. Or perhaps you got carried away and broke your silence in error, when I wasn't supposed to know you were there?"

I was in fact . . . well, speaking to myself, said the other, defensively. *We might even say that* you *eavesdropped on* me!

"Speaking to yourself?" Jake answered. "Deadspeak? In which case you're as new to it as I am. For a thought is just as good as the spoken word, Korath, to such as you and I."

And to all of the teeming dead, said the other. *Which makes you the odd man out.*

"But as for eavesdropping . . ." Jake continued, "it sometimes has its uses. What was it you said? That together we would make a very fine pair? What exactly did you mean by that? That we're alike in certain ways? No, I don't think so. Or did you perhaps mean that you'd like to team up with me?"

But that is precisely what I meant! Korath answered, just a little too eagerly. *For after all, if you're intent on tracking down and destroying the treacherous Malinari, who could possibly be of greater assistance than one who was as close to him as Korath Mindsthrall?*

"So close that he killed you?" Jake's sarcasm dripped.

Exactly! And I know what you are thinking: that the Necroscope Harry Keogh found it peculiar that The Mind should murder his first lieutenant out of hand, as if it were nothing to him. But it was in fact . . . something.

"He had good reason? Is that what you're saying?"

Well, he thought he had! said Korath. *He was concerned that one day I would usurp him, that I might have the means to usurp him!*

"Yet when Harry questioned you, you said it was just Malinari's nature. You were there to be used, and so he used you."

And so it was his evil nature, which caused him to so use and abuse his right-hand man, aye, Korath answered. *But in addition, there was this other thing. Something of his own making, which he feared would turn on him given time. And it might yet.*

"So why do you mention it to me—this thing, whatever it is—when you withheld it from Harry?"

Because it was my secret, said Korath. *And even a dead man should have something he can call his own—something private?—which might even be of value to the living, and with which he might seek to bargain. Ah, but Harry Keogh is one thing, while you are something else entirely, Jake. And it was never my intention to keep anything secret from you. Not if you require it, and if it should prove . . . useful to you?*

"Something you have," Jake mused, "Which might benefit me, but not Harry. . . ." And in a while, when Korath remained silent: "So what's the difference? Why would you help me and not him?"

The difference? But isn't it obvious? The Necroscope Harry Keogh can do nothing for me. And even if he could, he wouldn't—you have seen that for yourself. He is obstinate: despite that I never harmed him and he never knew me, still he hates me! But the greatest difference is this: that he is dead! While you—

"While I'm alive," said Jake.

And you walk among the living. My only possible instrument of revenge against him who put me here, and the others who have gone out into your world with him, aye.

"And that's all you'd expect out of it? All you'd want for yourself?"

All? But it is everything! said the other. *Through you, I would live again—er, metaphorically, of course. Through you, I would strike back from beyond the grave—or in my case from this dank and dreary pipe, in the bowels of a strange place, in a foreign land far from Starside. What more could I, poor dead thing that I am, ask of you? And what more could you give?*

"What more, indeed," said Jake, who hadn't forgotten Harry Keogh's warning, that even dead vampires are dangerous. And:

Well, and perhaps there is . . . something, said Korath.

"And now we get to it," said Jake.

Hear me out! said the other. *Is it too much to ask that in return for my gift to you, you shall give me your companionship—albeit rarely, however infrequently—when little else intrudes upon your time?*

"A word-game?" said Jake. "Is that what this is? The devious nature of vampires? For here I find myself bargaining—all caught up in it, beginning to go with it—when as yet I don't even know what's on offer!"

Then let me tell you! Korath was eager, barely able to contain himself. But in the next moment he slowed down, paused and said, *And yet . . . how best to explain? Now listen:*

Do you remember I told you, that in our Iceland banishment when food was short and Malinari thirsted, he supped on me? But it was no mere sip! He drank deeply, so deep indeed that I was weakened nigh unto death. Aye, that was how much my master took from me. But in taking, he also gave!

Now, Malinari is special even among the Wamphyri. His bite is virulent; well, so are they all, but his even more so. Under normal conditions a man is recruited, becomes infected, in the space of a single Starside night—or two or three days of your time—following which he is his master's thrall, in thrall to whichever Lord or Lady seduced his blood. But when Malinari bit deep it was a matter of hours! He could turn a man in hours!

It was in his essence, his strong Wamphyri essence. And it was the same with the making.

"The making?" This was a new one on Jake.

The making of creatures, Korath explained. *Monsters! Why, things waxed in the The Mind's vats of metamorphosis in days rather than weeks and months! I have seen flyers flop from their stone wombs in the space of a single day and a night—a Starside day and night, you understand—and even an ugly warrior wax mewling in its vat, its armoured scales hardening to chitin in little more than four sunups. So efficacious is Malinari's essence of metamorphism! And all of his men and creatures alike stamped with something of The Mind himself, imbued of his arts, made in their master's likeness. Do you see?*

"Imbued of his arts?" Jake repeated the other's words, and tried to fathom his meaning. "Are you saying you got Malinari's skills?"

Something of them, aye, said Korath. And, after a moment's pause:

And you will also recall the reason why my master found it so easy to talk to me: because as you have inherited the Necroscope Harry Keogh's mind-shields, so I had inherited my bestial father's. Malinari found little to fault in my thinking because I was able to keep him out. Which suited both our purposes: The Mind's because while by nature he's suspicious, still he needed a strong first lieutenant; mine because even the most loyal and obedient of thralls may on occasion harbour this or that small grievance against his master....

"Or, on occasion, a not-so-small grievance?" said Jake.

He sensed Korath's shrug. *In my case, not so much a grievance as an ambition. That was it: I harboured an ambition, and looked for an opportunity. For that time in the Icelands, Malinari had gone too far. Oh, he had glutted on me ... but what he had given back—albeit involuntarily, for in his hunger he was made careless—would soon be much stronger than what he took! From which time forward I knew that I was different. I felt the germ of a leech growing in me, but daren't disclose it. I could not admit that soon I would be ... Wamphyyyrrriii!*

The pain—the terrible longing—of Korath's cry shocked Jake to his very soul. Like a shovel in cold ashes, or chalk on a new blackboard, it grated on his nerve-endings, set his scalp tingling. And it brought him a new awareness, the certain knowledge that what he was dealing with here was far from a simple, uncomplicated creature. Dead it was, yes, but it hadn't by any means accepted that fact; it resisted death with every fibre of its long-since sloughed-away body, and would cling to life—to any life, to *his* life—with that same tenacity! And:

"I think . . . I think it's time you were out of here!" Jake said, his voice shuddering as the echoes of Korath's cry of anguish did a drum roll in his near-metaphysical mind. "You or me, but one of us has to go."

Aye, go if you will, said the other. *But best that you go bravely to your death, Jake, not whimpering as you whimper now. Go on, face Malinari the Mind, for you may be sure it is him in the mountains! Go against him with nothing but your puny human muscles, nothing but your puling, childlike mind—which even I can enter, as stealthy as a thief in the night. Oh? Oh really? And how do you think you'll fare against such as Malinari, eh? And this woman who you keep in your mind, this Liz of whom you sometimes dream—what, a mentalist, you say? But how unfortunate! For how will she fare against such as him? As for Vavara . . . ah, but she has her ways with pretty women, aye. Vavaaara! Oh, ha ha ha haaaaaaa!*

Korath's deadspeak laugh reverberated into a throbbing silence, but Jake knew that he was there, waiting. And Korath knew that Jake was hooked. To a point, at least. And he was right.

"How can you be sure that it's Malinari in the mountains?" Jake said in a little while. "What can you know of that?"

Ah, no! Too late! the other cried. *I was the fair one and told you a secret. Now you would have more. But what is my get out of all this?*

"But you still haven't told me what you want!" Jake answered. "Not *everything* that you want. And until you do, I'm not going to be signing any blank cheques, Korath."

And because deadspeak conveys more or other than is actually said, because it translates much as telepathy translates, Korath understood him well enough.

You are afraid that I would take advantage? But how may I take advantage? I'm only a dead thing drowned in a pipe! Korath Mindsthrall is no more except he acts through you. Ah, but Jake . . . the acts we can accomplish, and the things I have to offer!

"Such as?"

Everything I know about Malinari, Vavara, Szwart.

"You've already told me those things, both me and the Necroscope, Harry Keogh."

But can you remember them? When you're awake? I think not. For I have crept into your waking mind, too, Jake, and found it blank of all such knowledge, of everything I told you. Now tell me: Who do you suppose it was reminded you of how Malinari came by his name? Did you really think you were so clever as to work it out all by yourself that the name Aristotle Milan was a disguise, a pseudonym?

"But it . . . it was obvious," said Jake, caught momentarily off guard.

As it must also be obvious that I was there with you! Korath pounced. *Else how would I know it ever happened? And when we flew together, you and I, in that aerial machine, that helicopter with its twirling wings: did you once suspect that I was there with you? No, never, not for a moment. But I was. . . .*

Jake was shaken, but he was also Jake. "So you're a sneaky bastard!" he said. "What does that prove—except I can't trust you?"

It proves that I can help you—as I helped you with Malinari's name. And then, grudgingly: *Also, it proves that you are no slouch, no easy adversary, when it comes to word-games. More of the Necroscope's inheritance, I should think.*

And Jake wondered, *could* Korath help him? What harm

could it do to call on the vampire for advice in a tight spot? Surely it wouldn't be that much different from calling on Harry, whose help was uncertain anyway? And these thoughts, too—unguarded as they were—were deadspeak.

Exactly! said Korath. *And at all times I would be on hand to . . . to* advise *you, aye.*

"Not at all times!" said Jake, hearing warning bells. "For when we started this conversation you were happy with 'rarely,' or 'infrequently,' when little else was 'intruding on my time.' So how come you now arrive at being on hand 'at all times?' "

A figure of speech! Korath protested. *I meant whenever you called for me, of course.*

"And how would I do that? I mean, call for you?"

Why, by thinking of me, of my situation down there in that cruel conduit, and by calling for me by name, Korath.

But the dead vampire was getting ahead of himself; believing that he was winning Jake over, his deep "voice" had become semi-hypnotic, more phlegmy, glutinous, and sly than ever. Jake gave himself a shake and "woke up" to that fact.

"What, like rubbing a lamp to call out the genie?" he said. "And what happens when I've had my three wishes, eh?"

He sensed the sad shake of an incorporeal head. *Jake, Jake! Were you always this ungrateful, this misgiving?*

"No," Jake answered. "Not misgiving, not yet. Just cautious. But let's get on. What else is on offer? For after all, you did say 'things,' in the plural."

So, said the other, *esoteric knowledge is not enough. It is too ethereal—too* immundane—*for a clodhopper such as you. You would have something more physical.*

"No small feat," said Jake, feeling stung and retaliating, "for someone as far removed from physical things as you are."

Hurtful! said the other. *Hah! And you accuse* me *of taking advantage! But argument gets us nowhere, while what I'm proposing would be of mutual benefit. Very well, you ask what else is on offer, what other "thing" I have in mind.*

And that is exactly *where it is: in my mind. Now say, do you remember the Necroscope asking you about your numerical skills?*

"In connection with the Möbius Continuum? Yes," said Jake.

So then. And how are your numbers, Jake?

"I'm not innumerate, if that's what you mean."

Odd, said the other, *for I was. In my world, Jake, mathematics went no further than the count of a man's thralls or the beasts in his pens. Numbers? I had no use for them, nor have I even now, though I may have shortly. But in Starside, addition was a recruiting foray into Sunside. And division was what happened to the spoils.*

"What are you getting at?"

We come to it, said Korath. *Do you remember those numbers that the Necroscope showed you before he took his leave of us? And do you know what they were?*

"They were a formula," Jake answered. "They were the numbers that govern all space and time, Harry's gateway to the Möbius Continuum. But do I remember them?"

He thought back on it:

That incredible wall of numbers—like a computer screen run riot, evolving in the eye of his mind—its symbols, calculi, and incredible equations marching and mutating until they achieved some sort of numerical critical mass . . . and formed a door. A Möbius door.

Remember it? He would never forget it! It was like watching creation itself. But duplicate it?

No, you can't, said Korath. *But I can! I can make it, but I can't use it. Not without you. And you can't make it without me. And there you have my offer. . . .*

"Tempting, if it were true," said Jake.

It is.

"But how? You said yourself that numbers were practically unknown in your world."

Just so. But didn't I also say that Malinari's essence is strong in my blood?

And now Jake understood. "His photographic memory?

That's what you got from him! And it's why he killed you, because one day you might know as much as him."

Now you have it all, Korath said, *and I await your answer. What's it to be? Can we work together, for Malinari's downfall?*

"But there's something else." Still Jake was cagey.

And Korath sighed his frustration. *What now?*

"The secret that Harry Keogh was searching for, or in your own words 'the crux of the matter,' which is probably more important than all the rest put together. The Wamphyri—Malinari and the others—have been here for some time now, but it seems they've achieved very little. So like the Necroscope before me I'm asking you: what are they up to, Korath? What's their plan? You were one of theirs and so you must know."

Oh, I do, I do. But as you have repeated the Necroscope's words, now I shall repeat mine. That is for me to know, and for you and yours to discover—through me. It is my only remaining bargaining point, the last trick up a poor dead thing's sleeve. And before I give you that, we must be far, far better acquainted, you and I. That said, I can tell you this: there isn't too much time left, and what they have started will run its course. Unless it is stopped. Before you can stop it, however, you must know what it is.

Jake pondered that a while, then said, "I'll have to think it over. All of it."

But try not to take too long over it, said the other. *Your world hangs by a thread, and the thread is unwinding.*

"I'll keep that in mind," said Jake. "But for now leave me be. There's something I must do before I awake, or all this has been for nothing."

So be it, said the other without further comment. And Jake sensed his departure like a waft of fresh air, the way the shadows crept back from his mind.

Then, experimenting—making sure that Korath was gone—he attempted to close his mind to deadspeak and turned to telepathy instead:

"Liz, if you are there, and I think you probably are, try to remember this name: Korath. If it's possible, you might even write it down. But in any case remember it, and tomorrow remind me of it. It could be very important."

That done, Jake relaxed and let himself drift free on the tides of his own subconscious mind.

And in a little while he felt himself buoyed up, taken by far less ominous dreams, the disjointed, meaningless flotsam of his waking hours. . . .

30
The Lull . . .

SUNDAY WAS A BUSY YET PARADOXICALLY quiet time; work was being done, but in a kind of vacuum chamber. People moved about with purpose within an oddly surreal atmosphere of near silence. It was, Jake thought, a sensation similar to being on an airplane during its descent, in the moments before your ears pressurize, when sounds are flat and distant and you feel as though you've suddenly gone deaf. In short, it was the lull before the storm, when the hatches are battened down, and Jake (who seemed to be the only one with no hatches to batten) felt completely out of it. Apart from an O-group he'd been scheduled to attend in the evening, he had nothing to do.

Which was as well, for he didn't think he would be able to concentrate on anything much; there was something on his mind, in the back of his head, desperately trying to push its way to the forefront. It had to do with last night—something lingering over from his dreams, perhaps?—but apart from that he was at a loss.

Jake remembered his nightmare, of course. He *always* remembered that. It was a recurrent thing (a thing of conscience, he supposed) that came back to haunt him maybe two or three times a month. It had used to be far more frequent, but time is merciful and was doing its job. This thing in the back of his mind, however, was other than that; he found himself *listening* for an unknown something, and at the same time dreading it. So much so that he was shielding his mind to shut things out, and doing it consciously, holding at bay those whispering voices of which he was becoming ever more frequently aware . . . which might perhaps explain something of the eerie atmosphere: he was in fact isolating himself. And also from the living.

It was a shuddersome thought, and deadspeak was a terrible thing. Jake found himself wondering if perhaps that was it: Was it Harry he was listening for? Harry Keogh and the Great Majority? Was his neurosis growing, spreading out of control? Or was it something else, not fear at all but the simple need for privacy? Some kind of persecution complex, with Liz Merrick—his "partner"—taking on the role of the Inquisition, or of a spy at the very least? But in any case, she was giving him the cold shoulder this morning. Odd, because he also felt that there was something she might want to tell him.

Jake wandered about the safe house, through the ops room and other rooms, trying to interest himself in something—in anything—that was going on around him, and feeling more and more the outsider . . . at least until Lardis Lidesci joined him and Jake saw that he was in the same boat.

Jake really felt for Lardis, because he was a *genuine* outsider, not even of this world! On one occasion when they spoke to each other, the old man told him: "Don't fret so! We're men of action, you and I. That's all it is. But we'll get to it, never fear." Unlike Jake, however, the Old Lidesci made no complaint. Instead he prowled the safe house in tandem with the younger man, and kept his feelings to himself. . . .

The long hours passed slowly; hours of tactical and logistical planning and correlation, concentrated poring over maps, and the making of battle-plans in general. The techs were feeding questions to the computers, and supplying Trask and his SAS commanders with the answers; apart from catching the occasional break, they would probably still be working well into the eleventh hour. Surface plans of Xanadu—together with schematics of the resort's subsurface labyrinth—littered tables in the central ops room. Detailed diagrams, ordnance survey maps, and aerial photographs of Jethro Manchester's island in the Capricorn Group were scattered over the floor of a room with tightly drawn curtains.

Warrant Officer Class Two Joe Davis was on a radio in the ops room, logging in the task force's vehicles as they arrived in groups or as individuals across the mountains and down onto the coastal strip. They had kept radio silence until now; *even* now they voiced only their call signs—and then just the once—received coded grid-references of their destinations, verified their receipt, and disappeared again into the aether. Soon they would be arriving at the designated operational locations, in which they would maintain low profiles and wait for orders. The big articulated ops truck wouldn't be in until the dead of night or early morning. But everyone would be, and *must* be, in situ by midday tomorrow, Monday, the night of the full moon. . . .

By six in the evening Ben Trask was about ready to start pulling his hair out over his main problem with Xanadu. It was the one thing he couldn't request help on from higher authority (indeed, it was the one thing he dared not even *mention* to higher authority): how to evacuate the "civilians" from the resort before attacking the place. For Ian Goodly had forecast blood and thunder in Xanadu, and whether or not this was an accurate prediction or some scene from the past that the precog had somehow witnessed, Trask wasn't about to risk having his operation compromised, delayed, or possibly even shut down by the objections and vacillations of jittery political powers.

It was nerve-wracking; for from Trask's own point of view, and while it had been one thing to personally authorize, coordinate, and take part in a firefight in the badlands of the Gibson Desert, setting fire to Xanadu would be something else entirely. And since he didn't have time to argue the toss with the powers that be, it meant that should anything go wrong tomorrow night, he would be the one to carry the can.

Trask was desperately in need of a plan of evacuation, and it would have to be one that wouldn't alert Nephran Malinari to E-Branch's or any other enemy's hand in things. But with little more than twenty-four hours to go, no such plan seemed likely.

Then came the televised evening news report—of the first cases of Asiatic plague showing up in Brisbane and half-a-dozen other Australian ports—and with it the germ of an idea and a possible reprieve. It was Liz Merrick who heard the report, formulated the idea, and brought it to Trask's attention. At first he was doubtful; the notion seemed too devisive, contrived, too Hollywood . . . but it was the sort of idea that can grow on you. And as it grew on Trask, so he got to work on it.

For after all, it was all that he *had* to work on. . . .

Later, in the early hours of the night, when it was cooler and Liz went outdoors for a breath of fresh air, Jake took the opportunity to corner her and have a word in private.

"You've been avoiding me all day," he said. "Sort of peculiar behaviour for a partner, partner. Or is it wearing off?"

Seated together on a bench, they were close but not touching. Liz gave him a wary look, and said. "Umm? Wearing off?"

"I thought we had something special going," Jake said. "Er, business-wise, that is. I mean, psychically if not physically."

She smiled (a little ruefully, he thought) and said, "Perhaps physically, too, under different circumstances. So don't underestimate yourself, Jake Cutter. But you're carrying a lot of baggage around with you, and the extra weight is taking too much of a toll on you. You haven't been the most sociable type, you know? And even if you were, this isn't the best of times."

"Which disposes of physically," he said. "But there's still psychically to consider. I thought you were interested in that side of me, too—or should that be 'at least?' " With which he felt her shy away from him, as her expression became a lot more serious. But then she gave a shrug, and said:

"Out in the desert, that first job of ours was like an initiation, a baptism by fire—for both of us. As we were working together and it was part of our job, it seemed only fitting and sensible that we develop something of a rapport. But—"

"Which we did," he cut her off. "So, is that finished now?"

"—But," Liz went on, "for this thing tomorrow night we've been split up, and since we're not going to be working together there seemed little point in us, well, *working* together! I·mean, with this twin operation about to go down, Xanadu and the Capricorn Group island thing together, letting anything else get in the way would have been too much of a distraction. So I haven't been trying to avoid you, Jake. It's simply that we've all been very busy."

"*You* have all been busy!" said Jake, moodily. And abruptly: "I'm not . . . not having a good time of this."

"Of this conversation?"

"And of everything else," he answered. Then shook his head and said, "*Christ!* Do I come off sounding like a crybaby?"

And suddenly Liz found herself melting. It was the first time that Jake had shown any open wounds—in his waking hours, anyway—and here she was pouring salt in them with her deliberately detached, overly cool attitude. And so:

"What *is* the problem, Jake?" she said.

With which he felt that oh-so-tender telepathic aura probing in his direction, and immediately raised his shields.

She knew it, drew back from him, said, "Is that what it's about? But I can't help what I am, Jake If someone close to me is hurting, surely it's only natural that I should want to know why? And anyway, isn't it a contradiction? *You* were the one who brought up our telepathic rapport, this special 'thing' that we have going! But you can't expect anyone to be close to you, concerned for you on the one hand, while deliberately pushing them away on the other. You're shielding yourself—and from contact with me, Jake!"

He nodded, and said, "And if contact—I suppose we can call it that for now, instead of 'spying'—if contact gets to be a habit, what then? Look, Liz, last night I had a bloody awful nightmare, a piece of the extra luggage you were talking about, that's the result of something I've done. It was an act of vengeance, but a very terrible act. You say it's only natural you should want to know what's hurting, but please believe me, you really *don't* want to know about something like that!"

At which she scarcely managed to keep from biting her lip. For she already knew about that—all about it. But before she could say anything and perhaps give herself away, Jake went on: "I think . . . I *thought,* that maybe you were there with me, that you had seen, and that was why you were avoiding me."

"No," Liz shook her head. "I wasn't, I didn't, it isn't."

And she thought: *Damn you, Ben Trask! I know it's your job, but this is killing me!* And at the same time she knew how fortunate she was that it wasn't Trask himself she was talking to!

But even so (she tried to qualify her deceit), what she had told Jake was only a half-lie, or at worst a white one. For the real reason she had been avoiding him was because she knew that sooner or later she must remind him of that name, Korath.

It would be the right and proper thing to do after all, for with all the emphasis that Jake had placed on it, it might well be important to everyone. But now she had gone and complicated matters, making herself an even bigger liar. For as soon as she mentioned that name to Jake and he remembered it, he would know that she really had been there after all, sneaking in his mind, like a thief!

Right there and then she might have done it, blurted it out and accepted the consequences . . . except at that precise moment Ben Trask appeared in the door to the house, calling, "Liz? And is that you, Jake? O-group time. Come and get your orders."

Heading for the house, suddenly Liz found herself hating

it all. But especially hating her weird talent, her telepathy. And more clearly than ever she understood why most E-Branch espers thought of their skills as curses. Again and again her condemnation of herself rang in her mind, but she heard it as an accusation, as if spoken by Jake:

"Sneaking in my mind like a thief!"—*like a thief!—like a thief!*

And she hated it, yes. For the fact of the matter was that Liz valued him far too much for that. And not only psychically, either. . . .

Then it was Monday.

By midday an observation post had been set up on the single approach road that angled up the mountain to Xanadu. In a tree-shrouded lay-by, it looked like a party of picnickers was enjoying the view and the mountain air. A table had been set up, and a small barbecue stand sent up smoke from where it stood on the stump of a tree. Cubes of meat sizzled on skewers, and a camera and six-pack of beer sat on the table. Two of the cans had been opened, one of which lay on its side. All very "casual."

Three men in light summer clothes ran the show. One of them was sitting in the car with the windows rolled down, apparently listening to the radio. In fact he was *using* a radio, or would be when it was required. Another soldier sat at the table, "casually" watching the road where it zigzagged up into the wooded heights. He wore binoculars round his neck but only rarely used them. The third member of the team carried a guitar. He perched on a stool in the shade of a pine, his broad-brimmed hat giving him a little extra cover as he strummed an inadequate, mainly tuneless tune out of his instrument, which was in fact capable of far more serious music. He was the team's "minder," and the sound-box of his guitar housed a deadly 9-mm machine-pistol.

So far, the man in the car had registered their call sign and reported their situation only once, clearly and succinctly stating that they were "in situ. . . ."

*   *   *

Also at midday, Liz's Warrant Officer Class Two "Red" By-graves, and the tech Jimmy Harvey, had bought "day visitor" tickets at Xanadu's gatehouse reception desk. By one P.M., having "cased the joint" but oh-so-carefully, they were sunbathing on opposite sides of the main pool. Both men had taken an armful of local morning newspapers with them, with front-page spreads that dealt with the incursion of Asiatic plague; these had been left in strategic locations where they were bound to be picked up and read. Of course the resort had its own newsvending outlets; Trask's news-sheet ploy was intended as a supplementary incentive once his evacuation scheme got in gear.

As for the scheme: that was simplicity itself.

At precisely 1:15 P.M. Bygraves got up and strolled round to Harvey's side of the pool, stepping carefully around or over the many tanned bodies lounging there. The two men were "total strangers," of course. Jimmy Harvey saw Bygraves coming, adjusted his dark glasses, and stretched his arms up above his head, letting the sun caress the pale underarm areas. And:

"Christ!" said Bygraves, going down on a knee beside him, staring at the dark, purplish blotches under Jimmy's arms.

"Eh?" Harvey sat up. "What?"

"Sir," said Bygraves, would you mind if I examined those marks, that pustule?"

"Marks? Pustule?"

"Under your arms, sir. Because if they're what they look like . . ."

Harvey glanced under his arm, looked concerned. "Is that something new?" he said. And, "Who are you, anyway?"

"Dr. Bygraves," said the other, prodding beneath Harvey's left arm where he obligingly lifted it. And by now the people at the poolside were interested in what was going on.

"A doctor?" Harvey was starting to look worried.

"Specializing in communicable Asiatic diseases," Bygraves nodded. "I'm up here for the day, before reporting for duty in Brisbane. And while I don't want to frighten you, right now it looks like I'll have my work cut out!" He pushed Harvey's arm down by his side and asked: "How long have you been up here?"

"Just a fortnight," Harvey was on his feet now. "I'm taking my summer break. So what the hell's wrong?"

But "suddenly" Bygraves became aware of the people gathering to watch the show. And he leaned closer to Harvey, bending down to whisper in the smaller man's ear.

"What?" Harvey yelped.

"But haven't you heard the news, read the newspapers?" Bygraves looked astonished, and more worried than ever. "You say you've been up here for two weeks? Then it's here. It has to be here! Have you seen any rats? Have you noticed any other people with these marks? Jesus, it could be in the water!"

"Plague?" The word burst loudly from Harvey's mouth. "Hey, did you say plague? But how in hell can I have—?"

"Don't say it!" Bygraves cut him short, glancing anxiously at the concerned faces all around. "Listen, we have a serum. It isn't that serious if you get it seen to early—but I do mean right now! All of the medical facilities in this area have been supplied with the antidote. Unfortunately I don't have any with me, and this isn't a registered medical centre. So I can't give you any shots that will help here in Xanadu, but—"

As he set off in a hurry, with Harvey in tow, back around the pool to his sunbed, a small, anxious crowd began to follow on behind. Harvey caught up, grabbed his arm, and said:

"But?" His jaw was beginning to flap. "But what?"

Bygraves picked up a briefcase, went to open it and "accidentally" spilled some of its contents: pamphlets describing the symptoms of Asiatic plague, a new strain of bubonic. They fluttered to the crazy-paved pool surround and were quickly picked up by the gathering crowd.

And looking hopeless, frustrated, Bygraves said, "Look, I think we're probably too late to stop it spreading through this place, but *you* are already short on time." Pulling on a pair of shorts over his swim trunks, he said. "I have to get you out of this place now. And as for the rest of you people,"—he glanced at the milling, gawping faces all around—"this thing will work its way through this place like wildfire! So pass the message: you should all get out, go home, report to your hospitals, doctors, medical facilities— and you should do it now!" Then, to Harvey: "My car's this way."

"But my clothes . . . !" Harvey, whose clothes were in fact in their vehicle, started to protest.

"It's your clothes or your life!" said Bygraves, pushing a way through the crowd.

Ten minutes later they were out of there, and fifteen minutes after *that* the general exodus began. And Red Bygraves was right: the thing worked its way through Xanadu like wildfire. . . .

By that time Ben Trask and David Chung were at the observation point. They were on hand to greet W. O. II Bygraves and Jimmy Harvey when they came tearing down the road from Xanadu in a cloud of dust and heat-shimmer, pulled into the lay-by, and braked to a halt behind the other car.

"How did it go?" Trask was anxious; he sluiced sweat from his brow, glanced up and down the road. Up there the mountains, and down below the coastal plain reaching to the vastly curving horizon of the South Pacific. Normally it would be a beautiful, exhilarating view, but Trask had no time for that right now.

"Some people were piling into their cars even as we pulled out of the place," Jimmy Harvey said, keeping well down and out of sight inside the car. The dust was still settling. "I think we made a good job of it. Thank God for amateur dramatics, eh? Would you believe I once played Romeo?"

Trask looked down at him and couldn't help but smile. "No, but I'd believe a munchkin!"

"Eh?" Harvey grimaced as he pulled a blob of purplish cosmetic putty from under his left arm.

"The Wizard of Oz," Trask answered. "Probably before your time. How about the place? How did it look?"

"Like a resort?"

"Nothing odd about it?"

"No," the other shook his bald dome of a head. "Unless you consider all those well-heeled people and all that tanned flesh odd. But me? I felt like a right whitey from Blighty!"

Trask shook his head, chewed on his upper lip. "Why is it I'm not happy?" he asked of no one in particular. "Why is it so quiet? I don't know . . . but something doesn't feel right." And to Jimmy: "Time you got some clothes on, and wear a hat. We're out of here as soon as people start to exit the place, or we'll get snarled up in the traffic. That is, *if* people start to exit the place!"

The locator David Chung was at the side of the road. Lowering binoculars from his eyes, he called out, "Ben, here they come! A whole stream of cars on the high zigzag up there. Ten minutes and they'll be here." He came at a run across the lay-by's gravel surface.

W.O. II Bygraves had changed his T-shirt, put on a baseball cap and sunglasses. He slid out of the driver's seat and Trask got in. Now Bygraves would take over as the commander of this sub-section, making its numbers up to four. And they'd be here until they were ordered on up to Xanadu. There were sufficient armaments in their vehicle to start World War III.

Trask spoke to Chung. "What do you make of it?"

"He's up there, definitely," said Chung. "At this range I can't be mistaken. Mindsmog, and dense. But it's so steady—I mean, it registers like steady breathing, you know?—that at a guess I'd say he's asleep. Which at this time of day shouldn't come as a surprise. But Ben, hear me out: I think there's more smog than just his."

"Vampires!" said Trask, emphasizing the plural. "Lieutenants? Thralls? How many?"

"Him, and maybe two others. I can't be sure. But they're weak, too weak to be lieutenants. Again I'm guessing, but I'd say they're raw recruits, thralls."

Trask shook his head. "It still feels wrong. Too easy. I

have this feeling he knows about us, that this whole scenario is—I don't know—a lie?"

Chung shrugged, but not negligently. "That's your department, boss. I can't help you."

Trask gave himself a shake, tried to tell himself he was wrong. And anyway, there was nothing he could do about it now. Tonight was their window of opportunity, and it had been "foreseen" by Ian Goodly. So from now on it was all go, go, go.

"David," Trask said. "I won't be seeing you until I come in with Chopper One, after dark. Take care to stay tuned, old friend. And lead these people right to their target, right?"

"You've got it," Chung answered, as the first car out of Xanadu sped in a cloud of dust past the lay-by and on down the often precipitous road.

"You'd better be on your way," Chung nodded. "Good luck, Ben."

But then a strange thing. A car coming in the other direction, *up* the mountain road, pulled in sharply onto the lay-by's gravel surface and skidded to a halt.

The driver cursed out of his open window, said, "Did you see that? If it wasn't for this lay-by I'd be over the fucking edge! I mean, God damn it to . . . !" He had been forced off the road by someone trying to overtake the lead cars in the exodus from Xanadu. "What the fuck is going *on* up there?"

Trask stared hard out of his own vehicle's window at the speaker—at his angular, somehow spidery figure that seemed crammed into the seat of his battered, blue-grey, Range Rover–styled vehicle—and for a moment knew a sensation of déjà vu. The man wore an open-necked shirt and a wide-brimmed hat, and the way he crouched over the steering wheel like that, he had to be pretty tall.

Tall and spidery, and his vehicle was . . .

Trask stared harder, and the tall thin man stared back—but only for a moment. Then his eyes went wide and the back of his vehicle fishtailed as he slammed her in first, revved up, and slewed back out onto the road. And:

"Damn!" Trask shouted, getting out of his car as the dust

of the other's departure drifted back to earth. "Déjà vu nothing! That car, and that man—they fit Liz's description of the watcher at the airport where we came in!"

Even as the suspect car had fishtailed out onto the road, so the SAS type with the guitar had yanked open the boot of the observation post's vehicle and hauled out an evil-looking piece of artillery. Quickly assuming a firing stance behind a stunted pine, he rested the rifle's long barrel on the gnarled stump of a branch. And sweeping the steeply snaking road, he made adjustments to the telescopic sights. Then:

"Mr. Trask," he shouted. "Up there where the road zigzags. I can take him out as he rounds that last bend. The range isn't too much, maybe five hundred yards, and this weapon is lethally accurate to fifteen hundred. That's to assume a stationary target, of course. But I'm qualified with this gun and won't miss. Once he's over that ridge, though, he's gone with the wind. You have maybe thirty seconds to think it over."

Trask thought it over. He knew he was right—but what if he was wrong? What if the spidery man was an innocent? But then again, why had he taken off like that? And the look on his face—probably shock as he'd realized he was face to face with his master's enemy. In which case he'd be on his way to make report to Malinari even now. But if Trask was wrong . . . how to balance one life against the security of a world?

The man with the sniperscope yelled, "He'll be coming into view any time now!"

And Trask thought: *The die is cast. We've got Nephran Malinari trapped up there. He can't come out until sundown, and Ian Goodly has forecast shit and hellfire for tonight, the night of the full moon. So what difference does this make one way or the other?*

What was it that the precog was always saying— something about the future being as immutable as the past? "What will be has been," and all that? Yes, that was it . . . but it was always coupled with, "There's no way of telling *how* it will be, that's all. . . ."

Trask started towards the marksman's position, and in his mind's eye he saw the knuckle of the man's trigger finger turning white on the trigger. As if that were some kind of invocation, the marksman called out, "I have him in my sights now, Mr. Trask."

There was no time left, and Trask skidded to a halt shouting, "Do it! Take him out!" But:

"Shit!" said the other. His finger went slack on the trigger, and beads of sweat sprang into being on his forehead. Letting his weapon slump, he said, "Cars out of Xanadu, a fucking convoy! They were in my way, shielding him. Ordinary civilians. No way I was going to risk firing on them."

Trask had been holding his breath. Now he let it out in a long *"Phew!"* and then said, "Take it easy. It isn't your fault, and it wasn't meant to be. The future can be like that."

"What?" said the other, relieved but frowning. "Some kind of fatalism?"

"Forget it," Trask told him. "But tonight, if you see that car or its driver in the resort, then you can fire on them with all you've got. And ditto should they try to come back down out of there."

Then it was time for a final word with Bygraves and Chung, before the downhill traffic got too heavy. Even now the thunder of fleeing vehicles was becoming deafening.

"It looks like our little scheme is going to work," Trask told Bygraves. "Stay on it, and when the traffic thins out flag down a car. See if you can get some idea of how many people are still up there. As for that fellow who slipped through our fingers a moment ago: don't let it worry you. I'll do the worrrying for all of us. And anyway, what can he tell Malinari other than what he's already figured out for himself—or *will* figure out just as soon as he pops up from his hidy-hole?"

Then he turned to Chung. "David, stay tuned. If that mindsmog gets active, starts moving about, let us know at once. But whether it does or doesn't, and unless something really drastic happens, we'll probably be going in as planned. Okay?"

After the W.O. II and Chung had nodded their underst...ing, Trask got back into the car with Jimmy Harvey and drove to the side of the road. There he waited for a break in the stream of traffic, gave a final wave and set off downhill.

The vast bulk of the exodus was still to come. . . .

And in a Xanadu that would soon be empty of entirely human life, there were just three and a half hours of life-giving, or *un*life-threatening, natural light left. Then the sun would dip westward, the shadows of the mountain range would lengthen, and Xanadu's lights would blink on one by one, holding the darkness and the long night to follow at bay.

Or at least, that was how it would be under normal circumstances. . . .

It was some eighty miles back to the safe house. Along the way Jimmy Harvey radioed ahead to give the people back there their ETA. He also passed a brief, coded message concerning Liz Merrick's watcher, and likewise passed on the locator David Chung's expert opinion that Lord Nephran Malinari was indeed in Xanadu. At which the team at the safe house held a final O-group, then went into action to ensure that everything would be fully operational and ready for Trask on his return.

Radio messages went out. With the exception of the Xanadu observation post, the various SAS units began converging on the flying club where Chopper Two had been checked over, refuelled, and was warming up for the long flight to Gladstone. The other machine stood idle for the moment; its flight to Xanadu would be of much shorter duration. Meanwhile, in the harbour at Gladstone, a fully-fuelled coast guard vessel and pilot had gone on immediate standby. And every man who formed a part of the team was fully aware of the details of the job in hand. . . .

Five-fifteen P.M. in Xanadu, and for more than three hours now private eye Garth Santeson had been trying to get to see his employer, Aristotle Milan. But Santeson wasn't the only employee, and the two well-built young men who saw to Milan's privacy in daylight hours had been proving obstinate. For three hours and then some Santeson had prowled the casino and watched it emptying of punters, hostesses, croupiers and their overseers, and finally—and most tellingly—the tellers. For when the people who handled the cash moved out, then you knew for sure that something was about to go down.

Half an hour ago, turned back yet again by Milan's single-minded minders from his daytime sanctum sanctorum, Santeson had gone out from the almost deserted Pleasure Dome into the resort proper. By then the pools had been empty and the last cars were straggling out through the departure gate. The private investigator was no fool; he had long since found out what the alleged problem was, but he'd also made the connection between that and what he'd bumped into on the mountain approach road. And it was just too much of a coincidence. So how come Milan—who had definitely been on the alert for unfriendly visitors and suspicious activities for as long as Santeson had been with him—how come he wasn't up and about checking things out for himself?

Or was he simply unaware that there was a problem . . . ?

The trouble with Milan's goons was that they had insufficient grey matter between them to realize they should at least be doing *something,* if it was only to let their dodgy employer know what was happening here. This was Santeson's opinion, anyway, which seemed borne out by the dumb, unswervable obstinacy of the pair.

Normally he would have been able to contact Milan by telephone; the photophobic, night-dwelling boss of the resort would usually accept calls through the dark hours from four-thirty or five in the evening until nine in the morning, but not tonight. And when Santeson had tried to impress something of the urgency of an audience with Milan upon his watchdogs—the fact that he *must* see him, that his information was of the utmost importance—it had seemed to him that they couldn't care less! He'd simply been informed of Mr. Milan's instructions: that he wasn't to be disturbed under any circumstance until 6:30 at the earliest. And that had been that. But now, with the time approaching 6:00 P.M. and the resort already dark, cooling under the swift onset of a Tropic of Capricorn night, Santeson was determined to have his way.

He had last tried to call Milan just ten minutes ago from the deserted booth at the monorail boarding stage close to the casino's entrance, but the phone had only buzzed annoyingly at him, because by then there had been no receptionist to transfer the call! And now Santeson was very angry, for as the minutes had stretched into hours his sense of urgency—the anxious frustration of knowing that while something was definitely and dangerously out of kilter here, still there was nothing he could do about it—had increased in commensurate degree.

Garth Santeson had his own ideas as to what was happening or about to happen; it seemed obvious to him that the long arm of the law was reaching for Milan, and his oh-so-shady employer was about to get himself arrested (probably for skimming casino profits); in which case Santeson's monthly and more than adequate paycheque would disappear with him. It therefore followed that the longer he kept the boss out of trouble, the better his chances of collecting his next cheque, due in a few days' time. Which in turn meant he must speak to Milan about the people he had seen on the approach road, at least two of which he'd recognized from the party that had flown in a few days ago in those paramilitary jet-copters.

Santeson knew where Milan was—his approximate location, anyway—but couldn't get to him. On any ordinary night Milan might be found in the casino for an hour or two, but much preferred the privacy of his rooms in the solar-panelled bubble on top of the dome (which on rare occasions he would also use during daylight hours). Santeson had a special elevator key given him by Milan, which would take him to those topmost rooms when he was summoned into the man's presence. But generally, during the day, Aristotle

Milan stayed well out of sight, down in the subterranean bowels of the place. Santeson understood that his employer had private apartments down there, to which he wasn't and never had been privy. To his knowledge, only Milan's goons had ever got that close—

Well, until tonight, anyway....

31
...Before the Storm

IT WAS ALMOST AS DARK INSIDE THE CASINO when Santeson reentered the place. Some electrical failure, which had taken out most of the lights, and no one left to fix it. But even if it was black as night in there he would know where to find Milan's minders.

Surrounding the Pleasure Dome's central spindle, six elevators formed a hexagonal tube of glass and stainless steel. Four of these serviced the casino's upper levels, excluding Milan's bubble. The fifth was for the use of casino personnel only and gave access to the basement and the almost literally bomb-proof Fort Knox–like accountancy vaults. As for number six: that was exclusive to the persons of Milan himself, his minders, and anyone else who he might choose to entertain, either in the bubble or certain unknown regions in the belly of the place.

But associates? Visitors?

Huh! Damn few of those! Santeson thought as he approached the central area, where sure enough Milan's bouncers were waiting to intercept him. Flanking an elevator door marked PRIVATE (the door to Milan's elevator, of course), they were seated in pink-marbled leather armchairs beside slender, urn-shaped ashtrays. But as Santeson came hurrying between the unlit rows of sullenly silent slots, so the minders came smoothly yet indolently to their feet, and stood side by side, their arms folded on their chests, like a matching pair of eunuchs.

Their expressions remained blank, but the positions they had adopted said it all: they were blocking the elevator doors.

Santeson shook his head, wondering, *What is it with these two?* Apart from Milan himself, they were the only ones who had keys to that subterranean level housing what Santeson supposed would be sumptuous apartments. His key would only take him up, not down. But in any case he wasted no time in argument; these zombies always reacted precisely the same way no matter who it was who approached these doors.

"I have to see Mr. Milan," he told them. "And I have to see him now. So don't go fucking me about, because it's too important." They looked at him, then at each other, and back to Santeson. And he looked at them.

They could be twins, he thought, and changed his mind. No, it wasn't that they looked like brothers but that they had like looks. The way they stood there—smartly outfitted, well-built six-footers in their mid- to late-twenties, with sallow complexions that looked sort of grey in this indoor dusk—they could almost be tailor's dummies, motionless yet somehow threatening. Only their eyes moved, and their eyes . . . were weird.

Santeson was sure he'd never noticed it before, but now he saw a kind of yellowish, almost feral luminosity in those eyes. It must be the light, or lack of it, and he was further galvanized by that thought.

"Look," he said, "all shit could break loose any time now, and Mr. Milan has got to be told about it. Now, I don't want to see him on my own . . . hey, boys, if you're that concerned over security, you can escort me! I mean, you'll *have* to go with me anyway, 'cos I don't know where he is or how to get there. But you do. And believe me, if you don't take me to him right now tomorrow you could be out of work. . . ."

And then, losing it a little when their expressions didn't change: "Er, *hello?*" he said. "I mean, am I getting through to you, or would you like me to draw some pictures? Maybe your on-switches are off or something, or I don't know the secret code that could lead us to a basis for some kind of mutual, kindergarten understanding!"

But in fact he had never had anything of an "understanding" with them, not these two. The rest of the Pleasure Dome's workers were regular folks, but these two . . . everyone avoided them like the plague. *Hah, even an Asiatic plague!* Santeson thought.

It was a funny thing, because when they had come here looking for jobs a couple of months ago, they had seemed like regular people, too. But now: they never strayed far from the elevators, and Milan wouldn't go anywhere without them. But come to think of it, he never went anywhere much anyway! *And* there was the same kind of look about him, too. So maybe they were blood relatives, but Santeson didn't think so.

Finally one of them spoke. "Mr. Santeson," he said. "We've already told you three or four times—Mr. Milan won't see you. He isn't seeing anybody. He's expecting a busy night and wants to get some rest. If we take you to him, it won't be you he'll get mad with—*we'll* be in trouble. So why don't you take some good advice, and . . ." Pausing in mid-sentence, he gave a small but violent start, and a facial tic began jerking the flesh at the corner of his mouth. Then his face took on an odd attitude of listening.

From the first word out of the minder's mouth, the spidery Santeson had backed off a pace . . . mainly from his breath! The man had the worst case of crotch- or armpit-mouth that the private detective had ever come across. His breath was so vile it literally stank like a cesspit, or maybe a slaughterhouse? And now this. He stood there as if he'd been struck dumb, with his head turned a little on one side and his strange eyes rapidly blinking. But what was bothering him? What was he listening to?

It lasted for maybe twelve to fifteen seconds, until suddenly he gave his head a shake and straightened up. And smiling in a twitchy, nervous sort of way, he said, "Mr. Milan will see you now. We're to take you to him." His eyes had stopped blinking.

Earphone! Santeson thought. *Direct communication with the boss. This guy is wired, definitely, and in more ways than one! But at least it gets the job done.*

The other minder thumbed the button and the elevator doors opened. Santeson got in and the goons followed on. Then the one with the earphone used his key, and the glass cage descended—down past the basement level, then to a sub-basement level (the last stop marked on the internal indicator) . . . where to Santeson's surprise the elevator didn't stop! Not until the *next* sublevel, which wasn't even registered on the indicator. And Santeson had to admire the brilliance of it, for anyone who wasn't wise to the system wouldn't even know this nethermost level existed.

The elevator had lights, but as the doors hissed open Santeson saw that the corridor outside didn't. Well, it *did*, but so low-key, so subdued, he might easily be in some ultra-low-class Hong Kong brothel.

"This way," said one of the minders . . . and something else that had been niggling at Santeson at once crystalized. It was their voices. Voices that rumbled out of them; they coughed or growled their words. They fired them at you; speech came bursting from them, literally impacting on you, or at least that was how it felt. Up in the casino in some kind of decent light, the effect was lessened—lessened *by* the light, maybe, or the accustomed surroundings—but down here in the near-darkness . . .

. . . It was like these people belonged down here in the dark. Almost as if they were made for it.

The minders led the way. Santeson couldn't complain about that; it was oddly reassuring to have these two in front of him and not behind. But he'd only taken a few paces when he stumbled. And now that his eyes were growing accustomed to the gloom he saw why, and also why the place had reminded him of a brothel. It was the lighting.

The corridor was lit by a string of small red lightbulbs, well spaced out on a cable that was hooked up to a low ceiling. But the ceiling was of stone, likewise the walls and the floor. Natural stone, hewn stone. And this wasn't a corridor at all—except in the most primitive sense of the word—but a tunnel. A tunnel carved from the bedrock, and the floor was ridged and uneven.

So? Santeson asked himself. *What did you expect down here? You go far enough down and there's rock, for Christ's sake!* And as he stumbled a second time:

"Mind the floor," one of the minders grunted, half-turning to glance back at him. Only *half*-turning, but Santeson got a glimpse of his eyes. And he saw that they burned like sulphur in the dark! He began to panic, and immediately got a grip on himself. It had to be a chemical reaction, some kind of gas down here. For all he knew, his eyes might be burning yellow, too! Or perhaps—*again* perhaps—it was the lights. Like those fluorescent lights in the disco that made his false front teeth glow.

"How f-far is it?" He heard himself say. A stupid question, stupidly put. How long is a piece of string? But for no reason at all that he could give name too, Santeson's nerve was going, and all of the smart talk lay dead in him. And in front, one of Milan's minders chuckled like a file on broken glass, and answered:

"Not very f-far at all!"

The walls had widened out, disappeared into gloom; the ceiling was higher, and the light correspondingly dimmer. Ahead of Santeson, the broad backs of the minders were twin black silhouettes, moving unerringly, relentlessly through the darkness and leading him on like . . .

. . . Like what?

For suddenly, out of nowhere, there was this picture in his mind of a lamb with a noose round its neck, and in his nostrils a waft of slaughter house breath that stung like a slap. And as he tried to shut these scenes and sensations out, still he wondered: *How do these people see in the dark?*

"Now be very careful how you go," one of them said, and his voice echoed in what was obviously a large space, but one that was filled with a powerful musk and a strange rustling. And his colleague advised:

"Step where we step."

"I can't see a f-fucking thing!" Santeson husked, his voice a whisper in the darkness.

Abruptly the minders paused, so that he almost bumped into them; they looked at each other questioningly, then turned as a man to Santeson. "Would you *like* to?" One of them coughed a query.

"Eh?" Santeson stood there trembling. "L-like t-to?"

"Would you like to see a f-fucking Thing?" said the minder, tilting his head in inquiry, his face gaping into such a grin as Santeson couldn't believe.

"Lights," said his partner, moving swiftly—with a flowing motion—away into the darkness.

"Camera," said the one with the yawning cavern mouth, giving Santeson a small push in a certain direction. And:

"Action!" came the other's gurgling answer from some short distance away.

Santeson's balance was shot anyway. Weak as a baby, stumbling away from the one who had pushed him, he flailed his arms, fought to stay on his feet. But then he stepped on something—something that writhed or slithered underfoot— and at the same time was momentarily blinded as several neon tubes in the ceiling buzzed into life.

After that . . . madness!

Santeson no longer believed any of this. It had to be dazzle from the sudden glare, or his imagination, or anything. But it couldn't be real. What lapped at his feet . . . that couldn't be real. And what humped in one corner of the cave, tossing and heaving . . . *that* wouldn't interface with reality at all—

—Until it looked at him and said, "H-h-*help meeeee!*" And then he *knew* it was real!

As his eyes rolled up and he flopped, so the minders were there beside him, taking him under the arms, bearing his weight as easily as if he were a child. Tall, thin, and spidery as Santeson was, his knees scraped along the stony floor as they bore him up and away, out of the cave of the seething Thing, to Malinari. . . .

*   *   *

Three hours earlier:

Crouching low under the circular shimmer of the jet-copter's fan, and calling Jake's name, Liz Merrick was buffeted by a blistering whirlwind of heat where she ran across the helipad to where Chopper Two was making ready to take off. Jake shouldn't have been able to hear her over the high-pitched whining of the engine and vanes, but he "heard" her anyway.

Sliding a gunner's door halfway open, he clung to a strap, leaned out and down, and took the fluttering envelope that she passed up to him. And with a last long look into her eyes, seeing the pain in them, he felt the slight tremor that warned of imminent takeoff and closed the door to the merest crack. The chopper lifted off, rose up, and turned once, slowly, through 180 degrees.

Liz came back into view. She'd moved into a safe position at the edge of the helipad and was waving up at him. He opened the door a fraction more, waved back. But then, as the chopper gained altitude, keeled on its side a little, and headed north, she was lost to sight.

Jake closed the door and took his seat beside Lardis Lidesci. And thinking hard—thinking about Liz, and thinking *at* her—he said:

Take care of yourself, Liz. You be sure to take very good care of yourself.

You too, she told him, quite clearly. And also: *I . . . I'm sorry, Jake.*

It was in Jake's mind to ask her what about, but since he believed he already knew, there wasn't much point in it. Moreover, he knew that it wasn't her fault, that she really didn't have anything to be sorry about. It was the job that kept coming between them—Ben Trask and E-Branch—and E-Branch would always come first.

But a picture of Liz stayed in his mind—her night-black hair, cut in that boyish bob; her intelligent, sea-green eyes; her curves of course, and her smile like a ray of bright light—standing there at the edge of the helipad, waving, and gradually dwindling into the distance. And despite that it was all in his mind's eye, Jake knew that in fact she was still there, watching the jet-copter right out of sight.

He had put the envelope in his pocket. Now, as the rumble of the chopper's jets took over and he felt forward acceleration, he took it out to read what Liz had written on the single leaf of paper that was folded inside. But as he unfolded it:

"From Liz?" Lardis grunted.

"Mind your own business," Jake answered.

"She thinks a lot of you."

"That cuts both ways," said Jake. "Can you read our language?"

"Some," said Lardis. "When it's printed. But handwriting? Not a chance. It looks like spider shit to me!"

"Good!" said Jake. And despite the Old Lidesci's sideways squint, he read what was written:

> *Jake—*
> *It's a bit late, but you asked me to remind you of a name—the name was KORATH. You may not remember it, but if you do you'll probably think I'm a treacherous bitch. If so, well, there's not much that I can do about it. But it seemed to me you thought this was pretty important. And since we don't know what's coming, it could be a question of now or never, my one chance to put things straight—*
> *—Or to mess them up completely.*
> *I care for you more than you know, and a lot more than circumstances have let me show.*
>
> *Please take care.*
> *Liz*

Jake read it through again. Korath? The name rang a bell, but it was a far and almost forgotten clamour. Something he'd dreamed? Well, that was what she was talking about, obviously: the fact that she'd been snooping on him again, when he slept. But so what? It was her job and he would simply have to learn to accept it—and Liz would have to learn to accept whatever she found in there, in his subconscious mind, like it or not.

His recurrent nightmare? Well, that would explain yesterday's coolness, certainly. But Korath . . . ?

Again Jake heard the ringing of that distant bell—perhaps a warning bell? And this time more insistently—and he frowned as he tried to recall whatever it meant back into the focus of his memory. *Was* it something that he'd dreamed?

Jake had read a few things about dreams, and he knew that to many they were of special significance. To him, however, dreams had usually been trivial, easily forgotten things, the scurf or sloughed-off skin of more fully fleshed-out ideas and concepts from his waking hours. And he wondered: *How often does a man retain detailed memories of what he dreams, and for how long?*

Nightmares were one thing (for they left lasting impressions, if only through the emotion of fear), but common or garden-variety dreams? And again he thought: *Korath?* But this time it was a very deliberate thought, and unguarded.

And it was deadspeak.

Immediately there was someone—or some Thing—there in his mind. Shadows sprang into being, and *It* came with them.

You called! said a glutinous voice that was both surprised and pleased, causing Jake to start. *And you remembered. But how much have you remembered? It's all there, Jake, just waiting to come back to you. But I feel your sense of shock—the way you recoil from me—and I wonder, do you really remember? What is it, Jake? Why did you call out to me?*

"What in the name of . . . !?" said Jake, and at once, instinctively, brought mental barriers crashing down to shut whatever it was—this thing, this Other, this Korath—out of his mind.

The other fled or was banished at once, and Jake heard him go: his frustrated cry of rage, denial, as he disappeared into the deadspeak aether:

No, Jake, no! Don't send me away! You'll know soon enough how much you need me. And you must always re-

member: I have the numbers! I have the numbers, *Jake, and I know the waaayyy!*

Then he was gone.

"Eh?" said Lardis, staring hard at Jake, at a face turned pale and gaunt. "Eh, what? Is there something? You gave a start just then. You said something. And the way you look . . ." But:

"Shhh!" Jake shook his head, concentrated, and remembered! Remembered it all, but *most* of all that he'd almost made a deal with a vampire. And he remembered something else: Harry Keogh's warning that even a dead vampire is a dangerous thing that you should never, *ever,* let into your mind!

"You look peculiar," said the Old Lidesci.

Jake looked at him, swallowed hard, and slowly got a grip of himself. "It was . . . it was nothing," he said. "Nothing that I want to talk about now, anyway. Later, maybe—to Liz and Ben Trask—when tonight's business is over."

And between times . . . he dug out a ball-point and began to make shaky notes on Liz's scrap of paper.

For while he still hadn't quite come to terms with everything that was happening to him, and whether or not this latest manifestation was some kind of daydream, mental quirk, evidence of a dual personality, or whatever, still Jake knew that it was something he *must* remember in detail, something that he really couldn't afford to forget. . . .

Chopper Two disembarked its task force in Gladstone and refuelled. Earlier that day, three SAS men had made the long drive up to Gladstone to check that all was in order with the coast guard vessel. Now the two units met up for a final briefing.

The attack on the island would be two-pronged. Along with W.O. II Joe Davis and four NCOs, Jake and Lardis Lidesci would be airborne; four more NCOs would be in the boat.

Zero Hour—the time scheduled for the launch of simultaneous attacks on both the Capricorn Group island and the mountain resort of Xanadu—had been set for 6:30 P.M. The weather was good and the sea flat calm, and with just ninety minutes to go to Zero Hour, the boat cast off.

And an hour later, with the light failing as the sun sank down behind the Great Dividing Range, Chopper Two got airborne again.

At the same time, at the Brisbane flying club, Chopper One was warming up, ready to go. Ben Trask and the SAS major, joint operational commanders, were in a hangar using a radio in one of the vehicles. The precog Ian Goodly, Liz Merrick, and the rest of the SAS men were trooping out to the jet-copter, their combat suits fluttering in the bluster of night air that stank of hot exhaust fumes.

At 6:15 Trask transmitted: "Call signs One, Two, and Three, signals—over?"

And the answers came back: "One, okay—over." (The locator David Chung's voice, from the Xanadu approach road.)

"Two, okay—over." (Joe Davis's voice from Chopper Two.)

"Three, okay—over." (The senior NCO on the boat.)

"Sitreps," said Trask.

And three identical situation reports came back one after the other: "On schedule, and all systems are go."

"Synchronizing watches," said Trask, then waited a second. "Set your watches to 6:17. I say again figures sixer, one, seven. Counting down, I now have—three, two, one, zero—6:17 precisely. Good hunting, and good luck. Over?"

"Roger that, and out," from the same three sources. And:

"Let's go," said Trask. He and the major ran out under the gleaming vanes of the jet-copter and boarded her. Moments later she took off and headed south for Xanadu....

In Chopper One Trask had just minutes left to talk to Liz, Ian Goodly, and the major. "I'm concerned," he said. "There's something wrong and I don't know what it is. It's a feeling that—I don't know—that everything we've done or we're trying to do is somehow misguided, as if we're on the wrong track, or we've been misled, or there's something we've overlooked."

"That sounds like your talent at work, Ben," said the precog. And then he sighed. "Well, I'm glad that someone's talent is working!"

"And you?" Trask looked at him. "Nothing?"

"Just trouble," Goodly sighed again. "Just problems, frustration, confusion. But as you know, I can't force it; it comes when it comes. But in your case . . . is it anything specific?"

"No," Trask shook his head. "So it seems we're in the same boat—or airplane! It's a *feeling*, that's all. I had it today up at the observation post on the mountain road. When I looked up the road, toward Xanadu . . . it was all so quiet, so normal. Perhaps too quiet, too normal."

"A lie?"

"More like I was deceiving myself," said Trask. "This is a covert operation, but it didn't feel like one. Especially after that incident with Liz's watcher." He glanced at her—a guilty look, she thought—and said, "I should have paid more attention to you."

"But I wasn't that sure myself," Liz said. "And anyway, I'm the new kid on the block; I could have been wrong."

"That's what I mean," said Trask. "We all have our talents, and I should have listened to yours. If we had turned back and *I* had seen that fellow, I would have known at once. But we didn't, and I didn't. I blame myself."

At which the major, looking more than a little concerned, came in with, "Miss, gentlemen, I have some difficulty following you—these skills of yours, you understand—but are you saying the operation is in jeopardy?"

Trask shook his head, then changed his mind and said, "Any operation concerning these creatures is hazardous. But we have to go in no matter what. It's all set up, and we mightn't get a better chance. But with our weapons and providing everyone remembers the drills, I can't see what can go wrong."

Liz glanced at her watch. "Five minutes," she said. And as at a signal the intercom began buzzing.

The pilot was saying: "Message from Call sign One. The mindsmog has been 'awake' but more or less static for some time. Now it's on the move, but only locally. Call sign One is also mobile. His ETA on the target area is five minutes."

Trask answered, "Tell him roger that. We'll see him there, and not to forget his nose-plugs." Then, turning to the bulk of the helicopter party, "And you mustn't forget yours."

They hadn't forgotten. Aerosol sprays were hissing; a fine garlic mist filled the air, settling on everyone's clothing; it was almost a pleasure to insert filter plugs like fat cigarette tips deep into their nostrils.

In Xanadu, from a position some two hundred feet up the almost sheer rock wall of the mountainside, Lord Malinari of the Wamphyri looked down on the sprawling dark cobweb of the deserted resort, and at the single road that wound its serpentine route up the steep mountain contours to Xanadu's gates.

Malinari's vantage point was a roughly-hewn "room" carved from the solid rock at the head of a natural chimney. When Xanadu was being built, it had been Jethro Manchester's intention to create a special entertainment here. There was to have been a ski-lift or cable car from the gardens up to this point, and a series of aquachutes back down to the pools. The chimney had been fitted with a spiralling service-and/or emergency-staircase behind a facade constructed to match the flanking cliffs, so disguising the chimney's vertical fault, and work had commenced on this room or landing stage. At which point technical difficulties had caused the project to be abandoned.

Now the chimney was Lord Malinari's bolthole from Xanadu. From this window he would fly out on the night wind, and glide down to a place in which he had long since secreted a cache of clothing, money, and other necessaries to speed him on his way to his next venture. But *not* before he ensured that the chase ended here, and that this E-Branch had suffered such losses as to finish it forever, or at least slow it down until his, Vavara's, and Szwart's greater scheme was brought into play. . . .

Malinari looked down on Xanadu and smiled a hideous smile. If only he could be down there to see the mayhem. But that way he might find himself caught up in all of the destruction, and that was out of the question. As for Xanadu itself:

Oh, he might bemoan the waste of this place a very little . . . but not for very long. For the world was a wider place by far, and his plans of conquest of far greater scope.

A shame that his "garden" with its special "crop" must be discovered—especially now that it had been nourished so recently. Or then again, perhaps it would not be found; for it was after all hidden away, in the subterranean darkness that suited it so very well. In which case it would lie there, all unattended and dormant for now, only to flourish later in its own good time. For what Malinari had seeded would not die unless it were *put* down, deliberately and utterly destroyed. Ah, the tenacity of the Great Vampire, *and* of his works!

As for the last of Malinari's human watchdogs: the spider-like, gangling Garth Santeson was by now no more. He had served his purpose the moment he warned of E-Branch's arrival here, an intrusion that Malinari had been expecting ever since his lieutenant Bruce Trennier died the true death some few days ago far in the western desert, and of which he'd had warning apart from and *since* Trennier's demise, not alone from Garth Santeson.

A warning, aye, and delivered by a seeming idiot! But even an idiot may have his uses. Malinari had certainly found a good use for that one. . . .

But poor Trennier, the manner of his passing. Malinari remembered it well, those last few moments of the man's miserable life: the faithful servant crying his agonies, and Malinari the Mind, the master, feeling something of those agonies even here, in Xanadu:

The fire! That awesome, all-consuming, withering fire that melted even metamorphic flesh, exploded bone, liquefied sinew, and reduced all to ashes! It had lasted a while—the pain, too, Trennier's pain—until Malinari had been obliged to shut it out of his mind. But through the jet of blistering heat that stripped Trennier's flesh from his body and finally blinded and destroyed him, Malinari had recognized some of the faces of his lieutenant's tormentors. The face of Ben Trask, remembered from the mind of Zek Föener, and that of Ian Goodly, yet another man of weird talents . . .

But if only Malinari had had longer with the Föener woman. There had been so much more that he might have learned (such as the *nature* of their skills, these men of esoteric talents), and so *very* much more that he would have enjoyed . . . of that beautiful woman herself, perhaps, and not only her mind.

Well, too late for that now—too late from the moment he hurled her down that shaft into oblivion—but at least he had fathomed something of the dangers of this world. Especially the greatest danger of all, which was E-Branch.

And now they had found him . . . as he had known they would, against which inevitability he'd long since taken ingenious and even marvellous precautions.

On a board bolted to the wall close to Malinari's "window" (which was simply a large hole in the moulded concrete facade), a master switch stood in the off position beside a series of smaller electrical switches set in a roughly oblong array. The array was a precise match for Xanadu itself, its concentric pattern of switches duplicating the cobweb design of the resort in the gloom of the mountain saddle.

Now, waiting there in his secret bolthole, Malinari threw the master switch. There was a low, answering hum of power, but nothing more. And his slender fingers were impatient where they fluttered over the smaller switches—those electrical messengers of instantaneous death—as he gloatingly rehearsed a certain sequence:

"First the outer chalets, to close them in. Then the inner structures, to catch them where they run. And when finally they think they have me 'trapped' in my night-dark dome . . ." His hand trembled with pent anticipation over the central switch.

"A pleasure dome, aye. But for *my* pleasure, not theirs!"

He laughed a coughing laugh, long and low . . . then paused abruptly. Down there, coming into view along the approach road toward Xanadu's gates: a vehicle. The night was dark now—but night and darkness were Malinari's greatest allies—and that vehicle with its lowered, carefully probing lights; the coiled-spring tension in its vengeful passengers!

Malinari sensed it, their human bloodlust—or what passed for bloodlust in men—and laughed again. Bloodlust? Why, Nephran Malinari had *pissed* thicker blood than coursed through the veins of whelps such as these!

And with his telepathic probes concentrating on the vehicle, he felt what its occupants felt:

Fear, of the Great Unknown that was Malinari. Oh, he recognized and relished it! Primal fear of the night and what the night may bring, its roots burrowing like worms in every human fiber, revenant of cavern-dwelling ancestors. Fear in the face of an alien threat, the menace of the blood-beast!

But tempering the fear, holding it at bay, there was also a wall of grim determination. And bolstering that blind determination, the sure knowledge of vastly superior firepower.

Oh, really . . . ?

And again Malinari laughed, but a second later hissed and grimaced, and clasped his handsomely alien head in wildly trembling hands. It was the pain—those lightning flashes of terrible pain which ever accompanied any excessive use of his mentalism—the pain that came from searching out or listening to the thoughts of so many others, and of suffering the tumult of their massed emotions, their thronging dreams and fancies. For weirdly mutated minds were gathering here now, and the greater their talents the more piercing the pain in his head.

Cursing vividly, in the tongue of Starside, Malinari swiftly withdrew his probes. And as the pain receded, so he relaxed a little and gave vent once more to strained, broken laughter.

But strained? And broken?

He had thought often enough about that before—even he, Malinari—finding cause to wonder: *The laughter of a madman?* Well, perhaps it was at that, though he preferred to think of himself as merely . . . eccentric? And anyway, what of it? When a man is unique, surely he has a right to such small idiosyncrasies?

Drawing him back from his musing, the fading pounding in Malinari's temples was suddenly matched by a stuttering in the sky: the mechanical throbbing of jets, as their power diverted to whirling, fanlike vanes. And though momentarily startled—sufficiently so that he lifted his crimson gaze to the dragonfly shape that blurred the stars—still he felt no real concern or threat. His plans were laid, and every eventuality had been anticipated. Even this one.

Down in the gardens, in front of the casino, that was the most obvious of the few places where the jet-copter could land. But it was also one of the *many* places that Malinari had mined. And:

Hah! So be it! he thought. *Now let this game commence.*

The car at the gate issued a single man; equipped with a heavy, deadly automatic weapon, he crouched low and ran to the small, open-fronted chalet that housed reception. A rearguard, of course; also a guard against anyone trying to escape. These guileless fools! No one would be trying to "escape" from Xanadu—well, except for these ridiculous invaders themselves! As for Malinari quitting the place: but that was the plan. And in any case, what would it serve to stay? When this was all over, there would be nothing left to stay for.

And now the flying machine was settling towards the garden, its searchlight beams flickering over the dark casino, the chalets, the pools. And suddenly the car's lights were blazing bright, lighting the way as it sped to its rendezvous.

Its rendezvous with certain death . . . but not just yet.

First let Trask and these E-Branch people taste something of what they had brought down on themselves when, of their own free will, they had chosen to pursure Nephran Malinari.

Lord Malinari, aye, of the Wamphyyrrriiii!

The coast guard vessel made smoke where she lolled portside on toward the narrow strip of sandy beach that fronted Jethro Manchester's island. Apparently crippled, she rocked this way and that in the gentle wavelets of the night surf. On her starboard side, hidden by the cabin, an SAS man aimed his flamethrower at the sky and fired short-lived bursts of flame above the cabin's roof. As viewed from the island, it would seem for certain that the ruddily lit boat was on fire; even as her keel bit into the sand, so a signal flare made a starburst high in the sky.

Also in the sky, but not so very high now—indeed, wheeling in low over the ocean's horizon—Chopper Two's pilot saw the starburst and told his crew:

"We're over the island. I can see the boat 'burning' down there, and the lights of the villa in the trees. So this is it. Jump to it as soon as we touch down. I'll be airborne and waiting for you when you get done. You can whistle me down. I mean, you know how to whistle, don't you? Good luck, guys!"

Dark figures were running up the beach as the chopper came down, and a faint waft of garlic tainted the night air. . . .

32
The Storming

SITUATED 160 YARDS FROM WHERE THE COAST guard vessel had beached, and set well back from the high-water mark behind massively thick, fortresslike rock walls in four acres of landscaped rockeries and gardens watered from a small desalination unit, Jethro Manchester's two-storey villa was a luxurious, custom-built dwelling.

Standing central on a jutting promontory, the house was of timber and natural stone, mainly fossilized coral. It had been built from imported teak and dynamited rubble from a channel blasted through to a rocky inlet on the other side of the promontory. In style it was part sprawling Roman villa, part Austrian chalet. Manchester's yacht—by his standards a "modest" thirty-five footer—was moored in a roofed-over lock in the artificial channel, midway between the villa and the sea.

These features were visible from the air, where at five hundred feet Chopper Two's pilot stood his machine off like a hawk and viewed them through its eyes, sensitive night-vision scanners. Every few seconds he would flip a switch to convert his screen to infrared and thermal imaging. All of the men on the ground were wearing headsets; the pilot was able to talk to them individually or as a group.

All subterfuge had been thrown to the wind now; the air-borne party was safely down, and the boat had landed its crew without hindrance. Now the task force would deploy into a semicircle to isolate the promontory, and move in on the house. If the target group had seen the boat's "fire" or emergency flare—or if they had heard the chopper's low, prowler-mode throb and came out of the house to see what was happening or perhaps to take defensive action—then the men on the ground would be able to answer the threat without fear of firing on each other.

With his machine on autopilot, the pilot's attention was rapt on his viewers. For now, in addition to the central, gently fluctuating orange glow of the house, the dark-green terrain of his screen was lit by smaller blobs of human heat.

He saw two figures, fast-moving and crouching low, about to leave the narrow strip of beach and enter an area of land-scaped rocks and foliage east of the villa. They were heading for one of the regular breaks in the wall. And the pilot knew that the four-man boat party had split into two two-man teams. This was one of them; they would be equipped with their usual weapons, and one of them would be carrying a flamethrower.

But as the pilot scanned ahead of them, suddenly, as if from nowhere, he picked up two more figures. They were in the shrubbery or under cover of the trees, but they were making a *lot* of heat! The writhing, bloblike shapes on the screen merged, drew apart, melted together again . . . a repetitious, oddly sexual-looking activity. The men from the boat were heading directly toward it and at some speed, and the pilot was almost too late to advise them:

"Boat party east of the house. There's some fucking thing directly ahead of you!" He couldn't know it but he was absolutely right.

On the ground, the NCOs spied sudden, apparently startled movement. It was dark, but not that dark, and the almost luminous tangle of flesh on a blanket under the bowerlike branches of a tall, flowering shrub was unmistakable: the naked figures of a couple making love. Or they had been but now sprang apart.

"What the . . . ?" The man sat upright, and the girl tried to cover herself and gave a small, warbling cry. The scene was so authentic and natural, and the couple seemed so vulnerable, it was the SAS men who were taken by surprise.

"Bloody hell . . . !" said one of them, his jaw falling open. And his companion actually turned aside the barrel of his weapon a little, deflecting it from the pair and easing his finger off the trigger. Surprise, yes—momentary disorientation and confusion—the only advantage a vampire could ever ask for or require. And:

"Oh, thank *God!*" cried the girl, as she threw herself forward and sprawled at the feet of one of the soldiers. "Help me! Please help me! He was *raping* me!" A lie, which of course fell naturally from her lips.

But at the same time the naked man's arm swept up to aim and fire a short-barrelled, compressed-air speargun. The spearhead was a trident with four-inch tines; all three of them took the off-guard soldier in his throat. And gurgling, clawing one-handed at the short spear in his crimson-spurting neck, he fell over backward and let loose a burst of automatic fire uselessly into the sky.

The other soldier had reached down almost instinctively to lift the girl to her feet. But even in the act of gathering her up he saw his colleague shot, and simultaneously the feral yellow fire in the naked man's eyes as he flowed sinuously upright and drew back his arm to use the speargun as a club.

No further reminder was necessary. The soldier cursed and put the naked girl aside, then opened up with a burst of explosive shells that lifted the vampire from his feet, ripped into him in midair, and threw him backward into the shrub. There he hung in a tangle of crushed foliage, until branches snapped and he fell to the ground. And as he sat there— groping among his own intestines and mewling his undead agony—so the gibbering NCO cursed again and put a single shell right between his eyes. The contents of the vampire's head went every which way as the shrub collapsed on him.

Meanwhile the downed man had stopped writhing and tugging at the spear in his throat; he lay dead still, dead of shock or from choking on his own blood.

And the girl had disappeared into the night. . . .

Fleeing, sobbing, gasping for air—with her sliced feet leaving a trail of blood on the often jagged stones—Julie Lennox somehow managed to avoid the second pair of men from the coast guard vessel, and came across Jake and Lardis instead. With her night eyes, the eyes of a vampire, she saw them before they saw her: an old man and his younger colleague, in the garden, keeping low and making their way silently toward the house. And she remembered some advice that she'd been given:

"When they come, and they *will* come," (Martin Trennier had told Jethro Manchester and his small, family group just an hour or so ago), "there won't be any mercy. They'll come to kill you. And while you might not believe it now, you *won't* want them to! For you have a Great Vampire's blood in you, and in its own way it is alive, too. It *wants* to live, and it won't let you commit suicide—which means that you can't simply give yourselves up to these men. Ergo, you'll fight. And the more of them that you kill, the longer you'll stay alive."

With which he had rammed a handful of shells deep into the magazine of an ugly pump-action shotgun, and jerked once on its heavy wooden stock to arm it, before continuing:

"Now, while I know that some of you are still fighting the good fight, the fact is we can grow strong on our enemies— on the *blood* of our enemies—and the stronger we grow, the better our chances of survival. So that's it, now you know what to do. I have nothing more to say, except that I for one intend to survive. So go on, get busy. Prepare yourselves with whatever grit or cunning your vampire blood has bestowed, arm yourselves with whatever weapons you can find, and wait. It's just as simple as that."

But in fact it wasn't simple at all. Simple, perhaps, for Martin Trennier, one of the first taken by Aristotle Milan and utterly in thrall to him, but not for Julie; not now that Alan Manchester, Jethro's son was dead. Julie and Alan . . . how they had loved each other, and how desperately hard they had fought to cling to their humanity. But all in vain.

Alan had turned first, and now he was dead and gone, taken from her, and these merciless invaders were responsible—weren't they? Deep in her heart, she knew they weren't; and yet, as moment by moment Trennier's words made more sense, so the vampire essence in Julie's system worked on her, turning her, too.

Trennier had done it to her, done it to them all: a simple bite was all it took—and time. For Trennier was barely a lieutenant himself, and a weak one at that. Made by Milan, he had been given a minimum of essence, and so he'd been a thrall for long and long. But as the evil had grown in him, so he'd taken on stature, guile, strength. And thus he'd become Milan's lieutenant, to watch over the Manchesters on their island retreat. Or as it was now, their prison.

When they had known their end was near, Julie and Alan

had come out into the night, into the garden, to make love just one last time. They hadn't reckoned on being found so quickly, that was all. Not in their own secret place, in the garden, on their prison island. Their prison, yes . . . indeed their death cell.

Or perhaps not. For as the blood is the life, so there was plenty of hot blood in these two men. And without warning, suddenly Julie caught herself licking her lips in anticipation. At which she knew that it was too late for her, and that it always had been. But strangely—and as swiftly as that—she no longer cared, for she was now awake! As for what had awakened her:

Perhaps it had been the sight and salty smell of Alan Manchester's blood, or that of the soldier whom he'd shot with his speargun, or both. Which- or what-ever, it had acted on Julie as a catalyst, and now the "good fight" was over. She was what she was and would do what she must do. She moved like a wraith toward the two men, got behind them where they crept carefully forward, making for the villa's lights.

She got closer and closer to them, her hands raised, with nails like poisonous claws—indeed they *were* poisonous claws—poised and ready to strike. . . .

. . . But in that same moment Julie found herself betrayed, and by three things:

One—the full moon, emerging from behind fleeting clouds to sweep a silver swath over the sea and the land. Two—by the sharp stutter of automatic gunfire, sounding from a short distance to the west. And three—by a watchful, dragonfly spy-in-the-sky, hovering on high as it sent an urgent message to Julie's would-be victims:

"Central team. Why are there three of you? Do you have a tail?" Fading in and out, the pilot's words were hard to read.

Lardis didn't understand the message, but Jake, startled by the gunfire and the near-distant cries that accompanied it, turned and saw . . .

. . . A girl? A distraught, naked girl?

For seeing him beginning his turn, Julie had drawn back, shrunk down into herself, begun to sob and scream. "I was in the house," she sobbed, trying to cover herself as if ashamed of her nakedness. "They kept me prisoner there. But when they heard your helicopter they stopped watching me, and I . . . and . . . I . . . *oh!*"

She feigned a swoon, and Jake—forgetting all that he'd seen, all that he'd been told—put up his weapon and stepped forward.

She clung to him for a moment, this beautiful girl, who was naked and frightened and so pale in the flooding light of the moon . . . so pale and *so* cold. This girl whose grip on his combat suit was like iron, and whose nose was suddenly wrinkling suspiciously as she smelled garlic, and whose eyes were a reflective yellow, sulphurous in the night!

Julie held the front of his jacket bunched in one hand, drew back the other hand until Jake saw its nails, sharpened and bevelled to gouges that would cut bloody channels in his face as easily as a routing machine! And her awful smile: the way her lips curled back from gleaming teeth.

Jake tried to bring his machine-pistol to bear, to centre its muzzle on Julie's body. But she was faster; she knocked it away, out of his grasp. And now her "smile" was a fixed, nightmarish grimace—but of horror or pleasure in her own terrible strength, Jake couldn't say. Nor could he do anything about it.

But Lardis could.

An "old man," Lardis Lidesci had been ignored and almost forgotten by the girl. A mistake, for he was an old man with a difference. He was the Old Lidesci, and not nearly as naive as Jake. Not in the ways of vampires.

Jake saw that slender, incredibly strong hand lift up before his face, tried to draw back from it and couldn't. He saw the fingers crook, could almost feel their rake, and knew that he was *going* to feel it. But then, in a moment, the look on her face changed. And she sighed.

She sighed, then smiled again, but a real smile now. And a dribble of blood spilled from the corner of her mouth. Her hands straightened out—reached out to touch his face—but just a touch, almost a caress. Then her grip relaxed, her eyes rolled up, and she toppled away from him.

Lardis Lidesci stood ten feet away, but his machete stood much closer than that; it stood up from the girl's back, where it had split her spinal column.

"Get your gun," Lardis growled, and Jake began to breathe again after what had seemed like an hour of holding his breath. "Get your gun and put it in her mouth . . . and finish it."

Jake was numb; his hands were numb as he took up his machine-pistol. "But—" he started to say.

"But nothing!" Lardis snarled. "Do it, and be sure to turn your face away."

Just before Jake did it, Julie stopped her fitful, agonized writhing, saw the weapon's muzzle approaching her face, said something that Jake couldn't hear, just a breath of air. But he was sure that her lips formed the words, "Thank you. . . ."

By then there was plenty of shouting and shooting, the hissing of flamethrowers, great gouts of fire and columns of smoke, all of it toward the centre of the promontory, at the villa itself. And full moon or none, it would have made no difference; bright orange and yellow flames were leaping, and all the shadows cast back in Jethro Manchester's gardens and rockeries.

Lardis and Jake were the last to get there, but two of the SAS men would never get there. Close to the house, itself burning, they came across W.O. II Joe Davis and one of his men. The NCO had a flamethrower and was watching the house. Davis was on one knee, looking at a pair of crumpled figures. His hands kept reaching, and drawing back without touching. And his hands were trembling.

"Get up from there," said Lardis. "Back away. Let me see."

Davis looked up at Lardis through moist eyes; he was holding on, but only just, to would-be runaway emotions.

His Adam's apple rose and fell, rose and fell, as he fought not to betray himself. "Old man," he said, his voice on the point of breaking, "I trained this man, this boy. He was one of mine. But I didn't train him for this."

Lardis pulled him away, muttering, "What could anyone have taught him? There *is* no training for this kind of thing, except on the field of battle. The trouble with that is we only learn when we lose."

He looked at the mess on the ground. Part of it, the body of a mature woman in a once-white dress, was a mound of raw red flesh. Riddled with bullets—some of which had exploded—she had been torn apart from within. Her face wasn't there, and her lower body seemed to have burst outwards. Lying under her where she'd fallen, a young soldier in combat clothing stared blindly up into the sky. His brains had been split by a bright shining cleaver that was still buried in his skull.

But even as Lardis looked, the woman's arms twitched where they clasped her victim, and one foot shuddered and vibrated in a shoe with a broken heel. Jerkily, spastically, her chest rose and fell, as bubbles formed in the liquid red mask of her face.

"Did you touch . . . any of this?" Lardis looked up at Davis. The other shook his head. Then Lardis stood up, stood back, and turned to the man with the flamethrower. "Burn it," he said.

The man looked at his leader, who in turn looked at Lardis almost pleadingly. And Lardis said, "Their blood is mixed. Your man's corpse is contaminated. Take no chances. Burn it all."

As they moved away from the heat and the stench, Davis got hold of his emotions and said, "I've got men on both sides, in front and at the back of the house. No one's getting out of there. As far as I know that woman was only our second kill. *My* kill. God help me, I did that to her!"

"No," Lardis shook his grisly head. "Don't ask your god for help. *She* needed help, and you gave it to her. Also, it was the third kill. We've done one, too. A girl, back there in the garden. So you're not the only one who's feeling sick."

And Jake said, "Who was the other?"

"When I killed . . . that one," Davis answered, with a glance over his shoulder, "there was a scream from the house. A man in a gable window; he ranted and raved at us, tore his hair like a madman. Can't say I blame him. I think the woman must have been his wife. One of my lads fired a grenade in there with him, and it blew the gable to hell. Whoever he was, I'm guessing he went with it. But if he didn't he'll burn anyway. Look."

They looked back, and by then the front of the villa was an inferno. "It'll be the same at the back, said the warrant officer. "They have orders to raze it."

"But that still leaves three to go," said Jake.

"Two," a voice called out, as a man came stumbling from the shadows. He was very pale, and he was carrying his own weapons, someone else's, and a flamethrower. "I got a young guy—I blew the fucker's head off!—but not before he got Bill Powers. My old mate's dead! . . . But there was a girl, too. She got away."

"No," Jake shook his head. "She didn't."

"Two to go," said Lardis. "But where are they?"

Right on cue, their radio headsets came alive in a crackle of static like frying bacon. And: "Shit, shit, *shit!*" a frantic voice called. "Can't anyone fucking hear me?"

And Davis said, "Hawkeye, this is Road Runner. Where've you been?"

"Where've *I* been?" the pilot at once came back, his relief plainly audible, despite that his voice kept fading in and out. "I've been sitting up here listening to you! The radio's on the blink. I'm receiving but having difficulty sending. Now listen, I've also had problems with the thermal-imaging . . . the heat from that bonfire down there. I sorted that, but now there are life-signs at the boat, two of them. If they're not your people, they have to be the ones you're looking for."

"Show us the way to the yacht," Davis snapped, now fully in command again. "But if it gets away from us and makes a run for the sea, take it out. Bomb the bastard right out of the water!"

"Roger that," and the signal faded to nothing—

—But in another moment searchlight beams lanced down from on high, pierced the night and converged, swung west, and traced a path along the channel to the sea. . . .

In Xanadu, fifteen minutes earlier:

Malinari had been tempted from the moment Chopper One descended into the garden. The way it hovered, mere feet above the ground, with its pontoons occasionally touching down, while its task force contingent rapidly disembarked, regrouped into pairs and fanned out toward the casino; all it would have taken was a little pressure—literally the flip of a switch—and Malinari's worst enemies in this world would have been gone forever. Or most of them. Only the group from the vehicle would be left alive, to be dealt with at his convenience.

The way his fingers had caressed the array of switches— almost lovingly, certainly lustfully—it had been a moment of great temptation, yes. But no, it would have been too easy, and this Trask and his men would have learned nothing of terror, or the merest moment of terror, perhaps, before oblivion. And that just wasn't good enough.

Malinari wanted them to understand something of his superiority, wanted them to know they were trapped, even as they had thought to trap him. Then, if there were survivors of his holocaust, and when the flying machine returned to pick them up . . . time enough then for the grand coup de grâce, the final stroke of genius.

And meanwhile, things had progressed more or less as planned, and Malinari employed his mentalism (but as little as possible) to stay in touch with events as they unfurled.

For his telepathy wasn't without its own problems. Indeed, it was a two-edged sword. For one thing, it brought pain: *listening* to the thoughts of others was painful. And for another—and most importantly—Lord Malinari himself, his location in the face of the mountain, might be detected and jeopardized if he were to give full rein to his mentalism. For he had learned something (not enough by any means, but *something*) of the esoteric talents of Trask and this E-Branch from the Föener woman before he'd killed her in the sump of that watercourse. And he had found out a lot more since then, mainly by trial and error.

But it had been a *great* error to open his mind and accept Bruce Trennier's agonized communication—his final communication—when these people tracked him down to the Gibson Desert. For even as Malinari had felt the heat of his lieutenant's funeral pyre, so he'd known a different *kind* of heat: that of discovery, when a probe reached out from halfway around the world to seek him out, zeroing in on him like a Starside bat searching for a juicy moth, or a Sunside hawk stooping to its prey.

A mind had touched his, and left its fingerprint, its signature there, so that he would know it again. And in this last few days he had come to know it only too well. Now it was here in Xanadu, but if he studied it too closely, and if it were to lock on to his location—

—That flying machine, that jet-copter, was equipped with armaments that could cut through the false facade of this hollow chimney like a battle gantlet through the ribs of a disobedient thrall! But it all added to the excitement, the thrill of the game, what little it afforded him: their weird talents, and their puny human minds, against The Mind himself. . . .

So, this seeker, bloodhound, locator, or whatever he was, was one problem—and his talent was one that Nephran Malinari understood readily enough, for he had used just such skills in Sunside four hundred years ago to seek out the Szgany in their hiding places—but the locator's wild talent wasn't the only one that this E-Branch commanded, and it wasn't the only problem. Zek Föener's mind had been full of such things.

A man who could see the future, for example (though obviously he couldn't see it too clearly, else he would never have come here to die,) and Trask himself, to whom a lie was like a slap in the face . . . there would be no deceiving that one! And as for mentalists: no lack of those. Well, that last wasn't so rare; even the Szgany had something of *that* in them. It was in their blood, a legacy of their centuries under Wamphyri domination. But these E-Branch people weren't Szgany. No, they were adepts, much as Malinari was an adept, but lacking the advantage of his several . . . refinements? And of course without the ultimate advantage of being Wamphyri!

Take Zek herself, for instance. What? A woman who could reach out her thoughts across the whole world with such crystal clarity as to be able to speak to a man like Trask— not himself a mentalist—*and* make him to understand? Oh, he was a loved one, and so there had probably been an element of rapport in it, such as is found in twins. But still and all, *that* was a talent!

Or it had been . . .

Adepts, rivals, enemies, and bloodhound trackers who would never let go. All the more reason why *they* must go, and tonight. But it would have been so useful to know more about them first. Such people as this precog, and this locator, and Ben Trask himself . . . *and* this girl.

The girl, yes . . .

She wasn't an adept, not yet; she hadn't attained Zek Föener's level of achievement. But to another telepathic mind (for instance, Malinari's mind) she was like a small flame guttering in the psychic aether, and he had sensed her there from the moment these people arrived in Brisbane. But at such close proximity—*because* she was close now, and inexperienced—he might perhaps intrude for brief periods without fear of her detecting his presence. Of course, that would leave him open to the locator. But only introduce some small diversion into the game, and that would take care of that. Men, even talented men, when they are concerned for their own skins, have little time for casting about with their minds. Except that they look for boltholes, of course.

Very well then, a diversion. For in any case, the game was moving far to slowly.

From his high vantage point, Malinari looked down on Xanadu and the Pleasure Dome Casino (dark in the night but clearly visible in every detail to him) and chose a switch on his array. Down there, his enemies had deployed into first-phase positions. There were men held in reserve, four of them, evenly spaced out at the rear of the leisure area of gardens and pools that surrounded the casino. These four would believe they'd "secured" or "made safe" their strategic positions behind low walls just forward of the innermost circle of chalets. Equipped with superior, heat-seeking, image-enhancing weapons, they would consider themselves "ideally situated" to engage an enemy in flight from the central area.

And so they would be—if not for the fact that two of the four locations were mined.

Malinari's hand lingered over the chosen switch, while his scarlet night-vision eyes swept over, scanned, and committed to memory the second phase of the enemy's deployment.

In the last few minutes a large vehicle—an articulated truck marked with the symbols of a well-known beer manufacturer—had climbed the access road, entered through Xanadu's gates, turned about, and hissed to a halt in the otherwise empty parking lot. A party of four heavily armed men had issued from the rear of the truck and were hurrying forward into the resort in the direction of the Pleasure Dome.

Inwards—at the inner edge of the gardens toward the casino—five NCOs from the helicopter fanned out to surround the huge rotunda of the central dome itself. The men from the truck were now replacing the four in their rearguard positions behind the low walls, which allowed them in their turn to move forward and reinforce the assault force around the dome's perimeter.

Now, or when they were so ordered, three of these Special Forces men would go in through the Pleasure Dome's main doors; the rest of them, dispersed around the perimeter, would create individual points of entry. The casino's curving facade of interlocking concrete panels, glass, and reinforced plastic would scarcely suffice to stop them, Malinari was sure. It was after all a Pleasure Dome, not a fortress!

So much for the fighting men. And Malinari presumed correctly that their commander would be with Trask's E-Branch party where they were now gathered in a group behind the smaller vehicle on the main esplanade some seventy or eighty feet in front of the steps to the casino's canopied entranceway. He knew that this was they because of their mental emanations. *Hah!* But They might as well be carrying illuminated signs! They were as "visible" to him as they must be to the pilot of their flying machine . . . as indeed *he* would be, if he were down in the resort.

So, they were all set to go, and the onset of hostilities, which must be imminent, might create a sufficient diversion in itself, allowing Malinari to insinuate himself into the mentalist girl's mind without alerting the locator to his presence—but he thought not. Much better to be safe than sorry.

Let *them* be the sorry ones.

Earlier, before these people got here, Malinari had started a mist. His body and being—even his existence here in this or any world—these things were all contradictions of Nature. He was a poison that worked like a catalyst on and against any natural or mundane surroundings.

When he opened the pores of his metamorphic body and willed it, his pores would breathe a mist. Not only that but Nature would be made to respond, to answer his call. And even from the dry earth Malinari could call up a writhing mist like vile, airborne sweat, to disguise his presence. In Sunside it had served a dual purpose: to carry his probes more surely to their target (for the mist was like an extension of himself, or a medium for his mentalism), and also to hide him away should he have reason to make a covert exit—in short, a smokescreen.

But this time, so as not to draw attention to himself, he had merely started the thing, set it in motion. And now a fine, milky mist lay on the surface of the pools, and formed a barely visible ground mist in the gardens. But only let Malinari will it, it would spring into being at his command. And in the holocaust to come he would call it up in earnest to carry his mentalism, instill its primal terror, and add to the general confusion.

So then, it was time to set the wheels in motion. Time for his diversion. Time to let these fools know who he was.

He risked a quick, guarded probe, found one of his thralls inside the open doors to the casino, issued a command and withdrew . . . but with no time at all to spare! And even as Malinari felt his probe seized upon—and as he "heard" Chung's gasp of startled recognition: *"What the . . . ?"*—so he tripped the first of his switches. . . .

Six or seven minutes earlier:

Inside the innocuous-looking—but in fact armoured—estate car, Ben Trask, David Chung, Ian Goodly, Liz, and the SAS major were each in their own way concerned. The major because the articulated ops truck and its backup party were some minutes late.

Chopper One had relayed the reason for the delay: the big vehicle's engine had developed a fault; that and the steepness of the climb had combined to slow her down.

"The gradient," Trask said, "but it could have been any of a hundred and one other logistical problems. Well, we made allowances for this kind of last-minute difficulty. It's why we're made up of three contingents: chopper, car, ops truck. Okay, so we're four men short for the time being. But assuming our estimate of Malinari's manpower is accurate, we still outnumber him three or four to one. And our firepower is awesome."

And Chung said, "That bothers me a lot: what you just said about *our* estimate. For the fact is it's *my* estimate, so really it's all down to me."

"No it isn't," Goodly denied it. "It's *our* best estimate, and we're each of us equally involved in this. Or we should be. And anyway, it's like I told Ben earlier: at least your talents are working for you."

Trask looked at him. "Still nothing?"

"Just confusion," the precog answered. "And a feeling."

"You and me both," Trask said, and the others saw that

he was actually chewing his top lip. "A feeling, yes . . . that this is all wrong. Okay, in a deserted resort we'd expect the lights to be out—why waste the energy? But the *silence* of the place, this feeling of a pent-up something, and this inactivity . . ."

"Ours, or theirs?" said Liz.

Trask shook his head. "I don't know—really can't say—what I was expecting. But it certainly wasn't this. I mean, he must know we're here, he has to. So what the hell is he up to? David," he turned to the locator, "got any ideas? Is there any movement? What's going on?"

Chung's high brow was etched into deep lines of concentration. "It's weird as hell," he said. "I'm getting these momentary flashes. It *is* mindsmog, definitely, but from three or four different locations, and I can't pin them down. Up there in the dome, that's one of them for sure. But the others . . ." He looked out of his wound-down window at the night-shrouded cliffs where they climbed to the heights behind the resort, and frowned. "Up high, and down below . . . that's as much as I dare venture."

"Up high would be the bubble on top of the Pleasure Dome," Ian Goodly came in. But Chung only frowned.

"Well, possibly," he said, "for it's as strong a source as any. But there are shields in use, I'm sure of that." And:

"Malinari!" Trask grunted, grimly. "His aerie. Solar-panelled on the outside, painted black, and probably curtained on the inside, for his protection. Well, the murdering bastard will be needing all he can get of that!"

"So that's up high," said Liz, "but what about down below? It looks like Jake was right, and according to the plans of the place it's a real maze down there." And turning to Trask: "Ben, I wish you'd let me try to corroborate David's—"

"No way!" Trask snapped, turning to her at once. "That's right out of the question. No telepathic contact, not with Malinari. Only if it becomes absolutely necessary, *maybe* I'll use you then—but not until. Look, this is a mentalist who ranks alongside Janos Ferenczy. And it's one mind you *won't* be entering of your own free will!"

The E-Branch team had been offered radio headsets; Trask had turned them down, explaining to the major: "Now's the time when our talents come into play and we need clear, uncluttered heads. In the middle of a firefight, it would be too easy for Liz Merrick to confuse a voice in her ear with one in her mind. The same goes for Goodly: we can't afford to have him listening to a headset, so concerned to stay tuned in on what's going on this minute that he fails to see what's coming in the next! As for myself: I smell something fishy here, so when the truth becomes apparent I want to see it right away. I don't want to be distracted by all of that military jargon on the airwaves. And then again, we plan to stick close to you and your men throughout. So while I appreciate the offer, this is one time when the gadgets can really get in the way of the ghosts."

But they did hear the faint crackle of static as suddenly the major held up a hand. And a moment later: "The big artic is in sight." He sighed his relief. "They've had a long hard haul, but they're getting here." As he got out of the car he went on, "It's time we had a little fresh air, but take cover behind the vehicle. We're in a direct line of fire from the casino."

"Absolutely!" Chung agreed, coughing the word up from his suddenly dry throat—*made* dry by the mindsmog that he'd detected even as the major was speaking. "And up those steps, right in through those doors," he went on, "that's another source!"

"You're sure?" The major grasped his elbow.

"In there," Chung began to sweat. "Somebody—something—is waiting!" And in fact, and despite that it was cool and even chilly now, they were all sweating.

Abandoning radio procedure, the major spoke into his headset. "You men on the doors had better be aware. There's a reception party waiting for you. Before you go in there, a couple of stun grenades might help clear the way a bit. The rest of you: if you missed it from Hawkeye, here's a sitrep:

the backup has arrived. The next time you hear from me it will probably be the go ahead. Stand by for that, over?"

"Roger that," a multitude of terse, tense replies came in, then more static and radio silence. . . .

Seconds ticked by, but oh-so-slowly. Then:

There came the rumbling growl of a straining motor, a hissing of air-brakes, and finally the message that the major had been waiting for: "Zero, this is the backup squad. Sorry we're late. We're moving into our locations now."

The major turned to Trask, said, "The show's about to commence. Anything you'd like to say to them?"

"Your men?" Trask shook his head. "Just wish them the best of luck." And the major did it.

And Trask thought, *Damn it! I don't even know this bloke's name! Some of his men, but not him. But that's how it goes with these people. In their way they're much like E-Branch: the less we know about them, the better their security.*

There was swift, sporadic movement in the night: the shadowy figures of men, keeping low, moving forward, strengthening the assault force surrounding the casino. Using nite-lite binoculars, the major watched them take up their positions, turned to Trask and said, "Are we ready?"

Trask nodded. "Let's do it," he said. "Christ, the longer we wait, the worse it feels!"

"Right," said the major. And then, into his headset, "This is Zero to assault group. We're going in. *Attack! Attack! Attack!* At which all hell broke loose—if not exactly as expected—and it all seemed to happen at once.

The locator David Chung gave a massive start. As his eyes opened wide, he pointed at something—some nonspecific point high on the face of the cliffs at the rear of the resort—and gripped Trask's elbow. And as Trask looked at him in astonishment, Chung gasped, *"What the . . . ?"*

At the same time:

Fifty or so feet behind the group where they sheltered on the "safe" side of the armoured car, a ball of brilliant light lit the night; following hot on its heels, there came the deafening roar of an explosion, and the death cry of a soldier.

The savagery of the blast was such that it hurled them all against the side of the car and rocked the vehicle on its shock absorbers. All eyes blinked, and hands were thrown up to shield startled faces. Then, as debris began to rain down, they looked back. The SAS man was in midair, a human catherine wheel spinning there—torn almost in half, black and burning—and quite obviously dead.

Bricks from the low wall where the NCO had taken cover—which had at least sheltered Trask and his group from the worst of the blast—were showering down; a jagged half-brick struck Chung on the forehead, threw him a second time against the side of the car. He slid to the ground in a hail of lesser debris.

"Jesus Christ!" the major straightened up, went to stagger toward the spot where his man's body lay in a crumpled, smoking heap. Trask stopped him, croaked:

"You saw what I saw. You can't help him now."

"But what the hell . . . ?" The major asked helplessly, of no one in particular. "A mortar, a grenade—an accident? Jesus, it must have been a fucking accident!"

And meanwhile, the night had come deafeningly alive.

From the casino, a withering stream of automatic fire sent bullets ricochetting off the far side of the car, and from somewhere in the night a soldier shouted, "I'm hit! God—I'm hit!" It hardly sounded like the cry of a man, but more like a small, bewildered child.

Then the casino's entrance was lit by twin balls of brilliant white light—the blinding flashes and shattering reports of stun grenades—and figures were glimpsed briefly, silhouetted in the swift-dying glare.

There were explosions from all around the Pleasure Dome as two-man units hurled grenades to breach the outer wall and gain entry, and covering fire as men went in through smoking holes.

"We have to go in, too," said the major. "We need to know what's going on. But first let's see to your man."

They laid Chung on the rear seat of the car. Mumbling to

himself, the locator was already regaining consciousness. The major gave Liz a field dressing, said, "Staunch the blood. He looks okay, but stay with him. Where's your gun?"

Liz took out her Baby Browning, cocked it and laid it on the rear windowsill of the car within easy reach.

Trask leaned inside the car to touch her shoulder. "You'd better do as he says," he said. "And when we're gone, lock the doors." For the moment shaken, disoriented, and concerned for Chung, Liz did as she was told. Through the window, she watched the major, Trask, and Goodly move off toward the casino.

In a little while Chung opened his eyes, looked up at Liz and said, "He's up there . . . up high . . . Malinari!" He managed to lift himself up a little as she applied the field dressing. He was looking at (or perhaps looking beyond?) the casino. The way he rolled his not-quite-focussed eyes, it was hard to tell.

"The bubble on top of the dome?" Liz answered, and nodded an affirmative. "We know. They're going in after him now."

"No!" The locator tried to shake his head. "Not the Pleasure Dome, but up there! Up . . . up there . . ."

"Up there?" Liz had the dressing in place now. Tying off the bandage, she looked where Chung pointed a shaky hand. "The mountain?"

"The cliffs," he mumbled. "He's . . . *he's in the cliffs!*

After that it was all instinct, and almost instantaneous. Liz didn't think twice but sent out her telepathic thoughts to follow Chung's line of sight, to be guided like a laser-assisted missile to his target. Except that in this case the target was far more dangerous than the missile. And:

Ahhhhhh! said a voice in Liz's mind—a voice like steam escaping from a kettle, or the hiss of a volcanic vent—*It's the sweet little telepath herself!* And Liz could actually feel the patterns of her mind being scrutinized, fingerprinted, and memorized. She erected shields and felt the hideous, sluglike presence of Malinari withdrawing, dwindling, gone! Then:

"My God!" She exploded into frantic activity, grabbed her

gun, scrambled backwards out of the car. "I have to tell Ben!" But then, pausing to lean back inside: "David, I—"

"It's okay." Chung was really coming out of it now, beginning to make good sense. "Go find them, Liz, and tell them Malinari's in those cliffs. If they call the chopper down, and get the pilot to use thermal-imaging, he'll spot the bastard easily enough." He managed to sit up, however groggily.

"Lock the doors when I've gone," she told him. And crouching down low, she ran for the casino. . . .

33
Trapped!

CHOPPER ONE'S PILOT HAD HEARD THE MAJOR'S call for action, seen the explosions, heard something of the messages passing between the men on the ground. The assault on the Pleasure Dome was proceeding just a few minutes behind schedule; it was time to give the ground forces a little aerial support. Bright searchlight beams—aimed inwards on the casino, to blind anyone trying to escape from that place—swept down from above.

Like all the rest of the attacking force, Liz wore phosphorescent patches front and rear of her combat suit. It wouldn't do for anyone to be shot dead by "friendly" fire. Lit up like human neon, gun in hand, she ran toward the doors at the top of the steps. Hanging askew, the doors were still giving off smoke from the grenades. Of soldiers there was no sign, but she could hear the occasional burst of gunfire from within. . . .

A few minutes earlier, not far inside the same shattered doorway, Trask, Goodly, and the major had found a wounded NCO sitting on the floor with his back to a slot machine. He had taken a bullet in the leg but had seen to the wound himself. "This'll keep," he told them through gritted teeth. "I'm okay here—but you should take this with you." Trask accepted the man's flamethrower and pack, and the precog helped him into the gear. The wounded man retained his machine-pistol; when they left he was slapping a fresh clip into the magazine housing.

Then, moving deeper into the smoky gloom of the place, the major spoke into his headset: "This is Zero. My group is inside the main doors and advancing. Sitreps, over?"

And the answers came back:

"Zero, this is Alpha Group. We're on the stairs on the far side, going up one level. No opposition."

"Zero, this is Bravo Group. Stairs your side, going up one level. No opposition."

"Zero, this is Charlie. We're ahead of you toward the central spindle. We have a man down inside the doors—and we just found something nasty."

"Zero for Charlie, how nasty?"

"Charlie for Zero, not life-threatening—but nasty."

"Zero for Charlie, we saw your man," said the major. "He's okay . . . but you should have taken his flamer."

"Charlie for Zero, we couldn't stop. We're in hot pursuit. Our target is still in here somewhere. Toward the elevators, we think."

"Zero for Charlie, wait there," said the major, and moved on with Trask and Goodly close behind.

Throughout the casino's ground floor, mainly on the perimeter, several hissing phosphor flares had been lit; they gave light but also made smoke, which in turn made for a very eerie, shadow-etched atmosphere. Charlie group (which was now made up of just two men, W.O. II Red Bygraves and an NCO) was waiting midway between the doors and the central column of elevators. And indeed they had found something nasty. Zeroing in on their reflective patches, the major's group of three found the soldiers keeping well back from their gruesome discovery.

Hanging by its ankles, upside down from a chandelier, the corpse of a thin, spidery male figure turned slowly on a triple loop of electrical cable. The man's throat had been cut ear to ear, and his flesh was like snow, drained of blood. But on the floor, only a very few scarlet droplets had been spilled. . . .

Despite that the body was inverted, Trask recognized him at once. "Liz Merrick's watcher," he said grimly. "So much for working for a vampire! This will have to be burned. On our way out we'll burn this whole *fucking* place!" And the major turned to him and said:

"Trask, steady up now, okay? Now listen, all of you. This group is now five strong. We're all armed and we have a flamer. We have men climbing the perimeter stairs, closing them off. We know our main target's trapped in the bubble on top of the casino, and that he has at least one soldier, guardian, or—" He looked to Trask for help.

"Thrall," Trask told him hoarsely. "Call him a thrall."

"One thrall," the major went on, "—the one you men were pursuing—watching his back down here; which might mean that he was guarding the elevators to keep his boss safe. So that's where we're heading, the elevators. But remember: this guy has the advantage of being able to see in the dark; and your flak-jackets only give you so much protection. So spread yourselves out, but stay well within sight and sound of each other." As he finished, the major turned and headed deeper into the casino. And the others spread out on his flanks.

Shortly, the central hexagonal column of elevators became visible, and at the same time the stutter of automatic gunfire sounded from ahead. Ripping into a row of silent slot machines, the stream of bullets was like an invisible buzz-saw that gutted them and spilled their coins on the floor. Then the raking fire found Bygraves and lifted him clean off his feet. Shot in the right shoulder, injured, but by no means fatally, the W.O. went down in a stream of bright silver, a splash of bloodred, and his own cries of disgust and frustration.

And in the central area, close to an elevator door marked PRIVATE, there stood a flame-eyed Thing in human form, cradling a gun that spat fire one more time before the major sent a single bullet in through his left eye. Swatted, the vampire thrall thudded backwards against the elevator doors; his feet slid out from under him, and he sank down onto the floor in a seated position.

While Bygraves's subordinate went to his aid, Trask and the others approached the vampire thrall. One of Malinari's pair of minders, he obviously had to be dead . . . but wasn't. As his right eye opened, burning yellow in the gloom, so he toppled onto his side, turned himself facedown, and began to claw his way erratically away from the elevators. In another moment, however, the effort became too much for him. He came to a halt, coughed once or twice, and slurred out the words, "Oh, fuck it!"

He had dropped his gun and no longer posed any real threat. He looked up at Trask and his colleagues, and his clenched left hand jerked and twitched where he reached out towards them. His left eye was a gaping black hole oozing blood and pulped brains, and the rest of his face was a red-and grey-smeared mess.

But as the major stood back a little and took careful aim, so the thrall's hand opened and he dropped a metal key onto the floor. Then he gurgled, "This is wh-what you want, right? So go on, f-finish it. Then find *that* fucker and f-finish h-h-him."

The major didn't have to finish it. For as the man's head slumped to the floor, so a gush of blood and morbid fluid erupted from his ruined eye, and he jerked once more and was done.

Trask had called the elevator; as the doors opened, Goodly picked up the key, and the major called out to Bygraves's subordinate: "Try to get the W.O. out of here. And see if your number three is okay. We're going upstairs." He got in the elevator with Trask and Goodly.

The push-button control panel in the rear wall of the elevator had buttons for two basement levels, the ground floor, and floors one and two; plus two keyholes, one of which was marked PRIVATE–UP. The other keyhole was unmarked. The precog looked at the key in his hand and said, "Couldn't be simpler . . . could it?"

"Too simple by far," Trask growled. "And we've been losing men left right and centre."

"Your talent?" said the major. "You're still uneasy?"

"Worried sick!" Trask answered. "The whole thing is wrong. But we're committed now." He gave Goodly a nod, and the precog put the key in the UP hole and turned it. . . .

Liz had found the wounded NCO inside the Pleasure Dome's main doors and helped him out of the casino into the fresh air. She had thought he might be able to call down Chopper One, but his radio had been damaged when he was hit. When she'd left him to go back inside, he had told her that when he'd last seen Trask and his party they'd been heading toward the central elevators. Then he had warned her that for all he knew the vampire sniper who had shot him was still on the loose in there.

Going back into the casino, and knowing what might be waiting for her, Liz had not dared to call out after Trask. By that time some of the flares had burned out, leaving it much smokier and a lot darker in there. So that when she'd heard noises from deep inside—shouting, shots, and crashing sounds—she'd taken a circuitous route in the hope of avoiding trouble. In so doing, she had somehow managed to bypass Red Bygraves and his man on their way out.

But intent as Liz was on what she was doing—finding Ben Trask, and relaying Chung's message—her telepathic guard was down. Which was precisely the opening that Nephran Malinari had been waiting for.

Ben, where are you? she anxiously wondered, as she saw the hexagonal spindle of the elevator column looming ahead. But of course Trask wasn't a telepath, and Liz's probe (if she'd actually sent one, *if* she had even tried to, for in fact she'd simply been talking to herself, a natural response to her circumstances like whistling in the dark) would go unanswered.

Or it should have gone unanswered. But:

Liz? (it was Ben Trask's voice—his telepathic voice?—in her head!) *Is that you, Liz? But . . . can you hear me? If so, please listen. You've got to help us. We've got ourselves trapped down here, behind a bulkhead that only opens from the other side. Your side, that is. But there's been shooting and now the place is burning. We'll burn, too, Liz, if you can't reach us!*

She could actually feel the heat behind his mental S.O.S., could almost see the flames, it was so brilliantly clear. Clear like never before. So perhaps Jake was right: her talent really was growing stronger minute by minute! Yes, it must be so. And:

Ben, she sent. *But how can I reach you? Where are you?*

Down here, he answered. *Down in the guts of the place. You can reach us via the elevators. It's the only way.*

In the guts of the place? Underground in that maze of tunnels and pipes? At which she instinctively glanced at the floor . . . and at the ghastly figure of a dead man, who lay there with his brains trickling out through his eye.

Liz jumped a foot, but Ben had obviously seen through her eyes and quickly said: *We got that one, and followed the others down here. But you'll be safe because they're on the other side of the fire. Use the elevator, Liz, the one marked* PRIVATE. *But please hurry!*

She had already called the elevator, and anxiously watched the tiny indicator lights bringing it down to the ground floor. But bringing it down? Well, the military must have used it. For of course, the whole place would have to be checked out.

The doors opened and she got in, and the voice—Trask's voice, in Liz's mind—said: *Is there a key in one of the keyholes?* He sounded even more anxious, urgent now, and his voice was tinged with something else . . . anticipation, maybe? But of course it was! She had given him hope, and he was looking forward to being rescued.

A key, yes, she told him. *In the* UP *slot.*

Take it out, he said. *Use the other keyhole. Turn the key ninety degrees clockwise. But quickly, Liz, quickly!*

She did as instructed. And the cage descended, taking her down, down, down. . . .

On Jethro Manchester's island, Jake Cutter, Lardis Lidesci, and Joe Davis arrived at the open-ended, roofed-over section of the man-made channel that housed the millionaire's yacht—in effect a boathouse—midway between the villa and the sea. Hearing voices in heated argument, they split up and Davis took the far side of the structure, while Jake and the Old Lidesci crept up on that end of the boathouse closest to the burning villa.

The lock gates were open, but the yacht was still tied up. Both the boat and the ceiling of the flat-roofed structure were illuminated by their own lights. On the canopied deck, just aft of the cabin, two men faced each other down. The one was older, taller, white-haired and -bearded. Dressed in a khaki shirt and shorts, he looked almost military in his proud, upright stance. This was Jethro Manchester himself, Jake knew. The younger man, who was holding a shotgun on the first, was shorter, stockier; but his hard, leathery, sun-beaten features were very much similar to Bruce Trennier's, his older brother's, which Jake would never be able to forget.

"Martin," Manchester's voice rang out in the night, "can't you see it's all over and you can't run from these people? Man, you're like a walking plague, a pestilence—you and me both—but a far worse pestilence than any in the Bible! And would you take *that* among the people? I see that you would. Well, and why not, for you brought it down on me and mine! That was sheer *treachery,* Martin! So say and do what you like, you won't be taking my boat. She's mine and she goes with me . . . wherever."

Manchester had a jerrycan in both hands; as he had spoken, so he had been splashing its contents on the deck. The smell of diesel was unmistakable.

"Jethro, I'm not forgetting that I owe you," Martin Trennier spoke up. "It's the only reason you're still alive while we stand here and argue like this. But you're wrong to think this is the end of everything. It's only the beginning! You were the last to be taken—after he'd used your family to get his way—after he'd promised that he would give it all back, and cure us of this thing. Well, he's a liar, as we've seen, and he made me take you, too. But you were the last and it's still taking hold of you. When it does, and when it has fully taken hold—which it will!—then you'll know I was right. So stand aside and let me get on. Or better still, come with me and let's see what we can make of things together."

As he had spoken, Trennier had stepped to the port side of the boat to cast off a rope. But Manchester had taken the opportunity to pick up a second jerrycan. This time, before he could begin spilling its contents, Trennier stepped close and knocked it out of his hands. And now he trained his weapon dead centre on Manchester's body.

"I've no time for this, Jethro," he growled. "You can come with me now, or stay here. You can live or you can die. One way or the other, it's your choice. So what's it to be?"

Manchester took out a cigarette lighter from the pocket of his shorts. He flicked it once—and it failed to spark! Trennier cursed, but he wasn't about to give the older man a second chance. Sending the butt of his weapon crashing into Manchester's face, jostling him to the side of the boat, finally he succeeded in knocking him overboard. And as Manchester swam toward the side of the channel, so Trennier clung to the deck rail, leaned out over the water, and fired his weapon at almost point-blank range.

Which was as far as Jake was willing to let it go. He and Joe Davis acted together. Davis ran in under the far end of the boathouse, firing on the yacht as he came, and Jake ran to meet him, skidding to a halt on his knees to play the roaring, searing lance of his flamethrower on both the vessel and the man on her deck.

Trennier fired another shot, and another—fired blindly, through the shimmering fire that enveloped and ate into him—while the boat literally erupted in flames and he turned into a jet-black, shrieking silhouette, dancing in agony until finally he crumpled down into himself and lay still.

As Jake shut off his lance, there came the sound of feeble

splashing from the channel. It was Manchester. The flesh at the back of his head, his neck, and across his shoulders was a livid, liquid red. "Let me out!" he cried, climbing sunken steps. "Let me out and finish it then, but not in the water. I lived in the water—lived *for* the water—so I don't want to die in it."

And when he was out, and staggering on dry land, Jake told him, "Mr. Manchester, we heard everything. And we're sorry."

"I know you are," Manchester nodded his bloody head. "Yes, and I'm glad you came. My family . . . is no more, and I . . . have no reason or right to be here." With which he held out his arms in the shape of a cross, stood there and closed his feral eyes.

Then Joe Davis gritted his teeth, and cut the old man down with accurate, merciful shooting; the Old Lidesci went in close and used his machete; and finally, making *absolutely* sure, Jake finished it with roaring fire. By which time both the yacht and the structure that housed it were a mass of leaping flames, and the three backed away, leaning on each other while they watched it all burn.. . . .

In a little while Davis's radio crackled, and call signs began asking him, was it all over? He told them yes, called down Chopper Two, told everyone they could start mopping up. But as he and his party began to make their way back towards the villa:

"What?" said Jake, whirling on the balls of his feet. His eyes were wide and darting, searching here and there across the sculpted landscape of the gardens, and his ruddily-lit face was shocked and puzzled. "Liz?" But then his eyes went wider still, in sudden understanding.

It *was* Liz he'd heard calling for him, yes, but she wasn't here . . . she was in Xanadu!

Jake! Jake, if you can hear me (her telepathic voice was a tiny, terrified whisper huddling in a corner of his mind), *then please,* please *come and get me out of here!*

And behind her sweet voice another—but a loathsome,

gurgling thing—like hot tar bubbling in some medieval tor-
turer's cauldron: *Ah, no, my little thought-thief. No one can
help you now. You thought to use your mentalism against
me, but Malinari has used it against you! I have lied to Ben
Trask—impossible, but I have done it—and I've located and
lost your locator. As for your marvelous precog: he senses
nothing but confusion, for the death and destruction that he
foresaw was his own and yours and Xanadu's, but never
mine! And now there's this Jake—your lover, perhaps? But
where is he? Oh, ha ha haaaaaa!*

"Jesus!" Jake moaned. But he knew what he must do. *Korath!* he called out into the deadspeak aether. And:

About time, said that one. *But first tell me, do we have a
deal, you and I, as prescribed? Do you willingly give me
access to your mind?*

There was no way around it, and no time to argue. And
so: *Yes!* said Jake. *Anything! Only show me those numbers.*

So be it, said Korath. And Jake's inner being lit up like a
lamp, as those impossible numbers scrolled in not-quite-
endless progression down the computer screen of his mind.
But not *quite* endlessly, because he instantly recognized a
pattern and suddenly, "instinctively" knew where to freeze
it. Then:

A door! And:

Go! said Korath. *And I go with you. . . .*

Jake went—stepped in through the door—vanished from
the view of Lardis Lidesci and Joe Davis, and was gone.

"What?" Davis stood stock-still, frozen in his amazement.
And for a moment even Lardis was lost for words, astonished
as ever by this thing. But then he recovered and said:

"Pay no attention. It's a trick he does. Just an optic—er,
an optical—er . . ."

"An optical illusion?" Davis's jaw hung slack.

"Aye, something like that," Lardis said, gratefully. "Er, but
we needn't expect him back. He has his own ways of getting
about, that one." And once again, with a knowing, emphatic
nod of his grizzled head, "Aye!" he said.

*   *   *

In the ultimate, primal darkness of the Möbius Continuum, Jake whirled like a leaf in a gale. "BUT WHERE TO?" he said, and was nearly deafened as his words gonged like the clappers of a mad, gigantic bell.

The thought itself would appear to be sufficient, Korath told him, awed in his own right. *For I sense this place is the very essence of nothingness, wherefore physical speech— which is something—is forbidden here. But deadspeak, being as nothing, is permissible.*

Jake steadied himself—discovered that he *could* actually steady himself—and repeated, *Where to?* He could feel the Continuum tugging on him, and believed he knew where it would take him if he gave it the chance: Harry's Room, at E-Branch HQ. But that wasn't where he wanted to go.

Who is it you are concerned for? Korath remained logical.

Liz, of course! She had called out to Jake—asked for his help—and her telepathic voice had been a beacon. Now he remembered it, remembered its coordinates, and *went* to her. It was as simple as that. At least the *going* there was simple, but the rest of it wasn't.

When the door formed, Jake didn't know how to make an exit and so simply crashed through it. Into a living nightmare!

It was a room, shaft or cavern, but its lighting after the Stygian darkness of the Möbius Continuum was glaring, brilliant, blinding. Overbalanced as gravity returned (by the sudden, unaccustomed weight of the flamethrower), tripping and flying headlong into a wall, and rebounding, Jake landed on something soft and squirmy. . . .

. . . Something that cried its terror, and two seconds later wrapped its arms around him.

"Jake, oh Jake!" Liz gasped, holding tightly to him on the one hand, but wriggling and kicking desperately away from something on the other. Her Baby Browning was clenched in her fist, and she kept aiming it and pulling the trigger— *click! click! click!*—as the firing pin fell on blank space. A pair of empty clips lay on the sandy floor where she'd discharged and discarded them.

It was the strip lighting that had blinded Jake, that and his dizzying, head-over-heels emergence from the Möbius Continuum. Now, as his head stopped spinning, he saw what had turned this determined, self-possessed, assertive woman into a frightened little girl again: weird, morbid motion.

The floor of the place was alive . . . or undead!

Jake could scarcely take it in—scarcely believe what he was seeing—but he had to, and quickly.

The cavern was the size of a large room. A planked walkway crossed the centre of the floor and disappeared into tunnels at both ends. On the other side of the walkway, maybe fifteen feet away, the floor was . . . different. It was humped, veined, corrugated . . . and mobile. And it wasn't the floor!

Something tossed and turned—or *churned*—there. Something throbbed and gulped and gasped. It was a fleshy, flopping octopus of a thing; an immense doughy pancake of metamorphic flesh, throwing up purple-veined extrusions that groped blindly in the air before collapsing back down into the bulk of . . . of *It!* The colour of dead flesh in its main mass, it squelched, fumed, and stank like gas bubbles bursting in a swamp. And mindlessly, aimlessly, it worked at fashioning its ropy extensions.

Or perhaps not mindlessly. For as Jake sat there cradling Liz, so the thing extruded a tentacle that came whipping across the walkway to rear before them in a questioning, semi-sentient fashion. It pulsed, vibrated, *and an eye formed in its tip!* The eye was a uniform red, lidless, apparently vacant—yet it must be seeing or sensing something. For as Liz shrilled and started pulling the trigger again—*click! click! click!*—so a second tentacle emerged and lengthened in their direction.

As it came, a row of greedy, suctorial mouths rippled into metamorphic being along its length. They slobbered and grimaced those mouths—and they had human teeth! But far worse, some of them were reforming, shaping themselves into tumescent, purple-veined penises!

Jake felt rooted to the spot, for the moment paralysed. It seemed to him that the whole mass of the thing beyond the walkway was now on the move, edging towards him—and certainly towards Liz! And that was enough.

He unfroze, fought Liz off, brought up the flamethrower's nozzle and squeezed the trigger to get its pilot light going—then cursed vividly as nothing happened, and squeezed it again, and again, and yet again, before it lit—then gripped the firing lever and applied a steady, deadly pressure.

First Jake aimed down between his spread legs, aimed at the rearing pseudopods to drive them back, and his relief was immense as he watched them burst into flames and shrivel in the incandescent, pressured heat of his lance. Then he scrambled to his feet, and with Liz dancing close behind, clutching his combat jacket and urging him on, so he advanced toward the walkway and the bulk of the thing that hissed and steamed and shuddered its agony there.

And as the tentacles writhed, dripped their fluids, blackened and shrank—and as the main body withdrew into itself—there, sprouting in the floor where its bulk had protected them, clusters of small black mushrooms, dozens of them, were melting in the chemical fire. Their smell was nauseating, but Jake kept on firing; kept cursing, too, as Malinari's "garden" burned.

But this was vampire stuff, tenacious and defiant.

The shrinking body of the mass burst open, and a steaming head—a human, or almost-human head, and shoulders—grew out of it. Again Jake felt himself gripped by a paralysis of disbelief. Yet the nightmare was here and undeniably real.

But so was Korath here, and so was he real. And in Jake's mind as the livid vampire head took shape: *It is him!* Korath's deadspeak voice hissed. *Demetrakis Mindsthrall, who was Malinari's lieutenant, second only to myself! Because he had been a vampire for long and long, Malinari used him to make this garden. It must be so, for only the most contaminated flesh could ever have produced a crop such as this! Ah, but just think. If there had been no Demetrakis, then this would be me! And so it seems I got the better of the bargain after all . . .*

"Whoever it was, it's time he died," said Jake.

Aye, Korath agreed. *The true death. I know he would thank you for it.* And Jake hosed fire on the terrible thing where it mewled and melted, until his torch began to sputter.

Then he eased back on the flamer's lever, to see what damage he'd done, and if he had done enough. The cave steamed and smoked but was mainly still—except in one badly lit corner. There was some slight movement there, and Jake advanced across the smoking floor, making sure as he went that he stepped only where there was no sign of contamination.

But as he approached the corner: "H-help me!" the faintest of whispers reached out to him. "H-h-help me, *pleeeease!*"

A single short burst of fire from the flamethrower chased back the shadows, then a longer burst, to allow for confirmation of what Jake had seen. And indeed he *needed* such confirmation.

From the neck up the thing in the corner was a man . . . and from there on down it *had been* a man. But now the eyes in that purple, once-arrogant, once-querulous face were bulging, staring, terrified—and they were filled with such agony as Jake could only imagine.

As for the "body" of this thing: that was a slumped, naked heap of limbless, alien flesh similar to the composition of the monstrous guardian of Malinari's garden. And Jake couldn't stop his gorge rising—felt sick to his stomach—as it dawned on him in a sudden burst of loathing that this mutated abnormality was once a man, and that it or he had been converted into live *nourishment* for the garden and its guardian!

Finger-thick, pulsing, translucent arteries—like fleshy worms—even now connected the two forms, and toward the centre of the cave where Jake's fire had seared and split the guardian open, spurts of yellow and crimson plasma went to waste, fountaining uselessly in the smoky air.

All of which was bad enough, but worse by far was the fact that Jake knew who this travesty of a human being had been.

That Peter Miller "lived" in his condition—if this could

be called life—and that he was capable of realizing his fate and asking for help, was a miracle in itself. But it was also a curse that Jake would wish on no man, not even his worst enemy.

For this was worse than any death, compared to which death would be a blessing. And when Miller found strength to ask once more, "Please . . . please *help* me!" then Jake was happy to grant his request. It didn't take long, but it used up the last dregs of the flamer's fuel.

When it was over, Jake steadied himself and turned to Liz. But still his face was ashen as he asked, "Where now?"

"You can actually do it?" Almost back in possession of herself, still Liz clutched his jacket. "The Möbius Continuum?"

"Yes," he told her. "We . . . I mean I, can do it."

"The bubble dome," she told him. "Ben is up there. There's something I have to tell him. We walked right into a trap, Jake, all of us, and I think that we're still in danger. Malinari was in my mind, imitating Ben! But at the end—just before he left me in this place—then for a moment I was in *his* mind! Telepathy is a two-way thing, but my forte is as a receiver. And Malinari . . . he was oh so *sure* of himself! I think that maybe he's sabotaged this place! I sensed it there, in his mind."

"When you called out to me," Jake answered, "I heard something of what he said to you. You're right: he seemed very sure of himself. Perhaps too sure."

And Liz nodded and repeated, "The dome, on top of the casino. Take us there."

"Hold on to me," Jake told her, for he had flown over Xanadu and knew the coordinates. And Korath knew the numbers. . . .

In his vantage point in the cliff, Malinari allowed his fingers to drift over the array of switches and pondered his choice. By now the girl was being absorbed into his garden, and that was a shame . . . that he hadn't been able to stay with her, within her mind, to explain what was happening to her and feel her terror; but no, for he had other things to do.

His mist was up; it lay knee-deep, swirling through Xanadu from one end of the resort to the other. It was like a spider's web, that mist, carrying every faintest tremor back to its master and maker. A medium for his probes, it allowed him to touch the human flies that were "trapped" within it; he knew the location of every man in Xanadu. But there were those for whom no mist was needed.

The locator for one: injured, holding his head, he sat inside that car down there . . . such a pity the area wasn't mined. Then there was the so-called precog, and Ben Trask, together in the bubble. At this close range their talents were like magnets drawing Malinari's attention to the topmost dome; he could feel them there! But the bubble *was* mined; all it wanted was a touch on a certain switch in his array.

And again his hand hovered tantalizingly over that central switch. . . . But no, he must stick to the original plan, let them know the error of their ways before they died. First the perimeter, to let them see how truly he had trapped them, and then he would work inwards, leaving the bubble itself until the last.

And now his fingers were sure and fast, as one by one they tripped the outer ring of switches. . . .

Through the wound-down window of the car, the locator was suddenly aware of a strange figure approaching out of the mist. The mist was very bad here, drifting over the car and obscuring his vision. But Chung had been in far worse places, and he was equipped with a machine-pistol.

The strangely lumbering, mist-wreathed figure came closer, and the sights of Chung's weapon were centered upon it. Then he saw the blaze of a reflective patch, sighed, and allowed himself to slump a little. It was a soldier—an NCO, carrying another soldier in the fireman's lift position, which accounted for the many-armed, monstrous silhouette. As that fact dawned, so Chung was out of the vehicle, calling out:

"Over here! Bring him to the car." Then, behind the two, a third figure came weaving, on his feet but barely so.

Recognizing the staggering loner as Warrant Officer Red Bygraves, the locator went to meet him. "Are you okay?" He got under the other's left arm, took his weight. "Can I help you?"

"I'll live," Bygraves growled. And then, seeing the eagerness, the urgency in the locator's eyes: "What is it?"

"Your radio," Chung said. "Is it working, and can you call the chopper down? I know where the bastard is! I know where Malinari's hiding!"

Bygraves's eyes lit up with a fierce, fighting light. Gritting his teeth, and flicking his face mike with a fingernail to get Chopper One's attention, he told the locator, "Oh, I'll get him down okay. Just tell me where you want him to lay down his fire, that's all . . ."

From what little Trask, Goodly, and the SAS major could see of the interior of the bubble dome, it was a sumptuously appointed split-level affair of marble, chrome, and tan-coloured leather. Five marble-clad stanchions surrounded the single elevator tube and supported the high ceiling. The elevator opened into a central well, with concentric steps climbing to the living or work area. The place was lit, however dimly, by a sprinkling of tiny blue lights which formed, against the ceiling's jet-black backdrop, miniature constellations in a fair imitation of the night sky. Blue-tinged, the dusky-velvet atmosphere reminded Trask of nothing so much as a Starside night, which made the bubble seem even more an aerie.

That, however, was the extent of Trask's and his colleagues' knowledge of the place; for from the moment of their arrival when the elevator doors had hissed open, they had been under fire and pinned down. In fact their exit from the elevator cage—which in any event had been planned as a rapid deployment—had been hastened by a volley of shots that had sounded as soon as the doors were fully open, and a spray of bullets that chipped splinters from the marble columns where the three had taken shelter. All of which had felt very wrong to Trask.

He and the others had made such ideal targets in the elevator's confined space, he just couldn't imagine anyone missing his aim . . . especially someone who had been waiting for them to emerge from that precise spot! Yet no one had been hit, though for several nerve-wracking minutes now they had been obliged to keep their heads down to avoid sporadic single shots.

Thus, deep down inside Trask sensed (or his talent advised him) that he and his colleagues were being played with; or that they were simply being *played,* reeled in, like so many sardines on a single line. And he knew they dared not allow this stalemate to continue to the enemy's prearranged conclusion.

Now, as he glanced across the well of curving steps at the dark figures of the precog and the major crouching behind their individual columns, he wondered what to do next.

As for the sniper (if anyone so inept was worthy of such a title), it seemed that he must be a man or a vampire alone. All of his weapon's muzzle-flashes had been sighted in just the one location on the higher level, and there had been no other sound or movement from anywhere else. And Trask sensed, he just *knew,* that whoever this was, it wasn't Malinari.

But then it came to him that indeed there had been another sound: muted, repetitious music that came from one glowing spot, an antique jukebox, in the velvet darkness of the higher level. And the music—a plaintive song—was only repetitious in that it had been playing when first they'd arrived, had played again while they were pinned down, and was now into its second encore, curtain call, or whatever.

But curtain call? A farewell? Some kind of message, maybe? And for the first time Trask listened to the song. A moderately fast-paced and yet bluesy ballad, it was sung by Ray Charles, a favourite from Trask's youth:

"Sunshine, you may find my window but you won't find me. . . ."

And now it seemed to Trask that the coffee, sex, and cigarettes voice mocked not only the sun but also Ben Trask himself. For indeed sunshine might find the high blind windows of Malinari's aerie, but it certainly wouldn't find Malinari! Nor would Trask. The song *was* a message; but more yet, it was the mocking laughter of a monster! It mocked Trask, E-Branch, the military, and all their combined efforts.

So that now, in the heightened anxiety of this sudden knowledge, he used the temporary lull between shots to shout across to the major: "We have to get done here. So what's next?"

The major had not been idle; he'd been working out the sniper's position for himself, and now believed he'd got it right. Lighting a flare, and a moment later pulling the pin on a grenade, he called out, "This is what's next. Hit the deck— *now!*"

The warning was timely. Even with his eyes tightly closed and sheltered by the column, still Trask saw the blinding white light blossoming through the membrane of his eyelids . . . and at the same time he heard and indeed *felt* the terrific report that shook the floor and shattered glass fixtures into flying shards. Then there was a stunned silence and cordite stench, and at the last a mewling whimper rising to a scream.

A tattered male figure came staggering, wreathed in smoke, himself smoking. His eyes were feral in the gloom. And the major, Trask, and Goodly didn't wait to see what he would do or if he was capable of doing anything, but cut him down in a withering crossfire.

"We got him! We got Malinari!" The major stood up, started forward up the marble steps. But as the precog and Trask joined him, the latter was already shaking his head.

"That isn't Malinari," Trask coughed a denial into the now smoky atmosphere. "And this isn't over yet. The elevator's gone and we're trapped. Trapped by the very creature we're trying to destroy. . . ."

His words were portentous of the sudden thunder, the gouting fire and blazing light that at once rocked the night beyond the shattered windows. The three men looked at each other, then hurriedly crossed the floor to look out and down on a scene out of Dante's *Inferno*. On the far perimeter of

Xanadu, disintegrating chalets erupted in red and yellow ruin, and fireballs lifted their mushroom heads to the night sky. But Trask was right: it wasn't over yet.

For as the three stood there watching, impotent of action, so midway between the burning perimeter and the casino a second series of terrific explosions, then a third, ripped through the shattered resort. Concentric rings of destruction were closing in on the Pleasure Dome, hurling flaming debris aloft and turning night to day.

"Now he springs the trap," Trask husked. "Xanadu is no use to him now and he'll destroy it, and us with it. So this is it. We're next!"

"The place is wired, mined!" The major's face was ashen. "I should have known it from the very first explosion, the one that took one of my men."

"Don't blame yourself," said Trask. "We've all been equally stupid. And that bastard is sitting somewhere watching us, knowing that by now *we* know. I don't suppose there's any point asking you to call the chopper down?"

"Wouldn't if I could," the other shook his head. "No way—not into this lot. But in any case my radio's been out since we got into the lift. Some kind of electrical interference."

As he finished speaking, so Ian Goodly reeled and caught at the major's arm to steady himself. *"Jake!"* the precog gasped. "My God, Ben—it's Jake!"

"Jake?" Trask repeated him. "What about him?"

"He . . . he's on his way here," Goodly answered. "But so is the elevator!"

"Jake's in the elevator?" Trask failed to understand.

"No," Goodly shook his head. "Jake is in the Möbius Continuum. The bomb is in the elevator! When I staggered just now, it was because I'd seen it going off—but seen it at close range, even *this* close—and it's due to happen any time now!"

The major might have asked what they were raving about but didn't have time. In a sudden stirring of smoky air, Jake stepped out of the Möbius Continuum with Liz clinging to him like a leech—and at the same time the elevator pinged and its doors hissed open.

Jake and Liz were staggering, disoriented; the major didn't know what was going on; and the precog, knowing he was about to die, couldn't take his eyes off the elevator. Ben Trask was the only one who saw the "truth" of it and knew what to do.

"To me!" he shouted. "To me!" And without waiting he swept them into his arms, bundled all four of them close to himself.

"What?" Jake said, completely out of the picture.

"Make a door!" Trask shouted at him. "For God's sake, make a goddamned door! Make a big one, and I mean right now!"

And Jake, and Korath, they made a door.

The blast took them right through it, all five (or six of them, with Korath), through the door into the Möbius Continuum. And in the hot blast and the fire that followed them, Jake knew only one safe place to take them. He remembered those suntanned, near-naked bodies sprawling indolently, and the shadow of the helicopter dark on the sparkling water. And he knew the coordinates.

Down they went in one of Xanadu's pools, and coughing and spluttering they surfaced . . .

. . . In time to see Chopper One at altitude 150 feet, wheeling to face the backdrop of cliffs, steadying up and sitting like a hawk on the air, and opening up with its nose cannons on no clearly discernible target.

In his once-secret hiding place, Malinari saw it, too, and didn't believe it. But as cannon-fire ripped the chimney's facade to shreds he had to believe it. And while he still had time he tripped the rest of his switches. Then, with his thin clothing tearing under the pressure of madly metamorphosing flesh—and his bolthole hideaway collapsing around him—Malinari made a headlong dive through his window of observation, out into the night.

For a moment the pilot of Chopper One saw him: the jet-copter's thermal-imaging highlighted a shifting, flattening, morphing blob of a figure that at first plummeted, quickly adopted a manta-like shape, and finally glided from view. The pilot might even have taken a shot at the thing, but powerful updrafts from the blazing hell that was Xanadu were rocking his machine, forcing him to take action and climb out of danger.

And as Jake and the others left the pool, so Nephran Maliniari shot like an arrow overhead. He might easily have been some primal pterodactyl out of Earth's prehistory, but was in fact a predatory creature from an alien, parallel world. Trask saw him—his crimson eyes, the dark blur of his passing—and a moment later heard his taunting laughter echoing from on high.

Hearing that laughter, and remembering Zek—unable to forget her, ever—all Trask wanted was to stand there and let his hate out, and *will* this monster to a terrible death. He knew he couldn't, but he had never wanted anything so much in his life.

In close proximity like this—so intent upon each other—Malinari had "heard" Trask and sent back:

Hatred such as that is catching, Mr. Trask. It breeds hatred! As for willing me to death: we must see whose will is the strongest, eh? Not here and now, no, but in another place, another time. This was nothing but a skirmish, to get your measure. But if you would live to fight another day, first you must survive the night. Alas, I don't think so. If you survive, however, do not despair. For I shall be waiting, Mr. Trask, I shall be waiting. . . .

All of them with Trask heard it—that dark voice in their heads and its taunting message—but especially Liz. She heard it, and saw beyond it. Malinari's plan: flight, to safe haven in another place, another country.

She might even have discovered which one, but Nephran Malinari recognized her presence and withdrew snarling into mental obscurity. Where his evil telepathic voice had been, only mindsmog remained, spiralling after him into a mental void.

And Malinari was gone.

But to Trask and the others it seemed the danger was still present. Xanadu was burning end to end; a series of devastating explosions continued to rock the place; Malinari's bubble aerie on top of the Pleasure Dome was no more, and showers of plastic and glass were still raining to earth. Scraps of blazing debris drifted across the night sky, and clods of earth and grass were fountaining in the garden where Chopper One had made its initial landing. A lucky mistake on Malinari's part, that last. One of his few errors.

But the Pleasure Dome itself, the casino, was still standing, and now the precog Ian Goodly cried, "The big one is still to come. It's the casino. A set piece of delayed action—like the pause before the last big firework at the end of the show!"

Fortunately W.O. II Bygraves had taken the initiative. Thinking he'd lost his commanding officer when the major's radio had gone down, he had called the rest of the platoon out of the casino. Now they came running, gathering at the pool. But from the pool on outwards to the perimeter of the resort, it seemed that the whole of Xanadu was an inferno. Even if there were no more explosions, the sheer heat would certainly kill everyone before they made half the distance. And meanwhile the precog, in a fit of delirious anxiety, was turning this way and that, repeating, "It's going to blow! It's going to blow!"

Then a piece of burning debris from the bubble came drifting like a kite, weighed down by and trailing a length of electrical cable. No one noticed it until it struck the monorail's overhead power grid. There was a flash that sent blobs of molten copper skittering, and the kite and cable fell to earth.

Trask and the major glanced at each other, headed for the boarding platform no more than fifty feet away. The rest followed them, and Jake quickly caught up. "What are we doing?" he asked Trask breathlessly.

"The elevated monorail," Trask gasped. "It has power. Maybe we can drive out of this, or over the worst of it, at least as far as the main parking lot and the big ops truck."

His idea was as good as any other; in fact, it was the only

idea, for the armoured car had been blown over onto its side by the blast from the garden. Fortunately the locator David Chung, along with Bygraves and his men, had already vacated that area; like Jake they had seen the pool as the only sanctuary from the bomb blasts and the fires that licked closer with every passing moment. And by now the heat and smoke were suffocating.

Dragging Liz behind him, Jake was the first into the leading carriage of two articulated, open-sided cars. Climbing into the driver's seat, he hit the red power button and, as the motor throbbed into life, grabbed the drive lever.

The system could scarcely be simpler: push forward to go, pull backward to stop. And ahead the single overhead rail climbed and curved outwards towards the perimeter parking lot, the reception area, Xanadu's gates and safety. But while the motor warmed up, still the precog was shouting. "It's going any minute now!"

Men ran, limped, or were carried; they bundled each other into the cars. Until finally Trask yelled, "That's it. Now get us the hell out of here!" And Jake pushed the lever forward.

Slowly—agonizingly slowly, or so it seemed—the cars climbed to their elevated height and started along the spiralling, pylon-supported rail. Fifty feet, a hundred, and gathering speed. And then the Pleasure Dome went.

The blast was awesome as the casino literally lifted into the air, sank down into itself, split asunder under the irresistible pressure of expanding gasses, and blew apart in red and yellow streamers of flame. The whole thing disappeared in dust, rubble, and gouting fire, and in the next moment the hot blast of its passing reached out and rocked the monorail's carriages, causing its passengers to grit their teeth and hang on for dear life. But then the cars steadied up and the danger was past.

So everyone thought—

—Except Ian Goodly. "There's one bomb left!" he suddenly cried. "Its in the reception area, the gatehouse!" He was right—and just like the bomb in the Pleasure Dome, this too was a delayed action device. When it went it took a good man, their rear guard, with it—but it also took out the last elevated section of the monorail!

Liz was behind Jake, shouting, "Look! *Look!*" and pointing ahead. But he was already looking. All he could see through the smoke and the fire was a mass of slumping, buckled metal—the wreckage of the tower that had borne the weight of the monorail—beyond which there was empty space and a drop of some thirty odd feet into a red, roaring death!

Jake slammed the drive lever into reverse . . . and nothing happened. The power had gone along with the overhead gantry and power line, and the cars were freewheeling down a gentle gradient at some thirty miles an hour.

But Ian Goodly's talent was back in force. Suddenly he was there, leaning over Jake and shouting, "Jake, listen! There's a way out. I can see it. We're going to make it!"

And he told Jake what he had seen, shouted it into his ear as the articulated cars went lurching into empty space, heading for the inferno that waited below.

Korath knew what was required and set those fantastic formulae rolling yet again down the screen of Jake's mind—until Jake froze them and conjured a door that even Harry Keogh would be proud of. Then:

Darkness surrounded the cars—the Ultimate Darkness of a time before time—and in a single moment which might yet be as long as forever, light, gentle moon, and starlight, blinked into being as Jake made his first perfect three-point exit from the Möbius Continuum at well-known coordinates.

The cars were boat-bottomed. They didn't dig in but rode across the dry grass and sandy soil of the safe house's garden, quickly slowing until, with scarcely a jolt, they were brought up short by the stout wall. Then the rear car slewed a little—but not enough to spill anyone—and both cars rolled sideways through forty-five degrees and came to a rocking standstill.

For a long time there was silence. Until Jake and the E-Branch people climbed out of the lead car and, as a man, collapsed or plumped down on the withered grass and began to breathe again.

Then someone (it sounded to Liz like Red Bygraves) said, "Holy *fuck!*" And everyone started talking at once.

Epilogue

IN XANADU, JETHRO MANCHESTER HAD BUILT A Pleasure Dome. Now it was gone, and Manchester with it, to an end as undeserved as it was brutal and horrific. Likewise the alien author of Xanadu's and Manchester's ruin; he, too, was gone. But Lord Nephran Malinari was fled, not dead. And it grieved Ben Trask's heart that he must admit it: that the chase wasn't nearly over yet, but if anything was now more needful and deadly than ever.

For if the others, if Vavara and Szwart, were trying to do what Malinari had begun to do in subterranean Xanadu—if they, too, were nurturing "gardens" of loathsome, plague-bearing deathspawn—and if a single red spore, all unnoticed, inhaled like a speck of dust, could write *finis* on a human life and replace it with undeath, how then millions or billions of spores—and what then for the world . . . ?

On the second morning after the Australians cremated their four dead comrades in a quiet ceremony with full military honours—a ceremony which Trask and his E-Branch people felt privileged to attend, where in fact there were only three bodies in their coffins, for the fourth had burned on Manchester's island, and was represented by a photograph, a scroll of honour, and messages of farewell from his closest colleagues only—the second morning after that, the major and his two stalwart warrant officers were at the airport in Brisbane to see Trask and his people off.

After the British team had received their regulation new bubonic shots—for the Australian authorities were insistent that no one be allowed to enter or leave the continent without first being innoculated—then, over drinks in the departure lounge, Trask and the major had a quiet word in private. Jake, Liz, and the rest of the team sat at a table with Bygraves and Davis, where for the better part they commiserated in silence. Something of an aftermath, it seemed there wasn't a lot to be said. But Trask and the SAS major weren't willing to leave it at that.

"And so it goes on," said the major, "for you at least."

"For us it never seems to end," Trask answered. "Just when we think it might, there's always something new. Not always as bad as what we've just been through, but always bad."

"And you can't give up on it," said the major; not a question but a statement of fact.

"Never!" Trask growled. "This time, for me it's personal. But personal or not, it's always the same. We've seen all this before, and we'll see it again. Yes, and we'll see it through, all the way to the end. But myself . . . I for one will never be able to rest until this one is dead. Or until I'm dead. One or the other."

"Malinari?"

"The same," Trask nodded. "I want that bastard dead, dead, dead! And I intend to get him, no matter what it takes. As Lardis Lidesci might say, that's my vow. *Huh!* My Szgany vow, aye."

"Well, you have a good team to help you." The major glanced across the room at the people sitting with his men. "Weird as hell, but good. That David Chung, for instance. Such a quiet little man—with his built-in radar dish. And the tall fellow, Ian Goodly, who I'd hate to play cards with. And Liz, who hears people thinking? I definitely wouldn't play cards with her! And as for Jake . . . I just can't *believe* what he does! It may have saved my life, but I still don't believe it."

"I know," Trask answered. "And it doesn't help that it's something I can't talk about. Or something *we* can't talk about. But being what you are, SAS, I'm sure you understand that. Anyway—and if it makes it any easier—there are times when I don't believe this stuff myself. Times when I wake up and think I've been nightmaring. And the hell of it is, I'm the only one who really *knows* that it's true!"

The major shook his head and said, "Weird, weird people—but I'm glad to have known you."

"Same here," said Trask. "I'm only sorry that—"

"I know." The other cut him short. "The only consolation lies in what we've achieved. For let's face it, no sane people could ever suffer such as that to live. Those four lives might have saved thousands."

But Trask shook his head. "Think again," he said. "Thousands? There are over six billion people on this small planet. And that's how many we might have saved. Or that we've started to save."

And after a while the major said, "Hearing you put it like that, I know it was worth it."

At which Liz called across and said, "They're boarding."

"It's time we weren't here," said Trask, standing up. And as the major reached out his hand Trask looked at it, took it, and said, "I don't even know your name!"

"It's Tom," said the other.

"Just Tom? Major Tom?"

"That'll suffice," said the major, grinning.

Trask smiled, too, and said, "Well, Major Tom, ground control is calling for us."

The major had been carrying a fat, eighteen-inch-long parcel. Now he gave it to Trask. "This is for you," he said. "The men found it when they went down and burned out the underground rooms, tunnels and conduits in Xanadu. It got burned, too, so I can guarantee it's clean. I don't believe in trophy-taking, not after a job like that one. Maybe you'll find a use for it."

After that there was no time for anything other than handshakes all round, then Trask and his people went to board their Qantas VTOL Skyskip.

But as they queued at the boarding gate, Jake sensed someone's gaze upon him and glanced toward the reinforced flexiglass wall that secured the boarding area from the viewing

531

promenade. From the far side of the wall, distorted by the images of other passengers that moved across its reflective surface, a thin, pockmarked face looked back at him. And for a moment their eyes met before Jake looked away.

He looked away, but only for a moment . . .

. . . Until something went *click* in his memory and he gave a start and looked again. But the face was gone.

Standing just behind him, Ben Trask had noticed his reaction and said, "Is there something?"

Jake frowned, then shook his head. "No," he said. "I don't think so. But just for a moment then I thought I might have . . . recognized someone?"

Trask looked at him in a certain way, with his head cocked a little on one side, and said, "Or you're concerned that maybe someone recognized you?"

Jake shrugged uncomfortably, said, "That, too. But here in Australia? Unlikely."

Very unlikely, yes. For as Jake had said, what would that lousy, murdering, bastard thug—what would the face of a man who had featured in his worst nightmares for far too long now, one of Luigi Castellano's soldiers, unforgotten from a certain monstrous night in Marseille—what would he be doing here?

Then he shrugged again and put it out of his mind. It was part of his growing obsession, that was all, when from time to time he would see those faces wherever he looked; this despite that several of them were no more, dead by his hand. But still Jake looked again at the flexiglass partition before moving on into the boarding tunnel.

And of course there was no one there. . . .

As the VTOL Skyskip was rising vertically into the air, lifting its nose, and accelerating into the sky, the man with the pockmarked face was in a telephone kiosk, speaking long-distance to Palermo.

"No doubt about it," he said in Italian. "I'd know the guy

anywhere. He's alive and kicking, and there's been all kinds of shit going down around here, yeah! That Xanadu thing: they said it was a plague spot, and an accidental fire burned it out down to the foundations. But I can tell you, Luigi, some of the crew who were up there clearing up afterwards— like, you know, military types?—they were here at the airport to see Cutter and these British people onto their plane. Like pals all round, you know? Me, I'd like to know how you knew this Jake Cutter would be out here in the first place. . . .

"You didn't know? You were only interested in Xanadu. . . . ?

"And I . . . I ask too many questions. Yeah, I know. You're right, sorry. So what now?

"I should find out who the Brits were? Get after them, on the next plane? Sure, I can handle that. And I can use the account in England, have myself some fun? Hey, I like it!

"Er, yeah . . . ?

"But if I don't find out who they are, I needn't bother to go back to Marseille . . . or anywhere. Right, Luigi, I got that. But say . . ." And there he stopped short, scowling at the phone. For it was purring away vacantly to itself in his hand, and the oh-so-dark voice on the other end was gone.

On board the Skyskip, when they were indeed skipping across the outer atmosphere, Ben Trask started to open the parcel given to him by the major. But as gleaming metal hooks appeared, flexible fish-scale plates and sharp-pointed gouges, he stopped, went pale, and wrapped the thing up again.

Having seen its like before, on Starside in an alien world of vampires, he knew exactly what it was: a battle gauntlet, as used by the Wamphyri!

But then, looking up and across the central aisle at David Chung, Trask's colour returned and he smiled a mirthless, vengeful smile. And: "Lord Nephran Malinari," he murmured to himself, under the subdued rumble of the Skyskip's engines, "you can run but you can't hide."

And again, nodding to himself, "You can't *ever* hide, Malinari—not for long, not from me—and definitely not from E-Branch."

NEXT:

E-BRANCH:
DEFILERS

Jake and Korath struggle for supremacy. Vavara's Sisterhood of Evil. Szwart's Maze of Darkness. Malinari's Madness—and more . . .

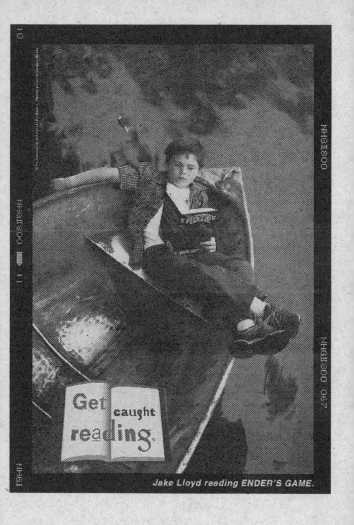

Get caught reading.

Jake Lloyd reading ENDER'S GAME.

A Message from the
Association of American Publishers